Monographs on Endocrinology

Volume 2

Edited by

A. Labhart, Zürich · T. Mann, Cambridge

L. T. Samuels, Salt Lake City · J. Zander, Heidelberg

K. B. Eik-Nes · E. C. Horning

Gas Phase Chromatography
of Steroids

With 85 Figures

Springer-Verlag New York Inc.   1968

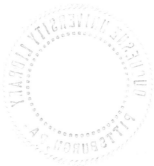

Preface

Few fields have advanced faster over the past quinquennium than separation and estimation of steroids by the technique of gas phase chromatography. A detailed and complete review of this topic would therefore be beyond the scope of the authors contributing to this monograph. It was, however, felt that a discussion of some of the highlights of this rapid advance might be of help for laboratories estimating steroids in biological samples. One of the difficulties in producing a monograph of this kind is that before it can appear in print it is likely that some of the methods it discusses will have been overtaken by better methods, so swiftly is progress now made.

No editorial power has been exercised in trying to make a uniform account of technology in this field, and the idiosyncrasies of each individual author have been left intact. Through this approach we hope that what has been lost in scholarly appearance is regained in general appeal.

Salt Lake City and Houston, May 1968

Kristen B. Eik-Nes
Evan C. Horning

Contents

Chapter 1

HORNING, E. C.: Gas Phase Analytical Methods for the Study
of Steroid Hormones and their Metabolites

Chapter 2

ADLERCREUTZ, H., and T. LUUKKAINEN: Gas Phase Chromatographic
Methods for Estrogens in Biological Fluids

Chapter 3

Chapter 4

EIK-NES, K. B.: Gas Phase Chromatography of Androgens in Biological Samples

Chapter 5

BAILEY, E.: Gas Phase Chromatography of Corticosteroids in Biological Samples

Abbreviations

ACTH:	adrenocorticotrophic hormone
BSA:	*bis*trimethylsilyl acetamide
CC:	column chromatography
CDMS:	cyclohexanedimethanol succinate
DC 200:	methylsiloxane polymer
DDT:	2,2-bis(p-chlorophenyl)-1,1,1-trichloroethane
Embaph:	Embaphase, a non-polar silicone oil
Epon 1001:	epoxy resin
F-60:	a methyl-p-chlorophenylsiloxane polymer
GLC:	gas liquid or gas phase chromatography
HCG:	human chorionic gonadotrophin
Hi Eff 8B:	cyclohexanedimethanol succinate
HMDS:	hexamethyldisilazane
id:	inside diameter
JXR:	a methylsiloxane polymer
17-KS:	17-keto steroids
MO:	methoxime
MU:	methylene unit
NGA:	neopentyl glycol adipate
NGS:	neopentyl glycol succinate
NG Seb:	neopentyl glycol sebaccate
od:	outside diameter
17-OHCS:	17-hydroxycorticosteroids
OV-1:	a dimethylsiloxane polymer
OV-17:	a methylphenylsiloxane polymer
PC:	paper chromatography
psi:	pounds per square inch
QF-1 (FS-1265):	a trifluoropropylmethylsiloxane polymer
RRT:	relative retention time
SD:	standard deviation

SE:	standard error
SE-30:	a methylsiloxane polymer
SE-52:	a methylphenylsiloxane polymer
SN:	steroid number
STAP:	a polyester (modified carbowax type)
TLC:	thin layer chromatography
TMSDMA:	trimethylsilyldimethylamine
TMSi:	trimethylsilyl ether(s)
vol:	volume
XE-60 (CNSi):	a cyanoethylmethylsiloxane polymer
Z:	a co-polymer of ethylene glycol, succinic acid and a methylphenylsiloxane monomer

Contributors

ADLERCREUTZ, H., Steroid Research Laboratory, Department of Clinical Chemistry, University of Helsinki, Meilahti Hospital, Helsinki, Finland

BAILEY, E., Sheffield Center for the Investigation and Treatment of Diseases, Nether Edge Hospital, Sheffield, Great Britain

EIK-NES, K. B., University of Utah, Department of Biological Chemistry, College of Medicine, Salt Lake City, Utah, USA

HORNING, E. C., Institute for Lipid Research, Baylor University College of Medicine, Houston, Texas, USA

LUUKKAINEN, T., Steroid Research Laboratory, Department of Clinical Chemistry, University of Helsinki, Meilahti Hospital, Helsinki, Finland

VAN DER MOLEN, H. J., Department of Obstetrics and Gynecology, University Hospital, Utrecht, Netherlands

Chapter 1

Gas Phase Analytical Methods for the Study of Steroid Hormones and their Metabolites

E. C. HORNING

I. Historical

The origin of gas-liquid partition chromatography is generally taken to be a 1941 comment by A. J. P. MARTIN indicating that it should be possible to use a gas and a liquid in a partition chromatographic separation (MARTIN and SYNGE, 1941). In 1948—1949 experimental work was undertaken, and the results of the first successful experiments were published in 1952 (JAMES and MARTIN, 1952). The separation of fatty acids was studied, and the theoretical basis of GLC separations was discussed. The separation of organic amines was investigated in later work. The need for gas phase detection systems became evident as soon as compounds other than acids and bases were studied. The separation of hydrocarbons, for example, was (and is) an application of great importance to the petroleum industry, but this separation problem could not be studied effectively without suitable detectors. During the next few years many types of detection systems were developed. The "gas density balance" of MARTIN and JAMES (1956) had moderately high sensitivity. The response was on a molar basis, and this detector was used extensively at Mill Hill (National Institute for Medical Research, London). Thermal conductivity detection systems (CLAESSON, 1946; RAY, 1954) came into wide use in studies where the sample was relatively large, while the argon ionization detector with a radium foil source was used as a sensitive detection system with microgram samples (LOVELOCK, 1958). The hydrogen flame ionization detection system was developed through work in several laboratories around 1957—1958, and this detector is now used universally in quantitative work with samples down to about 0.01 μg.

During 1959—1960 the possibility of achieving a separation of steroids by GLC procedures was under study in several laboratories. A report from the University of Glasgow (EGLINTON et al., 1959) indicated that several steroids could be chromatographed with an Apiezon phase under the usual conditions of that period but with the expected result: a retention time of hours, even at the highest temperatures in use at the time. A study carried out at Bethesda (National Heart Institute) showed that steroids could be eluted with short retention times when a polar (polyester) phase was employed at high temperatures; however, decomposition of some compounds occurred under these conditions (SWEELEY and HORNING, 1960). In Holland, a group at the Unilever Laboratories showed that with a thermally-stripped siloxane polymer phase it was possible to separate several steroids (BEERTHUIS and RECOURT, 1960). The problem was solved by the demonstration of VANDENHEUVEL, SWEELEY and HORNING (1960) that thin-film columns (1—3% of phase) prepared with a thermally stable liquid phase (SE-30, a methylsiloxane polymer) could be used for the separation of a number of steroids without structural alteration. The temperature range was moderate (210—230°) and the retention times were about 15 minutes to 1 hour.

From this work it became clear that thin-film columns, prepared with deactivated supports, were entirely suitable for GLC separations of steroids and many other compounds. The supposed requirement of 5% or more of liquid phase was not theoretically sound; this view was based on inadequate recognition of the practical problem of deactivation of the support. The fact that "non-volatile" steroids could be separated indicated that the range of organic compounds that could be separated by GLC methods was far wider than had been imagined. It now seems strange that practical problems were mistaken for theoretical limitations. Separations are based upon differences in the free energy of solution of the solute in the liquid phase under the conditions of the separation, and not upon boiling point relationships. The theoretical limit for the transfer of an organic compound to the vapor phase is about C_{70} for a hydrocarbon, and this limit has not been reached. The limitation in GLC work with respect to polarity is due to hydrogen bonding (excluding ionic substances), and derivative formation may be used to reduce or eliminate this effect. Almost the entire range of organic compounds of biological interest, with the exception of high polymers, are amenable to study by GLC methods.

During the decade 1950—1960, significant changes occurred in the field of mass spectrometry which are important to the further development of gas phase analytical work. The development of high resolution mass spectrometry resulted in analytical methods of very high precision and accuracy for the study of the composition and structure of organic compounds. These methods now require computer techniques for the analysis of the experimental data (BIEMANN et al., 1964). This work at first was of interest to organic, analytical and physical chemists, but not to biochemists. However, BERGSTRÖM. RYHAGE, STENHAGEN and their associates recognized the significance for biochemistry of combining gas chromatography with mass spectrometry. Valuable features of the combined gas chromatograph-mass spectrometer developed by RYHAGE (1964) at Stockholm included a high scan speed and a "molecule separator" that permitted the use of packed GLC colums. The most recent developments include mass marking and peak matching.

It is now clear that gas phase analytical work is emerging as a new field of chemistry. All of the steps of separation, identification, quantification and structural study are carried out in the gas phase. The methods, although not familiar to chemists trained in classical techniques, are fully as rigorous and as conclusive as past methods. They are well suited for the study of complex mixtures of organic substances on a microgram or submicrogram scale, and they are of particular importance for work in the fields of biology and medicine. The use of gas phase analytical procedures is not limited to steroids, but this is a highly important area, and it is the area of work from which many current methods are derived.

The key to new discoveries lies in new methodology. It is to be hoped that the field of endocrinology will benefit from these advances which are based on the physical sciences but which find their most important use in biological problems.

II. Analytical Methods

The traditions of analytical chemistry are derived largely from analytical problems pertinent to inorganic chemistry, and in early work the steps of separation and estimation were always carried out as sequential but separate operations. There is, however, no theoretical reason why a multicomponent analysis in which the separation and estimation steps are combined, or even in which the separation step is omitted, should not be satisfactory provided that an adequate discrimination procedure is employed at some point. In fact, methods of these kinds often offer the great practical advantages of time-saving and increased accuracy over sequential methods. GLC methods are an example of a way in which separation and estimation steps can be combined into a single operation.

Although distinct advantages are often attached to multicomponent analyses, there are many instances in biological work where single component analyses are required and where multicomponent analyses are unnecessary. Group analyses, where members of chemically or biologically related groups of compounds are determined, are by implication confined to a small number of compounds. The following brief discussion is aimed at contrasting the GLC requirements for these analytical methods.

1. Single Component Analyses

a) By High-sensitivity Non-selective Detection

The hydrogen flame ionization detector has a sensitivity limit of about 0.01 μg for most work. By using special conditions it is possible to extend this range by a factor of about 10. The detector, however, is relatively non-selective and it will respond to most organic compounds. It is therefore necessary to use samples of relatively high purity for high-sensitivity work. The major steps of purification are usually those of column chromatography (CC), thin-layer chromatography (TLC) or paper chromatography (PC). In effect, the separation conditions are designed to yield a fraction that contains only one steroid, and the function of the GLC column is to present a single component to the detector for quantification. There is little emphasis on the column as a means of separation; the requirements are nevertheless high in the sense that stable, low-bleed columns with low adsorption characteristics should be used. Isothermal conditions are employed in order to minimize base-line changes. The electrical components should be chosen for low-noise characteristics, and the area measurements should be made, if possible, by electronic integration rather than by recorder chart measurements. A "solid" injection technique should be used to avoid solvent fronts and solvent effects on the base line and on the detector. This technique also permits an entire sample to be used; when samples are injected in solution it is not uncommon to use 1—2 μl of a 100 μl sample (discarding 98—99% of the sample). Perhaps the best current example of this type of analytical method is the blood progesterone determination developed by SOMMERVILLE and his colleagues. References to his procedure are in a later chapter.

Procedures for the estimation of urinary testosterone also fall into this class, although high-sensitivity detection is not always required. Provision for the separation of epitestosterone must be made at some point, and the bulk of the urinary steroids must be removed by one or more high capacity, low resolution procedures. These, of course, might well be GLC procedures but at present they are more likely to involve CC and TLC methods. The sample injection may be carried out by liquid (solvent) or "solid" techniques, depending upon the size of the sample.

b) By High-sensitivity Selective Detection

Several selective detection systems are now available. Of these, the most useful for steroid work is the "electron capture" detector. This detector was developed as an off-shoot of early work on the argon detector, and it is particularly useful in pesticide work. The signal is noted as a lowering of the standing current of the cell. A few steroids are known to have "electron capture" properties (LOVELOCK et al., 1963), but it is customary to prepare derivatives for this purpose. Chloracetates have electron capture properties (LANDOWNE and LIPSKY, 1963) but derivatives containing perfluoroalkyl and perfluoroaryl groups with 5 or more fluorine atoms also show this property. In earlier work applications were limited by the fact that a foil-supported tritium source was used, with a temperature limit of about 220°. The temperature limitation has been removed by the development of the nickel-63 cell, although comparatively little information has been published about steroid analytical methods using this detector.

Extensive purification of the sample and all reagents and solvents involved in sample handling are required. The GLC column usually contributes very little to the separation and purification process; these steps are normally carried out by CC or TLC methods. Stable, low-bleed columns are used under isothermal conditions. The detection system usually does not give a response that is linearly related to the mass of the sample at all concentrations, although over a limited mass range linearity is observed (see later chapters). Measurements are usually made by comparisons of response for reference samples of the compound under study, and internal standards are recommended. Solvent injection techniques are usually employed.

The best current examples of these methods are the procedures developed by EIK-NES and his colleagues for the estimation of testosterone (as the chloracetate) and estrone (as the pentafluorophenylhydrazone). These methods are described in later chapters.

Chloracetates may be estimated in the range of 1—10 nanograms and the sensitivity of detection of some perfluoro derivatives lies well beyond this range. It is likely that considerable emphasis will be placed on selective detection methods in the next few years. There is a possibility that mass spectrometric methods may be developed for high-sensitivity work.

2. Group Analyses

Comparatively few GLC group analytical procedures have been developed. An example is the method of BROOKS et al. (1967) for the estimation of pregnanediol and estriol in pregnancy urine.

The usual detection system is the hydrogen flame ionization detector. Separations may be isothermal or temperature programmed. The sample injection may be by "solid" or solvent techniques. One or more CC or TLC separation steps are used to achieve a group separation, and the GLC column is used to separate individual members of the group.

The sensitivity is usually that of ordinary GLC work and there are no unusual requirements from the point of view of GLC techniques.

3. Multicomponent Analyses

The usual detection system for a multicomponent analysis procedure is the hydrogen flame ionization detector. Isothermal or temperature programmed conditions may be used; the latter condition is usually necessary for the study of highly complex mixtures with many components. Liquid (solvent) or "solid" injection techniques may be used. The GLC column is used for separation purposes to the maximum extent permitted by current techniques. Qualitative and quantitative data are obtained at the same time.

The objective of a multicomponent analysis is to provide significant information about a number of biochemically or biologically related substances. For example, the analytical method of GARDINER and HORNING (1966) for human urinary steroids provides a "steroid profile" which includes, as far as is known, all urinary steroids excreted at a level above about 100 μg per day. Compounds excreted below this level are also present, but these are seen as "compound noise" rather than as significant components of the sample. Another example of a multicomponent analytical method is that leading to the "urinary acid profile" described by M. G. HORNING, et al. (1966). An important property of these methods is that changes resulting from environmental alterations, pathological conditions or drug effects are readily apparent; patterns or relationships may be noted at the same time that individual values are determined.

The view is sometimes expressed that multicomponent analytical methods are lacking in precision and accuracy when compared with single component analytical methods. The chief problem is that levels of precision and accuracy can be determined easily for a single component analysis; a multicomponent analysis yields multiple analytical values which do not all show identical accuracy. However, it is possible to establish the characteristics of an instrumental system used for multicomponent analyses. It can be shown that the precision of a steroid GLC assay system with a flame detector is about 0.5% (standard deviation) and that the accuracy is about 1% (standard deviation) if automated sample addition and temperature programming is employed. The accuracy which may be achieved in an actual multicomponent analysis of a sample of biologic origin depends upon the effectiveness of the separation procedure; the accuracy for present methods will not be better than 1%, and "compound noise" may decrease the accuracy to about 5%. Major components are only slightly affected by "compound noise", while measurements for relatively minor components may be affected to a much greater degree. Each application therefore requires separate study and evaluation.

III. Instrumental Components

1. The Column and its Packing

a) Column Types

Steroid separations are usually carried out with glass columns 6 ft or 12 ft in length and 3.6—4.0 mm in internal diameter. The usual form is a U-tube (6 ft) or W-tube (12 ft), but coiled columns are also used for 6 ft or shorter columns. The length is important because this is related to column efficiency; a 12 ft column should show 5,000 to 6,000 theoretical plate efficiency. The usual closures are silicone stoppers or septa. Samples may be injected with a syringe, or provision may be made for "solid" injections.

The chief reason for using glass columns (which should be silanized before use) is to provide an inert surface in and near the vaporization zone. It is possible that metal columns (stainless steel) could be used for many separations, provided that a glass-lined vaporizer is employed.

When packed glass columns are employed, the maximum inlet pressure of the carrier gas should be about 30 psi. A 12 ft glass column, 3.6 mm ID, packed with a 1% SE-30 phase on 100—120 mesh diatomaceous earth support, will show a flow rate of about 40 ml/min of nitrogen at 200° when the carrier gas pressure is about 25 psi.

It has not yet been possible to prepare stable, long-lived thin-film capillary columns for use under the conditions required for steroid separations; the limitations, however, are of a practical rather than a theoretical nature, and more work on this problem is needed.

b) Supports

The usual support is a diatomaceous earth, processed to provide particles of small size with a large surface area. The usual mesh size for steroid separations is 80—100 or 100—120. Although highly polar phases may be coated directly on the support, it is usually necessary to deactivate the surface by silanizing before coating. This step should be used for all thin-film column packings prepared with polysiloxane liquid phases. The best deactivating agent is dimethyldichlorosilane; this is preferred over hexamethyldisilazane (HMDS). The use of other silylating agents (N-trimethylsilylimidazole (TSIM), *bis*-trimethylsilylacetamide (BSA) and related compounds) has not yet been evaluated.

Lowered resolution and adsorption (tailing) of samples are usually due to poor procedures in preparing column packings. The presence of "fines" always leads to poor resolution, and adsorption is due to inadequate deactivation of the support.

Many other supports including glass beads have been recommended. Diatomaceous earth supports may eventually be replaced, but at present they remain the best material for the purpose.

c) Liquid Phases

The requirements for satisfactory performance as a liquid phase for steroid work are met by very few materials. About a dozen liquid phases of those now known can be employed, but only a few of these are generally useful. The best non-selective phases are methyl-substituted polysiloxanes available under the trade names SE-30, JXR and OV-1. Thin-film (1—3%) columns with these liquid films show very low bleed rates up to about 300°, provided that a satisfactory deactivation process has been used for the support. Current samples of OV-1 are somewhat more thermostable than those of SE-30, although both polymers have the same basic structure.

The best "polar" phase for steroid work is OV-17; this material is a polysiloxane of the methylphenyl type containing about 50—55 mole-% phenyl groups. The polymer may be used up to about 300°. Selective retention effects are shown for carbon-carbon unsaturation and for hydroxyl groups; the latter effect is useful when working with trimethylsilyl (TMSi) ethers of polyfunctional steroids since with OV-17 steroid TMSi ethers are eluted before the corresponding parent hydroxyl-substituted steroids.

Other phases that have been recommended for steroid separations include cyanoethylmethyl polysiloxanes (XE-60), polyesters (NGS and CHDMS), fluoroalkylmethyl polysiloxanes (QF-1) and p-chlorophenylmethyl polysiloxanes (F-60). Several of these phases are useful for special purposes. The polysiloxane QF-1 shows a high degree of stereospecific selectivity in the retention of hydroxyl- and keto-substituted steroids. Polysiloxanes of the XE-60 type (containing cyanoethyl groups) have been recommended for some applications, but they have limited thermal stability. The polyester NGS is useful for steroid work involving compounds of relatively simple structure; the chief disadvantage of polyesters is their relatively poor thermal stability. Polymer F-60 is essentially non-selective and it is not particularly useful in steroid separations in comparison with SE-30 or OV-1.

Table 1 contains a list of phases that are suitable for steroid work, together with an indication of the approximate upper limit of temperature for sustained use. All of these phases may be used for brief periods of time at temperatures about 30—50° above those listed in Table 1; this leads to a greater bleed rate and shortened column life.

Table 1. *Liquid phases suitable for steroid separations**

Chemical Nature	Abbrev.	Max. Temp. ** °C
Non-selective:		
Dimethylsiloxane polymer	OV-1	320
Dimethylsiloxane polymer	SE-30 ***	320
Dimethylsiloxane polymer	JXR	300
p-Chlorophenylmethylsiloxane polymer	F-60	250
Selective:		
Methylphenylsiloxane polymer	OV-17	320
Fluoroalkylsiloxane polymer	QF-1	235
Cyanoethylmethylsiloxane polymer	XE-60	235
Neopentyl glycol succinate	NGS	225
Cyclohexanedimethanol succinate	CHDMS	235
Epoxy resin	Epon 1001	230

* These materials are commercially available as synthetic polymers.

** The limits cited are for stable columns and low bleed rates. Most phases may be used at temperatures 30—50° higher, but with increased bleed rates and greatly decreased column life.

*** Improved form.

d) Preparation of Column Packings

The following procedure for the preparation of column packings has been in use for about five years. We concur with the view of SUPINA et al. (1966) that "fines" in the packing are to be avoided, and that dichlorodimethylsilane is better than hexamethyldisilazane as a deactivating-silanizing reagent.

Gas Chrom P or its equivalent, 80—100 or 100—120 mesh (the size depends upon the application; 80—100 mesh is used for all packings with more than 3% of liquid phase; 100—120 mesh is used for 1% liquid phase packings for 6 ft and 12 ft columns where superior resolution is required) is size-graded by sieving in small quantities. Since continued dry sieving breaks down the support, the time of sieving should be relatively short and constant. The size-graded material is acid-washed in the following way. Concentrated hydrochloric acid is added to cover the support in a beaker or flask, and the mixture is allowed to stand for 24 to 48 hours. The acid is decanted or removed with the aid of a filter stick, and fresh acid is added. This is removed (a one-hour treatment is adequate) and the washing is repeated two or three times. The support is then washed well with deionized or distilled water. This should be done by decantation; all fines should be washed out of the slurry by alternate flooding and decantation. (Some fine particles are produced by the acid wash, and these must be removed by water decantation-washing.) The support is separated by filtration and washed well on the filter with acetone to remove most of the water. The support should be spread on a smooth-surface filter paper and dried, first at room temperature for about 15 minutes and then for at least 2—3 hours or overnight at 100—110°.

The washing process may be varied in the following way. After acid washing, followed by flooding and decantation to remove fines, the support is separated by filtration. It is then resuspended in a 0.5% solution of potassium hydroxide in methanol, and again separated by filtration and washed thoroughly with deionized water and with methanol to remove the water. The support is dried at 100—110°.

The silanization step is carried out with a 5% solution of dimethyldichlorosilane in toluene. The warm support is removed from the drying oven and added immediately to the dimethyldichlorosilane solution in a side-arm filter flask. The flask is placed under reduced pressure for a few minutes with swirling and shaking to dislodge entrapped air, and the mixture is then allowed to stand for 15—30 minutes. The support is removed by filtration and washed on the filter with an equal volume of toluene. The support is slurried on the filter with methanol (300 ml for each 25 g of support). A final thorough washing with methanol is carried out. The silanized support is air-dried for about 15 minutes and then dried for at least 2—3 hours at 100—110°.

For the preparation of a 1% SE-30 packing, a 1% solution of SE-30 in toluene is prepared. About 125 ml is used for the treatment of 20—25 g of support; best results are obtained when relatively small amounts (20—50 g) of packing are prepared in a single laboratory operation. The relation of the 1% solution to a 1% packing is fortuitous, and when different supports are used the relation between the concentration of the solution and the amount of phase deposited on the support should be determined by direct experiment. The dried support is removed from the oven and added to the SE-30 toluene solution in a side-arm filter flask. Suction is applied briefly and the mixture is swirled and shaken to dislodge entrapped air. After about 15 minutes the support is removed by filtration, but without washing. It is important to bring the entire mixture on the filter, and to allow the solution to drain evenly through the bed of support. When the excess solvent has been removed on the filter (filtration is continued for about 5 to 10 minutes to remove the solvent) the packing is air-dried for about 15 minutes. A recent improvement in drying consists in the use of a "fluidizing" drying process in which the packing is dried in a stream of hot nitrogen for 30 min. Oven drying at 100—110° for several hours may also be employed. A free-flowing powder should result.

Other phases may be applied in the same way, with appropriate solvents. Polyesters are usually soluble in chloroform, and QF-1 is soluble in acetone and in methyl ethyl ketone.

Perhaps the most important points in the procedure are the removal of fine particles by decantation in the acid-washing stage, and the immediate addition of the acid-washed support to the silanizing solution after removal from the drying oven. The deleterious effect of fine particles is well established although rarely mentioned in the literature (SUPINA et al., 1966). The alteration of silicate surfaces by adsorption of water vapor from the air is relatively rapid, and the time factor involved in the treatment of the dried support is important for this reason.

All glass surfaces should be silanized. This includes the columns and the glass wool used as plugs. A satisfactory method is to fill the column with a 5—10% solution of dichlorodimethylsilane in toluene. After about 15 minutes the column is emptied, and then washed several times with methanol and air-dried. Glass wool may be treated in the same way, but it should be oven-dried (80—100°) before use.

2. Detection Systems

a) Hydrogen Flame Ionization

In the hydrogen flame ionization detector, the carrier gas stream (nitrogen is usually employed) is directed into a hydrogen-air or hydrogen-oxygen flame. It is customary to mix hydrogen and the carrier gas stream in the burner base, and to surround the flame with a continuous flow of air or oxygen. One electrode is situated around or above the flame; the second may be the burner tube or a separate electrode. The conductivity of the flame is measured continuously with the aid of a suitable picoammeter (electrometer). The current flow is small (10^{-9} to 10^{-12} amp range) and the usual power supply is a 240 or 300 v battery. The major advantages of the hydrogen flame detector are its sensitivity and its relatively great linear range.

Not all organic compounds give identical responses, and "response factors" should be determined by the use of reference compounds of high purity. However, a response factor should not be a correction factor.

Although the detector is in theory flow-sensitive, it is found in practice that temperature programmed separations may be carried out for quantitative purposes with a constant inlet pressure (the gas flow decreases during the separation) when appropriate ratios of nitrogen/hydrogen/air are employed.

When this detector is used in steroid work, it is customary to calculate mass-area relationships for methoxime (MO) and TMSi ether derivatives on the basis of the structure of the parent steroids, rather than on the basis of the steroid derivatives.

b) Electron Capture

There are differing views with respect to the design and operation of electron capture detectors. Summaries of these views may be found in a number of texts and brochures. The entity which is measured is the conductivity of the carrier gas stream in the cell; this may be nitrogen or an argon-methane mixture. A source of electrons of relatively low energy is required, and at present this is usually supplied by a foil-supported radioactive source (titanium tritide or nickel-63). A constant or pulsed (square wave) direct current is applied across the cell. As the name implies, the capture of electrons by sample components results in the formation of negative molecular ions; these ions are relatively slow-moving and they are likely to undergo recombination with positive ions which are also present. The overall result is a decrease in conductivity when a compound with electron capture properties is present in the cell.

A few halogenated compounds, notably DDT and its relatives, can be detected with very high sensitivity by the "electron capture" detector. A few steroids show direct electron capture properties, but the usual practice is to convert the compounds under study to derivatives of special structure. These may be chloracetates, heptafluorobutyrates or pentafluorophenylhydrazones. Other types of derivatives have also been recommended, including chloromethyldimethylsilyl ethers and chlorodifluoracetates.

The tritium detector is limited in operation to about 220° (loss of tritium occurs above this temperature) but a nickel-63 detector may be used to 350—400°.

There are many difficulties associated with the use of the electron capture detector for quantitative purposes. However, since high sensitivity may be attained there is a great deal of interest in the use of this detection system. A later section of this Chapter contains a summary by EIK-NES of the present state of knowledge of the use of the electron capture detector in steroid studies.

c) Other Systems

Thermal conductivity detectors are not used in gas phase biochemical work because of their relative insensitivity. The gas density balance of MARTIN is rarely used; only a few functioning detectors of the original design are in existence. Selective detection systems for halogens, sulfur and phosphorus are available, but these are not used at the present time in steroid studies. The LOVELOCK argon detector is rarely used in quantitative work because of its relatively small linear range.

3. Sample Introduction

a) Samples in Solution

Syringe injection methods are widely used; the usual sample size is about 1—2 μl for isothermal work and about 2—8 μl for temperature programmed separations. A variety of solvents may be used. For free steroids, these may be isooctane, benzene, ethyl acetate or methanol, depending upon the solubility of the compounds. When derivatives are employed, the reaction mixture is usually injected directly. For example, when steroid TMSi derivatives are prepared with *bis*-trimethylsilylacetamide (BSA), the reagent also acts as the solvent and the mixture is injected directly. Pyridine or acetonitrile is added as a solvent for some reactions with BSA, and in these instances the solution is also injected directly. Carbon disulfide is often recommended as a solvent because of the low response observed for this material with a flame detection system, but in fact this solvent is not widely used.

The advantages of liquid injection methods are many; simplicity, speed and usefulness with many solvents and reaction mixtures are among them. The chief disadvantage in analytical work is that a large portion of the sample is often unused. For example, a reaction mixture may have a volume of 0.1—0.2 ml, while the sample withdrawn for GLC analysis may be 2—5 μl. The remainder of the sample, after one or two GLC samples are removed, is usually discarded. If blood steroids are under study, this may represent an unacceptably large waste of sample, and in these instances a "solid" injection technique is preferable.

b) Solid Injection

Several forms of "solid" injection have been described. The most useful is the introduction of the sample on a small portion of stainless steel or platinum gauze. This technique (MENINI and NORYMBERSKI, 1965) permits an entire analytical sample to be introduced into the chromatographic system, and it is also useful for sample introduction in automated systems. In the usual method, the sample is evaporated in a depression in a Teflon plate to a low volume; methylene chloride is added and the evaporation is repeated. This is done while a gauze roll is in the plate depression, and the sample is effectively transferred to the solid support. The gauze is introduced manually or by automatic means into the chromatographic system.

For high-sensitivity work an advantage of this method is that the solvent front is not present (it is not desirable to carry out analytical measurements on or near the solvent front).

IV. Derivatives

1. Reactions of Hydroxyl Groups

The most useful derivatives for GLC work with hydroxyl-substituted steroids are TMSi ethers. It is important to recognize that the rate of reaction of a steroid hydroxyl group is dependent on the silylating conditions and on structural features of the steroid. For practical purposes the reaction conditions may be classified as non-catalyzed exchange with a silylating agent, and catalyzed reactions proceeding by as yet unverified mechanisms.

An exchange reaction occurs when a hydroxyl-substituted steroid is treated with a silylating agent in the absence of a catalyst; the reagents which are available include trimethylsilyldimethylamine (TMSDMA), HMDS, BSA and TSIM. A fairly rapid reaction ensues when a hydroxyl-substituted steroid is treated with BSA; pyridine or acetonitrile may be added as a solvent, and the following reaction occurs:

$$\underset{\substack{| \\ \text{ROH} + \text{CH}_3\text{C}=\text{NTMSi}}}{\overset{\text{OTMSi}}{}} \rightarrow \underset{\substack{\| \\ \text{CH}_3\text{CNHTMSi} + \text{ROTMSi}}}{\overset{\text{O}}{}}$$

At room temperature the time required for completion of the reaction with an hydroxyl group varies from minutes to hours. Hindered hydroxyl groups do not react; for example, the 11β-hydroxyl group does not form a TMSi ether with BSA at room temperature. This circumstance permits the quantitative conversion of the MO derivatives of steroids like THE and THF to TMSi ethers with unreacted 11β- and tert. 17α-hydroxyl groups. The formation of these derivatives was described by E. C. HORNING, et al. (1967). The use of HMDS or TMSDMA is not recommended because of their slower reaction rates.

The mechanism of the catalyzed silylation reaction is unknown, but it is possible that the first step is the formation of an imonium ion from BSA:

$$\underset{\substack{| \\ \text{CH}_3\text{C}=\text{NTMSi} + \text{TMSiCl}}}{\overset{\text{OTMSi}}{}} \rightarrow \underset{\substack{| \\ \text{CH}_3\text{C}=\text{N}}}{\overset{\text{OTMSi}}{}}\overset{+}{\underset{\diagdown\text{TMSi}}{\diagup\text{TMSi}}} + \text{Cl}^-$$

and that the reaction which then occurs is:

$$\underset{\substack{| \\ CH_3C=N}}{OTMSi} \overset{+ \quad \diagup TMSi}{\underset{\diagdown TMSi}{}} \rightarrow \underset{\substack{\| \\ CH_3C}}{O} -N(TMSi)_2 + (CH_3)_3Si^+$$

$$(CH_3)_3Si^+ + ROH \rightarrow ROTMSi + H^+$$

The HMDS-TMCS (hexamethyldisilazane-trimethylchlorosilane) sily-lation method of MAKITA and WELLS (1963) is also an example of a catalyzed silylation reaction, and this may proceed through a substituted ammonium ion. The reacting species may be a siliconium ion.

The usual procedure for carrying out a BSA-TMCS catalyzed silylation reaction is to dissolve the steroid sample in BSA alone or in pyridine-BSA and to add TMCS. Unhindered hydroxyl groups are converted immediately into TMSi ether groups, and sterically hindered groups may also react. For example, the 11β-hydroxyl group is converted into a TMSi ether group (E. C. HORNING et al., 1967). This is an excellent silylating condition for many steroids. A special problem exists for steroids of the adrenocortical series containing a 17α-hydroxyl group. MO derivatives of compounds E, F, THE and THF are converted to fully silylated MO-TMSi derivatives. This reaction may be carried out in quantitative fashion to yield thermally stable adrenocortical hormone (cortisone, cortisol) derivatives.

No precipitation of salts is observed in BSA-TMCS reaction mixtures. When HMDS-TMCS reaction conditions are used, a precipitate of ammonium chloride is always present. The TMCS-catalyzed HMDS reaction is usually carried out in pyridine, and the products are the same as those observed under BSA-TMCS reaction conditions. TMCS-catalyzed TMSDMA silylation reactions can also be carried out, but these have not been studied extensively for steroids.

TMSi ethers have excellent properties for GLC work. They are thermally stable, and the bulky TMSi group provides steric shielding for the oxygen atom. With non-selective phases, TMSi ethers are eluted after the parent steroids, but the order is reversed with selective phases. For example, when OV-17 is employed TMSi ethers are eluted before the parent hydroxyl-substituted steroids. A minor disadvantage is that use of silyl derivatives leads to silica "whiskers" in flame ionization detectors; these, however, are easily removed by mechanical or chemical cleaning of the electrodes.

Dimethylsilyl derivatives may be prepared by the reaction of hydroxyl-substituted steroids with *bis*-dimethylsilylacetamide or with tetramethyldisilazane-dimethylchlorosilane. These reagents and the derivatives contain a silicon-hydrogen bond, and the silicon hydrides act as reducing agents. This may account for the fact that most dimethylsilyl ethers of steroids are not very stable, in contrast to the TMSi ethers.

The chemical uses of TMSi ethers of steroids have not yet been explored thoroughly. TMSi ethers are highly soluble in non-polar systems. Their hydrolysis occurs under mild conditions, although not as rapidly as is implied by most literature descriptions. For example, TMSi ethers are used in the column chromatographic group separation of steroids (pregnanediol-estriol) according to BROOKS et al. (1967).

Acyl derivatives may be prepared easily for many hydroxyl-substituted steroids. The usual reaction condition is to add an acyl anhydride to a pyridine solution of the steroid sample. (Acetic anhydride-pyridine mixtures contain 10—30% of the anhydride, and the reaction is usually carried out at room temperature or at 60—80°.) Reaction mixtures may be injected directly. The usual reagents are acetic anhydride, for qualitative and quantitative work with ordinary flame detection systems; trifluoracetic anhydride, for special studies of structure; and heptafluorobutyric anhydride, recommended for electron capture work (CLARK and WOTIZ, 1963).

Phenolic ethers may be prepared by classical methods. The most useful reaction is the methylation of a phenol with dimethyl sulfate in alkaline solution. Diazomethane in ether-methanol solution reacts rapidly with a few phenols with special structures, but under ordinary circumstances the reaction is too slow to be useful. The reactions of TMSi ether formation and acylation occur readily for phenols.

2. Reactions of Keto Groups

Many steroid ketones, including progesterone and androstenedione, may be separated by GLC methods without derivative formation. However, if hydroxyl groups are present and if it is desired to prepare TMSi ethers, it is often helpful to convert ketone groups to methoxime (MO) groups. This is done in order to prevent enol ether formation, to decrease the polarity of the ketone group, and in the case of steroids of adrenocortical origin with a tert. 17α-hydroxyl group to provide thermally stable TMSi derivatives. The reaction of methoxime formation was first described by FALES and LUUKKAINEN (1965). This is usually carried out in pyridine solution with methoxylamine hydrochloride. The reaction mixture may be injected directly, or the derivatives may be treated further to form MO-TMSi ethers.

Geometric isomers of the syn/anti type may be formed from some ketones:

$$\begin{array}{c}R_1 \\ \diagdown \\ R_2 \diagup\end{array}C{=}O \rightarrow \begin{array}{c}R_1 \\ \diagdown \\ R_2 \diagup\end{array}C{=}N\diagdown_{OCH_3} + \begin{array}{c}R_1 \\ \diagdown \\ R_2 \diagup\end{array}C{=}N\diagup^{OCH_3}$$

The formation of two isomeric derivatives is not desirable in analytical work, but fortunately not all steroid ketones give two products. The 17- and 20-ketones of the human urinary steroid series do not form isomers, but Δ^4-3 keto steroids give two isomers. The problem is discussed in a recent paper by M. G. HORNING et al. (1967).

Methoximes are more stable to light and air than the N,N-dimethylhydrazones described by VANDENHEUVEL et al. (1965 a). In general, hydrazones can be prepared easily by reaction of the steroid ketone with a substituted hydrazine in pyridine solution; acetic acid is added as a catalyst. Reaction mixtures can be injected directly. N,N-Dimethylhydrazones have good GLC properties and they are useful in structural studies. Pentafluorophenylhydrazones have been used by EIK-NES in high-sensitivity electron capture studies.

The rate of reaction of ketones with oxime and hydrazine reagents is strongly affected by steric influences, and by the presence or absence of an acid catalyst. The usual reaction is acid-catalyzed, but 11-keto groups do not react under conditions where reaction will occur for 3-, 7-, 16-, 17-, and 20-keto groups.

3. Reactions of Acids

Acids are not of general interest in endocrine studies, although the formation of bile acids from cholesterol is an important metabolic transformation. Steroidal acids are never subjected directly to GLC separation conditions. The carboxylic acid group is converted to an ester group for GLC studies. Methyl esters (ME derivatives) are prepared by the addition of diazomethane (in ether solution) to the steroidal acid in methanol-ether solution (or suspension). Trimethylsilyl esters may be prepared easily by reaction with BSA in pyridine solution. The reaction mixture may be injected directly.

β-D-Glucosiduronic acid conjugates are discussed later. These acids may be converted to ME-TMSi derivatives by reaction with diazomethane to form the methyl ester, followed by reaction with BSA. The TMSi ether-esters may be formed by reaction with BSA alone; the carboxylic acid group and the hydroxyl groups react at the same time to form ether-ester derivatives.

4. Steroid Hormone Derivatives

Testosterone and other androgens. Testosterone and related steroids may be chromatographed directly by GLC methods. When a non-selective phase (SE-30, JXR or OV-1) is used, epitestosterone and testosterone are eluted together; this is a disadvantage in both qualitative and quantitative work. It is not advisable to employ the free steroid in quantitative methods if the sample size is small, as is usually the case when working with biological samples. Derivatives which have been used for quantitative work include the TMSi derivative, the MO-TMSi derivative (two isomers) and the acetyl derivative. The derivatives of epitestosterone and testosterone may be separated with selective or non-selective phases.

The heptafluorobutyrate and the chloracetate have been recommended as derivatives for use with electron capture detection systems (CLARK and WOTIZ, 1963; BROWNIE et al., 1964).

Estrogens. The classic estrogens and their metabolites are not usually chromatographed directly. Derivatives which have been used in quantitative work include the TMSi derivatives, the phenolic methyl ether-TMSi derivatives and acetyl derivatives.

The pentafluorophenylhydrazone of estrone and the chloracetate of estradiol have been used by EIK-NES and his coworkers in quantitative procedures employing an electron capture detection system.

Adrenocortical steroids. Stable derivatives of the adrenocortical steroid hormones and their metabolites containing a 17α-hydroxyl group may be prepared by the MO-TMSi procedure; the preferred method is to isolate the MO derivative(s) and to carry out an uncatalyzed silylation reaction with BSA. The 11-keto group and the 11β- and tert. 17α-hydroxyl groups do not react under these circumstances.

If a catalyzed BSA-TMCS silylation reaction condition is used, it is possible to convert both cortisol and cortisone (as MO derivatives) into fully silylated stable derivatives.

Cortol and β-cortol may be converted to fully silylated derivatives by the use of TSIM-BSA-TMCS reaction conditions.

If compounds of the adrenocortical series with a tert 17α-hydroxyl group are subjected directly to GLC conditions, without derivative formation, the side chain is lost and the compounds which are eluted are the corresponding 17-keto steroids (VANDENHEUVEL and HORNING, 1960).

RAPP and EIK-NES (1965) used the C_{21} acetate of deoxycorticosterone for electron capture detection of this hormone.

Aldosterone presents special problems, and the most satisfactory derivative at present is the oxidation product (γ-lactone).

V. Separation Methods

1. With Non-selective Phases

Separations with a non-selective phase are more dependent upon molecular size and shape than upon the presence of specific functional groups. Fig. 1 shows the separation under isothermal conditions of 5α-cholestane and 5β-cholestane with a 1% OV-1 column. The 5α-steroid structure is more nearly planar than the 5β-structure, and this leads to an increase in retention time. Fig. 2 shows the effect of an increasing number of functional groups added to the 5α-androstane structure. The magnitude of the retention time increase is not identical for hydroxyl and keto groups, and it is not the same for all positions of substitution. Epimers are rarely separated, apparently because the change in shape of the molecule is relatively small. However, steric effects can be accentuated by derivative formation, and one of the most effective ways to separate epimers is to prepare TMSi or acyl derivatives and to employ a non-selective phase.

Increasing the molecular size results in an increase in retention time. As the bulk of a derivative increases, the separation of epimeric structures becomes more marked. For each pair, axial structures are eluted before the equatorial isomers. These effects are illustrated in Fig. 3.

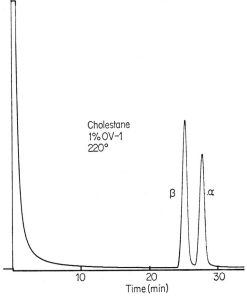

Fig. 1

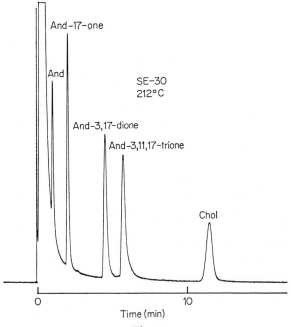

Fig. 2

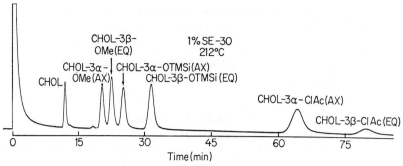

Fig. 3. Isothermal separation of cholestane (CHOL) and several types of derivatives of cholestanol epimers: 3α-hydroxy-5α-cholestane methyl ether (CHOL-3α-OMe AX), 3β-hydroxy-5α-cholestane methyl ether (CHOL-3β-OMe EQ), 3α-hydroxy-5α-cholestane TMSi ether (CHOL-3α-OTMSI AX), 3β-hydroxy-5α-cholestane TMSi ether (CHOL-3β-OTMSi EQ), 3α-hydroxy-5α-cholestane chloracetyl ester (CHOL-3α-ClAc AX) and 3β-hydroxy-5α-cholestane chloracetyl ester (CHOL-3β-ClAc, EQ). Conditions 6 ft 1% SE-30 (on 100—120 mesh Gas Chrom P) column; isothermal at 212°; injector, 260°; detector, 260°; nitrogen, 16 psi; flame detector. The separations are based upon molecular size and shape. Derivatives of 3α-hydroxy-5α-cholestane (axial) are eluted before those of 3β-hydroxy-5α-cholestane (equatorial)

It is usually possible to predict the effect of a structural change on retention time, although unexpected steric factors sometimes have a relatively great influence on retention behavior.

Fluorine substituent groups do not follow these general rules. The fluorine atom has a small radius and hydrogen bonding effects are weak. For example, trifluoracetyl esters are eluted before the corre-

---

Fig. 1. Isothermal separation of 5α-cholestane (α) and 5β-cholestane (β) with an OV-1 column. Conditions: 12 ft 1% OV-1 (on 100—120 mesh Gas Chrom P) column; isothermal at 220°; injector, 260°; detector, 300°; nitrogen, 26 psi; flame detector. The separation is based upon a difference in molecular shape; the more planar 5α-isomer is eluted after 5β-cholestane

Fig. 2. Isothermal separation with an SE-30 column of 5α-androstane (And), 5α-androstan-17-one (And-17-one), 5α-androstan-3,17-dione (And-3,17-dione) and 5α-androstan-3,11,17-trione (And-3,11,17-trione). Cholestane (Chol) is included for comparison purposes. Conditions: 6 ft 1% SE-30 (on 100—120 mesh Gas Chrom P) column, isothermal at 212°; injector, 260°; detector, 260°; nitrogen, 16 psi; flame detector. The separation is based upon increasing molecular size

sponding acetyl esters, although the molecular weight is much higher. An increase in chain length for perfluoralkyl groups has almost no influence on retention behavior; a heptafluorobutyryl ester, for example, may have about the same retention behavior as the corresponding trifluoracetyl ester.

2. With Selective Phases

The retention behavior of a steroid observed with a selective or polar phase is due to a combination of effects. The size and shape of the molecule is important, just as in separations with a non-selective

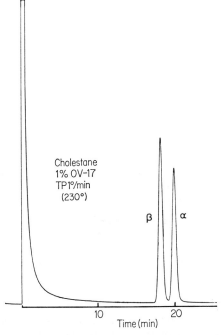

Fig. 4. Temperature programmed separation of 5α- and 5β-cholestane with on OV-17 column; see Fig. 1 for an OV-1 separation. Conditions: 12 ft 1% OV-17 (on 100—120 mesh Gas Chrom P); temperature programmed at 1°/min from 230°; injector, 260°; detector, 300°; nitrogen, 26 psi; flame detector. The separation is based upon a difference in molecular shape, but the MU value difference is slightly greater for OV-17 than for OV-1 (see Table 2). This is due to a "polar" effect which is discussed in a later section

phase. This is apparent in Fig. 4; the separation of 5α- and 5β-cholestane occurs with OV-17 as well as with OV-1. The number, nature and stereochemical arrangement of the functional groups is an important matter as well, and as the polarity of the phase increases the functional group retention effects also increase in magnitude. Phase QF-1 has perhaps the greatest degree of stereochemical specificity of all phases now in use, but positional isomers and epimers may also be distinguished with polyester phases. Hydroxyl and keto groups lead to major increases in retention time; the acetyl group also has polar properties, while ethers are relatively non-polar. Aromatic systems show polar retention effects. Unsaturation (double or triple carbon-carbon bonds) usually leads to selective retention effects; the

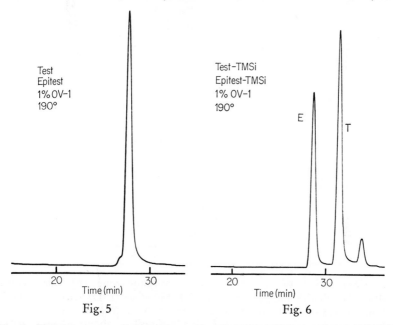

Fig. 5   Fig. 6

Fig. 5. Testosterone and epitestosterone (free steroids) are not separated with an OV-1 column. Conditions: 12 ft 1% OV-1 (on 100—120 mesh Gas Chrom P); isothermal at 190°; injector, 260°; detector, 300°; nitrogen, 26 psi; flame detector. The difference in molecular shape of the epimers is not sufficient to bring about a separation with an OV-1 column

Fig. 6. Separation of testosterone (T) and epitestosterone (E) as TMSi ethers with an OV-1 column under the same conditions used for Fig. 5. The difference in molecular shape of the derivatives leads to a separation; this is in distinction to the result found for the parent steroids

molecular shape may also be modified when unsaturation is introduced.

An expected corollary to these generalizations is that conversion of a polar functional group to a non-polar derivative leads to a decrease in retention time when a selective phase is employed. For example, the di-TMSi derivative of pregnanediol is eluted before the parent steroid with an OV-17 phase. Methoximes are generally eluted before the corresponding ketones. Dehydration, through loss of an alcohol group, reduces the retention time both because of a molecular size change and because a polar functional group is lost.

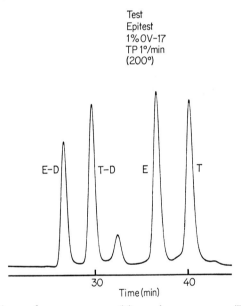

Fig. 7. Separation of testosterone (T), epitestosterone (E), testosterone TMSi ether (T-D) and epitestosterone TMSi ether (E-D) with an OV-17 column. Conditions: 12 ft 1% OV-17 (on 100—120 mesh Gas Chrom P) column; temperature programmed at 1°/min from 200°; injector, 260°; detector, 300°; flame detector. The separation of the free steroids is due to a difference in selective retention with an OV-17 phase. The secondary 17β-OH group of testosterone is less sterically hindered than the secondary 17α-OH group of epitestosterone, and this leads to selective retention of testosterone compared with epitestosterone. The TMSi ethers are eluted in the same order, but the separation is based on a difference in molecular shape, just as observed for OV-1. The derivatives (E-D, T-D) are eluted before the free steroids (E, T) as a consequence of the selective retention effect of the phase for hydroxyl groups

Some of these effects are illustrated in Fig. 5, 6 and 7. Testosterone and epitestosterone (free steroids) can not be separated with an OV-1 phase (Fig. 5). Fig. 6 shows a separation of the TMSi derivatives of the steroids with the same column. Fig. 7 demonstrates the separation of testosterone and epitestosterone, both as free steroids and as TMSi derivatives, with an OV-17 phase. Epimer separation of the free steroids occurs with a selective phase, but not with a non-selective phase. The derivatives, however, are separated with both types of phases, and the separation is based upon a difference in molecular shape.

Fig. 8 and 9 show the separation pattern observed for the MO-TMSi derivatives of testosterone and epitestosterone with OV-1 and OV-17 phases. The *syn/anti* methoxime isomers are not separated with a non-selective phase, and only two peaks are observed. However, when a selective phase is employed, the isomers are separated and four peaks are observed, two from each parent steroid.

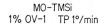

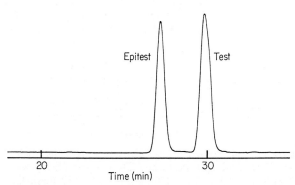

Fig. 8. Lack of separation of methoxime isomers for the MO-TMSi derivatives of testosterone (TEST) and epitestosterone (EPITEST) observed with an OV-1 column. Conditions: 12 ft 1% OV-1 (on 100—120 mesh Gas Chrom P) column; temperature programmed at 1°/min from 200°; injector, 250°; detector, 300°; nitrogen, 26 psi; flame detector. The geometric *(syn/anti)* isomers are not sufficiently different in molecular shape to permit a separation, although the shape of the testosterone peak indicates that two compounds are present. The epitestosterone peak has an approximately theoretical shape, but two isomers are present. This is shown in Fig. 9

The chromatographic relationships between androsterone and pregnanediol, both as free steroids and as TMSi derivatives, are

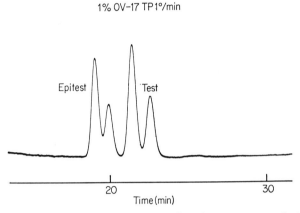

Fig. 9. Separation of methoxime isomers for the MO-TMSi derivatives of testosterone (TEST) and epitestosterone (EPITEST) with on OV-17 column. Conditions: 12 ft 1% OV-17 (on 100—120 mesh Gas Chrom P) column; temperature programmed at 1°/min from 200°; injector, 250°; detector, 300°; nitrogen, 26 psi; flame detector. The pairs of geometric isomers are separated with a selective phase

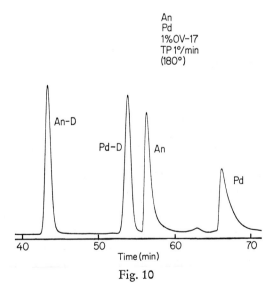

Fig. 10

illustrated in Fig. 10. The derivatives are eluted before the parent steroids because of the selective retention effect arising from the presence of the functional groups (hydroxyl and keto).

3. Column Efficiency

Ordinary columns of 3.5—4.0 mm ID and 6 ft length with 80 to 100 mesh packing usually show an efficiency of about 2000—2500 theoretical plates. A 12 ft column with a 100—120 mesh 1% phase packing should have about 5000—6000 theoretical plates. In general, an increase in length and a decrease in column diameter leads to an increase in efficiency; however, this approach can not be employed with great success with systems containing glass columns and silicone rubber closures because of the increase in pressure needed to maintain a suitable gas flow. The usual aim for practical purposes is to attain 500 theoretical plates per foot of column length.

Column efficiency is important because it determines the separations that are possible with a given phase. For example, a difference in methylene unit (MU) value of about 0.2 will lead to a base-line separation with a column of about 6000 theoretical plates. If the column length is reduced, the degree of resolution will also be reduced. However, for some purposes a 3—4 ft column may provide adequate resolution along with a lower bleed rate, lower temperature of separation and shorter retention time than would be obtained with a 12 ft column.

The highest efficiencies are needed for multicomponent separations. Where extensive purification of the sample has been carried out by other methods, a low efficiency column may be satisfactory.

Fig. 10. Separation of androsterone (An), pregnanediol (Pd), androsterone TMSi ether (An-D) and pregnanediol di-TMSi ether (Pd-D) with an OV-17 phase. Conditions: 12 ft 1% OV-17 (on 100—120 mesh Gas Chrom P) column; temperature programmed at 1°/min from 180°; injector, 260°; detector, 300°; nitrogen, 26 psi; flame detector. The TMSi derivatives are eluted before the corresponding free steroids. Both peaks for the parent steroids show trailing due to the presence of free and relatively unhindered hydroxyl groups; very little trailing is usually observed for ketones, and none for TMSi ethers. The peaks for the derivatives are of approximately theoretical shape. The order of elution for derivatives with an OV-17 column is dependent on molecular size and shape and on functional groups other than TMSi ether groups

Mathematical treatments of column efficiency and problems of resolution may be found in texts. The simple formula that is usually employed for the calculation of plate efficiency is:

$$n = 16 \left(\frac{t_r}{w_b} \right)^2$$

where n = the number of theoretical plates, t_r = retention time measured from the time of injection, and w_b is the base width obtained by triangulation. An isothermal procedure must be used. It is often implied that column efficiency is a property of the column which is dependent only on mechanical or physical characteristics. This is not entirely correct, in the sense that the calculated efficiency also depends upon the sample size, the conditions of the separation and to some extent on the structure of the solute.

The GLUECKAUF graph (GLUECKAUF, 1958) may be used to estimate the plate efficiency needed for a given degree of resolution of two solutes.

While it is often stated that two solutes may occur in a single peak, the precise nature of this effect is rarely mentioned. With a low degree of resolution, two solutes may be eluted with a peak of nearly theoretical shape. The observed retention time will be between the retention times observed for the pure solutes. It is usually possible to detect an effect of this kind by mass spectroscopic analysis, or by changing the phase to one of different polarity. *The appearance of a single peak in a GLC record, in the absence of further information, is not a proof that only a single compound is present. The appearance of two peaks, or a shoulder, is sufficient to indicate unequivocally the existence of a mixture.*

VI. GLC Characterization of Steroids

1. Relative Retention Time

The most popular method of GLC characterization at present is through calculation of relative retention time. The most attractive aspect of this method is that the numerical value can be determined with high precision. Unfortunately, these values, which are based upon a comparison with the behavior of a single reference substance, are temperature dependent and for this reason they are not highly useful in interlaboratory comparisons of data. (Most GLC equipment is manufactured with relatively poor temperature control, and the "observed column temperature" is usually based on a single thermo-couple reading which will vary with the placing of the thermocouple.)

GLC retention behavior should be described through comparison with retention time values for two reference substances. This was first suggested by Kovats (1958), who proposed the use of saturated unbranched aliphatic hydrocarbons as reference substances. Two hydrocarbons were used for reference purposes in an isothermal separation, and the "Retention Index" was calculated as a four-digit value. Somewhat later Woodford and Van Gent (1960) used the "carbon number" concept in connection with the treatment of retention data obtained in a study of fatty acid methyl esters. These values were based on the use of unbranched aliphatic saturated fatty acid methyl esters as reference compounds, and two reference sub-stances were used in each determination of "carbon number".

The Woodford-van Gent technique was based upon the use of reference substances which were structurally related to the compounds under study. The Kovats approach was based upon a need for a universally useful set of reference compounds. The similarity in these methods lies in the use of two reference substances, rather than one, for the calculation of a numerical value.

In a series of studies mentioned in the next sections, it was deter-mined by Horning and coworkers that the use of two reference substances in a GLC separation provides comparative retention values that are independent of small changes in temperature, flow rate and amount of liquid phase. The use of methylene unit (MU) values was proposed for general use (MU values are equivalent to the Kovats retention index values divided by 100) and SN (steroid number) values were proposed for structural correlations within the steroid field. A temperature programmed procedure is currently used for the determination of these values.

One of the confusing aspects of GLC retention behavior, to those who have not employed these methods, is the abundance of contra-dictory retention data in the literature. For example, the order of elution of the TMSi derivatives of androsterone, etiocholanolone, dehydroepiandrosterone and pregnanediol with a 1—3% NGS phase does not seem to be reproducible. The origin of this difficulty lies in varying treatment of the support. The treatment, or lack of treatment, of the support influences the polarity of a selective phase to a considerable extent. This problem has been discussed by VANDENHEUVEL et al. (1966). It is therefore necessary to specify the nature of the support treatment as well as the nature of the phase if meaningful comparisons of retention data are to be made.

2. Methylene Unit (MU) Values

Fig. 11 shows the retention time relationships for a series of aliphatic unbranched saturated hydrocarbons observed in a temperature programmed separation with an OV-1 phase (1%). Although a uniform linear relationship in retention time with respect to the number of carbon atoms is not observed, the time interval between adjacent hydrocarbons after the first two can be treated on a linear basis, and retention values for other compounds can be obtained by interpolation between values for the nearest neighboring hydrocarbons. These values may be expressed as "methylene unit" (MU) values.

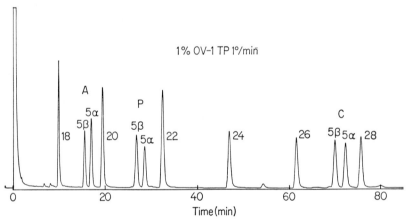

Fig. 11. Temperature programmed separation of long chain saturated aliphatic hydrocarbons (alkane reference hydrocarbons) and steroid hydrocarbons (sterane reference hydrocarbons). The alkanes are those with 18, 20, 22, 24, 26 and 28 carbon atoms. The steranes are 5β- and 5α-androstane (5β, 5α A), 5β- and 5α-pregnane (5β, 5α P) and 5β- and 5α-cholestane (5β, 5α C). The MU values for the steranes may be determined by linear interpolation between the alkane peaks, or by use of a chart similar to Fig. 12. Conditions: 12 ft 1% OV-1 (on 100—120 mesh Gas Chrom P) column; temperature programmed at 1°/min from 160°; injector, 260°; detector, 300°; nitrogen, 26 psi; flame detector

For example, an MU value of 26.15 indicates that the compound would be eluted at a time 0.15 of the interval between the reference hydrocarbons with 26 and 27 carbon atoms in a linear temperature programmed separation carried out as indicated in Fig. 11. Reference substances now available are mostly in the even-numbered series but odd-numbered hydrocarbons should be employed as well when they become available.

It is also possible to define MU values in terms of an isothermal separation. When this is done, the MU value is equivalent to the KOVATS "Retention Index" value divided by 100. However, current studies suggest that the temperature programmed method is superior to the isothermal method.

Table 2. *MU values for steroid hydrocarbons of the androstane, pregnane and cholestane series determined by temperature programming with OV-1 and OV-17 liquid phases*

Steroid hydrocarbon	OV-1 *		OV-17 **	
	MU	5β-5α	MU	5β-5α
5β-Androstane	19.20		20.53	
5α-Androstane	19.50	−0.30	20.87	−0.34 ***
5β-Pregnane	21.12		22.46	
5α-Pregnane	21.42	−0.29	22.80	−0.34 ***
5β-Cholestane	27.18		28.56	
5α-Cholestane	27.50	−0.32	28.94	−0.38 ***

* 1% OV-1 column, temperature programmed at 1 °/min from 160°.
** 1% OV-17 column, temperature programmed at 1 °/min from 160°.
*** These values are greater than the corresponding OV-1 values, indicating that a "polarity" effect occurs when the A/B ring relationship is altered. "Polar" effects arising from the steroid hydrocarbon structure are discussed in the text.

Table 2 contains MU values for the steroid hydrocarbons androstane, pregnane, and cholestane, in both the 5α and the 5β configuration, determined with OV-1 and OV-17 liquid phases. Fig. 12 shows a typical experimental record for the separation (temperature programmed) of the steroid hydrocarbons and aliphatic reference hydrocarbons with an OV-1 phase.

Tables 3 and 4 contain MU values for a number of steroids and steroid derivatives determined with OV-1 and OV-17 liquid phases.

Table 3. *MU values for a group of human urinary steroids and their MO derivatives determined by temperature programming with OV-1 and OV-17 phases.* *

Urinary steroid	OV-1 **		OV-17 ***	
	Free	MO	Free	MO
3α-Hydroxy-5α-androst-16-ene	21.29	—	23.96	—
Androsterone 3α-Hydroxy-5α-androstan-17-one	24.00	24.72	28.44	28.70
Etiocholanolone 3α-Hydroxy-5β-androstan-17-one	23.73	24.48	28.15	28.33
Dehydroepiandrosterone 3β-Hydroxyandrost-5-ene-17-one	24.00	24.72	28.58	28.77
Epiandrosterone 3β-Hydroxy-5α-androstan-17-one	24.04	24.84	28.51	28.83
Androstenediol 3β,17β-Dihydroxyandrost-5-ene	24.19	—	28.37	—
11-Ketoandrosterone 3α-Hydroxy-5α-androstan-11,17- dione	24.85	25.77	30.07	30.46
11β-Hydroxyandrosterone 3α,11β-Dihydroxy-5α-androstan- 17-one	25.91	26.70	31.31	31.58
11-Ketoetiocholanolone 3α-Hydroxy-5β-androstan-11,17- dione	24.55	25.43	29.64	29.97
11β-Hydroxyetiocholanolone 3α,11β-Dihydroxy-5β-androstan- 17-one	25.55	26.22	30.89	31.09
Pregnanediol 3α,20α-Dihydroxy-5β-pregnane	25.85	—	29.72	—
Pregnanediol-20β 3α,20β-Dihydroxy-5β-pregnane	25.53	—	29.45	—
Pregnanolone 3α-Hydroxy-5β-pregnan-20-one	25.44	26.37	29.71	30.20
Cholesterol 3β-Hydroxycholest-5-ene	30.00	—	32.94	—

* This table includes only those steroids that are likely to be subjected to GLC separation in free form for identification purposes. Compounds with a greater number of functional groups are best converted to derivatives before separation.

** 1% OV-1 column, temperature programmed at 1 °/min.

*** 1% OV-17 column, temperature programmed at 1 °/min.

Table 4. *MU values for TMSi and MO-TMSi derivatives of human urinary steroids determined by temperature programming with OV-1 and OV-17 liquid phases.* *

Urinary steroid	OV-1 **		OV-17 ***	
	TMSi	MO-TMSi	TMSi	MO-TMSi
3αHydroxy-5α-androst-16-ene	21.61	—	22.73	—
Androsterone 3α-Hydroxy-5α-androstan-17-one	24.21	25.01	26.81	27.15
Etiocholanolone 3α-Hydroxy-5β-androstan-17-one	24.41	25.22	27.12	27.32
Dehydroepiandrosterone 3β-Hydroxyandrost-5-ene-17-one	24.90	25.63	27.85	28.17
Epiandrosterone 3β-Hydroxy-5α-androstan-17-one	25.02	25.71	27.85	28.19
Δ^9-Androstenolone 3α-Hydroxy-5α-androst-9-ene-17-one	23.89	24.72	26.42	26.89
Δ^9-Etiocholenolone 3α-Hydroxy-5β-androst-9-ene-17-one	23.97	24.78	26.52	26.84
Androstenediol 3β,17β-Dihydroxyandrost-5-ene	25.86	—	26.80	—
11-Ketoandrosterone 3α-Hydroxy-5α-androstan-11,17-dione	25.03	26.00	28.46	28.86
11β-Hydroxyandrosterone 3α,11β-Dihydroxy-5α-androstan-17-one				
3α-trimethylsilyloxy	25.90	26.67	29.47	29.73
3α,11β-ditrimethylsilyloxy	26.43	26.93	28.31	28.55

* These steroids are present in human urine in varying quantity. Estrogens, testosterone and metabolites of aldosterone are not included in this table.

** 1% OV-1 colume, temperature programmed at 1 °/min, starting at 180° or 200°.

*** 1% OV-17 column, temperature programmed at 1 °/min, starting at 180° or 200°.

Table 4 (continued)

Urinary steroid	OV-1 **		OV-17 ***	
	TMSi	MO-TMSi	TMSi	MO-TMSi
11-Ketoetiocholanolone 3α-Hydroxy-5β-androstan-11,17-dione	25.15	26.10	28.59	28.85
11β-Hydroxyetiocholanolone 3α,11β-Dihydroxy-5β-androstan-17-one				
3α-trimethylsilyloxy	26.00	26.18	29.70	29.79
3α,11β-ditrimethylsilyloxy	26.68	27.12	28.60	28.70
16α-Hydroxydehydroepiandrosterone				
3β,16α-Dihydroxyandrost-5-ene-17-one	27.26	27.32	29.18	29.04
Androstenetriol 3β,16α,17β-Trihydroxy-androst-5-ene	28.40	—	28.80	—
Pregnanediol 3α,20α-Dihydroxy-5β-pregnane	27.58	—	28.32	—
Pregnanediol-20β 3α,20β-Dihydroxy-5β-pregnane	27.30	—	28.05	—
Pregnanolone 3α-Hydroxy-5β-pregnan-20-one	26.20	27.08	28.63	29.16
Pregnenediol 3β,20α-Dihydroxypregn-5-ene	28.18	—	29.19	—
Pregnanetriol 3α,17α,20α-Trihydroxy-5β-pregnane				
3α,20α-ditrimethylsilyloxy	29.05	—	30.14	—
3α,17α,20α-tritrimethylsilyloxy	28.00	—	28.42	—
Pregnantriolone 3α,17α,20α-Trihydroxy-5β-pregnan-11-one				
3α,20α-ditrimethylsilyloxy	30.00	—	31.75	—

Table 4 (continued)

Urinary steroid	OV-1 **		OV-17 ***	
	TMSi	MO-TMSi	TMSi	MO-TMSi
Tetrahydrodehydrocortico-sterone (THA) 3α,21-Dihydroxy-5β-preg-nan-11,20-dione	29.88	29.71	32.65	31.85
Tetrahydrocorticosterone (THB) 3α,11β,21-Trihydroxy-5β-pregnan-20-one				
3α,21-ditrimethylsilyl-oxy	30.68	30.17	33.74	32.57
3α,11β,21-tritrimethyl-silyloxy	30.59	29.94	32.00	31.02
allo-Tetrahydrocorticosterone (allo-THB) 3α,11β,21-Trihydroxy-5α pregnan-20-one				
3α,21-ditrimethylsilyloxy	30.77	30.45	33.82	32.75
3α,11β,21-tritrimethyl-silyloxy	30.58	30.11	32.00	31.08
Tetrahydrocortisone (THE) 3α,17α,21-Trihydroxy-5β-pregnan-11,20-dione				
3α,21-ditrimethylsilyl-oxy	—	31.21	—	33.77
3α,17α,21-tritrimethyl-silyloxy	—	29.60	—	30.92
Tetrahydrocortisol (THF) 3α,11β,17α,21-Tetrahydr-oxy-5β-pregnan-20-one				
3α,21-ditrimethylsilyl-oxy	—	31.82	—	34.54
3α,11β,21-tritrimethyl-silyloxy	—	31.79	—	33.16
3α,11β,17α,21-tetra-trimethylsilyloxy	—	30.23	—	30.52
allo-Tetrahydrocortisol (allo-THF) 3α,11β,17α,21-Tetrahydr-oxy-5α-pregnan-20-one				
3α,21-ditrimethylsilyloxy	—	31.96	—	34.78

Table 4 (continued)

Urinary steroid	OV-1 **		OV-17 ***	
	TMSi	MO-TMSi	TMSi	MO-TMSi
3α,11β,21-tritrimethyl-silyloxy	—	31.86	—	33.25
3α,11β,17α,21-tetratri-methylsilyloxy	—	30.36	—	30.64
Cortolone				
3α,17α,20α,21-Tetrahydr-oxy-5α-pregnan-11-one				
3α,20α,21-tritrimethyl-silyloxy	32.07	—	33.25	—
3α,17α,20α,21-tetratri-methylsilyloxy	30.50	—	30.77	—
β-Cortolone				
3α,17α,20β,21-Tetrahydr-oxy-5α-pregnan-11-one				
3α,20β,21-tritrimethyl-silyloxy	32.35	—	33.79	—
3α,17α,20β,21-tetratri-methylsilyloxy	30.79	—	31.73	—
Cortol				
3α,11β,17α,20α,21-Penta-hydroxy-5α-pregnane				
3α,20α,21-tritrimethyl-silyloxy	32.66	—	33.91	—
3α,11β,20α,21-tetratri-methylsilyloxy	33.07	—	33.06	—
3α,11β,17α,20α,21-penta-trimethylsilyloxy	31.22	—	31.43	—
β-Cortol				
3α,11β,17α,20β,21-Penta-hydroxy-5α-pregnane				
3α,20β,21-tritrimethyl-silyloxy	32.85	—	34.17	—
3α,11β,20β,21-tetratri-methylsilyloxy	33.13	—	33.24	—
3α,11β,17α,20β,21-penta-trimethylsilyloxy	30.79	—	30.15	—
Cholesterol				
3β-Hydroxycholest-5-ene	30.79	—	32.09	—

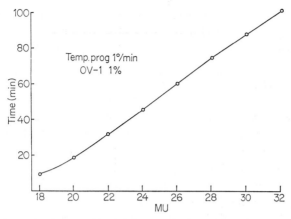

Fig. 12. Chart showing relationship between number of carbon atoms for alkane reference compounds (MU reference values) and retention time for the separation shown in Fig. 11 (the original separation extended to $C_{32}H_{66}$). An approximately linear time relationship is observed between successive peaks except for the first two. The separation of a compound in 10—15 min with a temperature rise of 1°/min resembles that seen with a combination of isothermal and temperature programmed conditions. The flow rate decreased during the separation (a constant inlet pressure was maintained). The useful range for a separation under these conditions is usually 100—150°. MU values are calculated by interpolation or from the chart. It would be desirable to employ odd-numbered alkanes as well when these become available

3. Steroid Number (SN) Values

The retention behavior of a steroid may also be defined by using two of the three steroid hydrocarbons of the 5α-series as reference compounds. The original papers (VANDENHEUVEL and HORNING, 1962; HAMILTON et al., 1963) described an isothermal procedure; this method is illustrated in Fig. 13. Values of 19.00, 21.00 and 27.00 are assigned to the steroid hydrocarbons (5α-androstane, 5α-pregnane and 5α-cholestane) and relative retention times are plotted on a logarithmic scale. Although the slope of each line varies with the temperature of the separation, the SN value, determined through the use of two reference substances, is independent of the temperature.

It is also possible to determine SN values by a temperature programmed procedure. The steroid hydrocarbons 5α-androstane, 5α-pregnane, and 5α-cholestane are employed as reference substances, and their MU values are determined in a temperature programmed separation (Fig. 12 and Table 2). When this is done, it is found that saturated steroid hydrocarbons have polar properties (VANDENHEUVEL et al., 1967). This effect is shown in graph form in Fig. 14. As the polarity of the phase increases, the MU values for the steroid hydrocarbons also increase. The observed retention of a steroid with a selective or "polar" phase is therefore due to a combination of three effects: 1. a retention effect due to the molecular size and shape and based on non-bonded interaction of the LONDON type, 2. a retention effect due to the "polarity" of the saturated polycyclic steroid system (this type of non-bonded interaction has not been previously recognized) and 3. a retention effect based on interaction of the functional groups of the solute and the phase; these forces are primarily due to hydrogen bonding.

The relationship of SN to MU values is described by the following equations based on theoretical considerations outlined by MARTIN

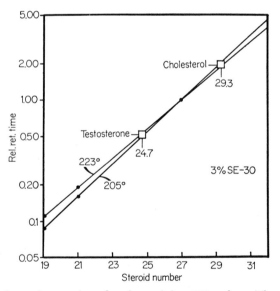

Fig. 13. Isothermal procedure for determining SN values. The relative (to cholestane) retention times are determined for a second reference sterane (5α-pregnane or 5α-androstane) and the compounds under study. Although the slope of the line relating the log RRT value to the SN value is temperature dependent, the SN values are the same when measured at 205° and 223° (SE-30 column)

and by many others who have dealt with the nature of partition chromatography.

   (i) $SN = S + F_1 + \ldots + F_n$

   (ii) $MU = S + S_p + F_1 \ldots + F_n$

In (i), SN is the steroid number, S is the number of carbon atoms in the steroid nucleus and $F_1 \ldots F_n$ are values characteristic of the type and position of the functional groups which are present in the steroid. For (ii), MU is the methylene unit value, S is the MU value for the steroid nucleus and $F_1 \ldots F_n$ (MU values) have the same significance as in (i). S_p is the contribution due to the effect listed as 2. in the previous paragraph.

Ways of relating structure to retention time are of considerable practical and theoretical interest. This may be done through use of SN or MU values. Another useful method is to contrast the retention behavior of a steroid before and after treatment with reagents leading to derivative formation. "Group retention factors" have been proposed as a useful index in this connection. However, the most effective means of studying structure is by the use of gas chromatography-mass spectrometry. These methods are summarized in a later section.

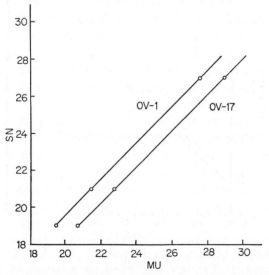

Fig. 14. Relationship of SN and MU values for sterane reference hydrocarbons of the 5α-series determined with OV-1 and OV-17 columns. The increased MU value observed with an OV-17 column is due to "polar" properties of the steroid hydrocarbons

VII. Problems of Quantification

1. Precision of GLC Systems (Flame Detection)

A precision of 0.5% (standard deviation) was found for steroid separations carried out with an automated GLC system (HORNING et al., 1966). The column was a 12 ft glass W-tube containing a 1% SE-30 packing; temperature programming was employed with a hydrogen flame ionization detector. The sample components were representative human urinary steroids converted to TMSi and MO-TMSi derivatives. Peak areas were calculated as the product of the height of each peak and the width at half height. This is a widely used method for area measurement. It is necessary to realize, however, that the least precise part of the entire operation is the measurement of the peak width, and that a magnifying scale should be used for this purpose. In the study cited, the width was measured to the inside of the chart pen line, and the height was measured to the outside of the pen line. Since the observed precision was that of the peak width measurement, it may be surmised that the use of electronic integration methods (with base line drift corrections) would give still higher precision. However, the observed precision is adequate for most work.

There are many variables associated with the operation of a GLC system and with the calculation of results from a chart record. The fact that a precision of 0.5% can be attained is not unexpected, but in every application potential sources of error should be recognized. The major difficulty in the past has been the occurrence of "column loss" through two effects: inadequate deactivation of the support, and failure to prepare suitable derivatives. The practice of "priming" the system should not be used. This recommendation found in the literature arises from an effect that is seen whenever unsatisfactory columns are employed. If active sites are still present on the support, loss of hydroxyl-substituted steroids will always occur, and ketonic steroids may be lost as well. If a large sample is used, a temporary deactivation of the support by the sample will occur. The "priming" effect leads to cyclical improvement in precision (and accuracy) with use. When a suitably deactivated support is used for the column, this effect is no longer noted. It is now a general practice to use deactivated supports and to use TMSi ethers or other derivatives for sterol separations, although derivative formation is not always necessary if the samples are large and satisfactory column packings are employed. Highly hindered hydroxyl groups may resist derivative formation, but such groups rarely lead to adsorption and column loss. Column loss can be estimated by the methods described by HORNING et al. (1963); a hydrocarbon is used as an internal standard and peak area ratios are measured with samples of decreasing size.

Peak height measurements are sometimes used as a substitute for area measurements in quantitative work. This procedure is not recommended when the highest possible precision is desired.

2. Accuracy of GLC Systems (Flame Detection)

A discussion of the accuracy of an instrumental measurement usually requires information of two kinds. It is necessary to know the limiting accuracy of the measurement; this is the highest accuracy that can be obtained under conditions that represent optimum performance of the instrumental system under study. It is also necessary to know the accuracy attainable in specific applications, since this varies greatly as a consequence of variations in experimental procedures and usually with composition or size of the analytical sample.

At the present time the hydrogen flame ionization detector is universally used in quantitative analytical biochemical work for the quantitative measurement of sample components in the range 0.01 to 1 or 2 μg. From a theoretical point of view the detector is flow sensitive and therefore not well-suited for use in temperature programmed separations; in practice, however, gas flow rates can be found that will permit the detector to be used in quantitative fashion in temperature programmed separations. The linear range is relatively great, and column "bleed" does not usually lead to detector problems (although the electrodes must be cleaned regularly because of silica deposits formed when silyl derivatives are under study). The response of the detector is not the same for all organic compounds, although within a given series of compounds the ratio of response (peak area) to mass may be constant (calculations are based on the mass of the parent compound rather than on the mass of the derivative). "Response factors" may therefore be needed in calculations for some analytical methods.

A study was recently carried out to determine the accuracy attainable with an automated GLC system with temperature programmed separation conditions. The test samples were hydrocarbons (in order to avoid adsorption problems) and the conditions were those previously found to result in a precision of 0.5% (standard deviation). The accuracy was found to be 1.0% (standard deviation) (HORNING et al., 1966). This limiting accuracy is satisfactory for most work.

An accuracy of 1% is not usually attained in GLC steroid analyses. There are two major reasons for this circumstance. Column packings often show undesirable adsorption characteristics, and when steroids containing free hydroxyl groups are present tailing and "column loss" due to adsorption are likely to occur. Supports and packings are improving, and adsorption losses are now less common than in an earlier period. Derivatives that show very low adsorption characteristics (MO-TMSi derivatives, for example) should be used in quantitative separations of polyfunctional steroids.

A second problem arises from "compound noise". Samples of biologic origin frequently contain many compounds which are present in low concentration, and when a separation is carried out the base line may show an almost continuous background of low-level compounds. It is not possible to generalize about the accuracy which may be attained under these circumstances, since this will depend upon the magnitude of the effect, which is particularly marked for samples of urinary origin. Columns of greater resolution, or extensive purification of the sample prior to GLC separation, must be used if the effect is unacceptably large.

An example of this problem is shown in Fig. 15. A number of human urinary steroids can be estimated in this analytical separation without undue loss of accuracy due to "compound noise". The determination of THA, however, is not possible for this sample because of an interfering peak, and it would be unwise to estimate several other steroids present at low concentration. It is usually stated that the accuracy is about 5% in a urinary separation of this kind, although both higher and lower figures could be cited for specific components.

Single component analyses are less subject to this difficulty, although the inclusion of a number of fractionation or purification steps prior to the GLC separation may result in lowered precision and accuracy for the entire determination. Estimations requiring GLC separations at high sensitivity are, of course, likely to be less accurate than those carried out with somewhat larger samples. Examples of specific methods are cited in later chapters.

Although it has been suggested at times that GLC methods are inherently lacking in precision and accuracy for steroid work, this is not true. At the present time, the steps required to obtain an analytical sample from urine or blood usually have a much greater effect on the precision and accuracy of the determination than the final GLC procedure.

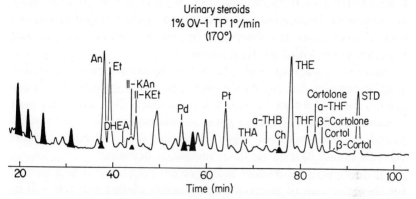

Fig. 15. GLC separation of human urinary steroids (24 hr collection) as TMSi and MO-TMSi derivatives with an OV-1 column. The steroid sample was obtained by enzymic hydrolysis (Glusulase); the solid peaks are from the enzyme preparation. The derivatives were prepared by reaction with methoxylamine hydrochloride, followed by reaction with *bis*-trimethylsilylacetamide (BSA) in an uncatalyzed reaction. The steroids which have been identified are derivatives of androsterone (An), etiocholanolone (Et), dehydroepiandrosterone (DHEA), 11-ketoandrosterone (11-KAn), 11-keto-etiocholanolone (11-KEt), pregnanediol (Pd), pregnanetriol (Pt), tetrahydro-11-dehydrocorticosterone (THA), *allo*-tetrahydrocorticosterone (a-THB), cholesterol (Ch), tetrahydrocortisone (THE), tetrahydrocortisol (THF), *allo*-tetrahydrocortisol (a-THF), cortolone, β-cortolone, cortol and β-cortol. The internal standard is cholesteryl butyrate (STD). Conditions: 12 ft 1% OV-1 (on 100—120 mesh Gas Chrom P) column; temperature programmed at 1°/min from 170°; injector, 260°; detector, 300°; nitrogen, 26 psi; flame detector

3. Radioassay of GLC Effluent

Methods have been developed for the measurement of radioactivity for steroid hormones and their derivatives in effluents from gas phase chromatography columns. Two general approaches may be employed. The radioactivity can be measured in the effluent gas using a gas flow counter (Wölfgang and Rowland, 1958; Mason et al., 1959; Collins and Sommerville, 1964) or the effluent com-

pounds may be condensed on a suitable medium followed by estimation of radioactivity (KARMEN et al., 1962; KARMEN et al., 1963 a).
Simultaneous quantification of a compound and its content of radioactivity can be done when the column effluent gas is passed through
a non-destructive mass detector and a proportional counter which
are placed in series. Alternatively, if the effluent gas is divided, any
type of mass detector (destructive or non-destructive) may be used
in combination with a gas flow counter.

Gas flow radioactivity detection systems are somewhat limited in
their application because of the requirement for quench gases which
cannot always be used with all GLC detectors. Thus argon-methane
mixtures which can be used in gas flow radioactivity detection systems
placed in series with an argon ionization or an electron capture
detector cannot be used for flame ionization detection.

The proportional counter technique has been applied in a method
for the estimation of progesterone in human plasma and this will be
discussed in detail in a later chapter. High efficiency scintillators
(STEINBERG, 1959) with high efficiency for condensation (KARMEN
and TRITCH, 1960) have been used in steroid assays based on the
principle of derivative ratio analyses (KARMEN et al., 1963 b). In these
methods, GLC serves as a final step of purification. In methods
estimating submicrogram amounts of steroids in biological samples
by isotopes of different energy spectra (double isotope assay), the
sample used for the final measurement of radioactivity must be in a
high state of radiochemical purity. It has been observed that such
methods often have a relatively high background in spite of repeated
chromatography on paper or on coated glass plates. The use of GLC
for final purification in these methods may decrease the H^3/C^{14} ratio
in the plasma blank as well as in the steroid sample by as much as
13% (BARDIN and LIPSETT, 1967). Such purification cannot be obtained by conventional chromatography. GLC will therefore decrease
the time and cost per assay (KLIMAN, 1965) and also give samples of
high purity, thus increasing the precision of the assay. In order to
apply adequately the discontinuous method of collecting radioactive
vapor to the problem of purifying biological samples, the amount of
steroid chromatographed must give rise to sample signals in the
ionization detector. Since sample size often is a limiting factor in
biological work, the use of detectors of high-sensitivity could provide
opportunities for wider application of the discontinuous method of

vapor collection to biological problems. This technique has not been explored in GLC with electron capture detectors.

A procedure for calibrating flow-through detectors of C^{14} in GLC systems has been described by KARMEN (1967).

One should be aware that isotope fractionation has been observed during GLC (KIRSCHNER and LIPSETT, 1965, KLIMAN and BRIEFER, 1967). Displacement as well as dispersion (KLEIN et al., 1964) of the labeled species may occur. These phenomena can also be seen in liquid partition chromatography (CC) (CEJKA et al., 1966) and in PC (GOLD and CRIGLER, 1966). No theory has been formulated to describe why isotope fractionation takes place during chromatography (KLEIN, 1966).

VIII. Analytical Applications with High-sensitivity Selective Detection (K. B. EIK-NES)

LOVELOCK and LIPSKY (1960) observed that certain organic vapors may capture electrons. This was also the experience of WENTWORTH and BECKER (1962). Subsequent to these observations it was suggested that detection of submicrogram amounts of steroids should be possible by electron capture following gas phase chromatography (LANDOWNE and LIPSKY, 1963; LOVELOCK et al., 1963). A general approach to this problem was laid down in the publication of LOVELOCK (1961) and since few natural steroids contain electron absorbing groups (Table 5), steroid derivatives containing such groups must be made prior to quantification by an electron capture detector. By 1964, it was clearly evident that extremely low levels of pure cholesterol haloacetates (LANDOWNE and LIPSKY, 1963), pure steroids reacted with heptafluorobutyric anhydride (CLARK and WOTIZ, 1963) and the chloroacetates of synthetic testosterone and of 20α-hydroxypregn-4-ene-3-one (BROWNIE et al., 1964) could be detected by electron capture following GLC. These findings were used in methods for the submicrogram detection of testosterone (BROWNIE et al., 1964), progesterone (VAN DER MOLEN and GROEN, 1965) and estradiol (AAKVAAG and EIK-NES, 1965) in biological samples. Details of these methods will be given in later chapters. Moreover, from preliminary communications it is evident that the observation of CLARK and WOTIZ (1963) concerning heptafluorobutyrates can be extended to the estimation of estrogens (CHARRANSOL and WOTIZ, 1966) and tes-

Table 5. *Affinities for thermal electrons of compounds of biological interest. All values are relative to the electron affinity of chlorobenzene, which is taken to be unity*

Compounds with high electron affinity	Electrophore	Affinity	Compounds with low electron affinity	Affinity
Ethyl pyruvate	—CO·CO—	1,700	Ethyl acetate	<0.01
Diacetyl	—CO·CO—	2,000	Acetylacetone	1.2
Dimethyl oxalacetate	—CO·CO—	1,300	Ethyl acetoacetate	0.7
Diethyl fumarate	—CO·CH:CH·CO—	1,500	Ethyl acrylate	0.1
Diethyl maleate	—CO·CH:CH·CO—	1,700	Diethyl malate	0.01
			Diethyl succinate	<0.01
Quinone	Q	5,000	Hydroquinone	0.1
Dimethylnaphthaquinone	Q	4,100	Benzyl alcohol	0.05
Benzaldehyde	—CO·P	48		
Cinnamaldehyde	—CO·CH:CH·P	310	Styrene	<0.01
cis-Stilbene	P·CH:CH·P	1		
trans-Stilbene	P·CH:CH·P	4		
Acetamide	—CO·NH·	12	Methyl amine	0.01
Azobenzene	P·N:N·P	9		
Diacetyldihydropyridine	Q	4,000	Pyridine	0.02
Anthracene		12	Phenanthrene	0.05
Azulene		340	Napthalene	<0.01
Cyclo-octatetrene		210	Cyclopentadiene	<0.01
Carbon tetrachloride	—Cl	7,000	Ethane	<0.01
Chloroform	—Cl	800		
Hexachlorobenzene	—Cl	1,100	Benzene	<0.01
Chlorobenzene	—Cl	1		
Bromobenzene	—Br	6		
Iodobenzene	—I	370		
Nitrobenzene	—NO₂	390		
Dinitrophenol	—NO₂	1,450		

P, phenyl radical.   Q, quinone structure.   The data are from a publication by LOVELOCK (1961).

tosterone (EXLEY, 1966; VERMEULEN, 1967; VAN DER MOLEN, 1967) in small volumes of human plasma.

RAPP and EIK-NES (1965) studied the electron capture affinity of corticosteroid derivatives and observed that the 21-acetate of deoxycorticosterone and the γ-lactone of aldosterone would capture electrons. These authors published a detailed method describing the measurement of deoxycorticosterone and aldosterone in biological samples (RAPP and EIK-NES, 1966 a). The final concentration of aldosterone in the purified sample must be rather high and the sensitivity of the method of RAPP and EIK-NES (1966 a) would not permit adequate estimation of aldosterone in physiological volumes of human plasma (BRODIE et al., 1967). AAKVAAG (1967) has used this method for the measurement of conjugated aldosterone in human urine. Since the γ-lactone of aldosterone has good gas chromatographic properties (RAPP and EIK-NES, 1966 a), it may be possible to measure submicrogram concentrations of aldosterone in biological samples using the pentafluorophenylhydrazone of the γ-lactone.

The observation that adrenosterone and the 21-acetate of 11-dehydrocorticosterone also will capture electrons (RAPP and EIK-NES, 1965) has been used for the submicrogram estimation of cortisol and corticosterone in blood (LLOYD et al., 1967), but the sensitivity for adrenosterone detection by this technique is low compared to that for the other steroid derivatives discussed.

Recently, our laboratory (ATTAL et al., 1967) made the observation that estrone-3-methyl ether-17-pentafluorophenylhydrazone will capture electrons. This steroid derivative has more sensitivity for electron capture than steroid chloroacetates, but probably less sensitivity than the derivatives obtained following the reaction of steroids with heptafluorobutyric anhydride. There is, however, no agreement in the literature on the relationship between electron capture affinity of a steroid and its concentration of atoms other than carbon and hydrogen (LANDOWNE and LIPSKY, 1963; NAKAGAWA et al., 1966). Recently we have observed (WASSERMANN and EIK-NES, 1967) that the electron capture affinity of the 3-acetate-17-pentafluorophenyl-hydrazone derivative of dehydroepiandrosterone is higher than that of its 3-chloroacetate-17-pentafluorophenylhydrazone.

Steroid monochlorodifluoroacetates (RAISINGHANI et al., 1966), chloromethyl dimethylsilyl ethers (THOMAS et al., 1966) and bromomethyl dimethylsilyl ethers (EABORN et al., 1967) will all capture electrons and show adequate stability during GLC. The use of these derivatives for the estimation of steroids in biological samples has not been fully explored.

Technological progress in this field has been hampered by two factors: 1. instrumentation, and 2. purification of compounds from a biological sample.

Most investigators prefer to apply a pulsating voltage to the electron capture detector. This results in a lower noise level than the use of direct voltage and will thus increase the sensitivity of detection and decrease baseline drift (LOVELOCK, 1961; LOVELOCK, 1963). It is also possible that the non-pulsed cell is more sensitive to column bleed than the pulsed electron capture cell (LOVELOCK, 1963; OAKS et al., 1964) though this point is not settled (RAPP and EIK-NES, 1966 b).

In most commonly used electron capture detectors, the electron environment is created from a tritium foil. The highest permissible temperature for the operation of such detectors is 220 °C. In most work short columns (2—3 ft) must be used and this may severely limit steroid separations. On a 12 ft XE-60 column, the retention time of steroid chloroacetates is too long to be of practical use even if the column is operated at 220 °C (VAN DER MOLEN et al., 1965). One should therefore look forward to publications on the use of the Ni-63 electron capture detector, since this would permit gas phase chromatography at much higher temperatures than is possible with the tritium foil detector (VAN DER MOLEN et al., 1965; ATTAL et al., 1967). The Ni-63 detector would probably be less sensitive than the tritium foil detector; the latter can detect about 10^{-9}—10^{-8} gram of a steroid chloroacetate with good precision. The electron capture detector of the Beckman GC-5 instrument may also permit estimation of extremely low concentrations of steroid chloroacetates. Few communications have, however, appeared on the estimation of picogram concentrations of steroids with this detector.

With few exceptions (VAN DER MOLEN et al., 1965), the steroid chloroacetates are stable compounds and can be purified by conventional TLC. This is imperative in order to get rid of excess reagents prior to GLC. Purification by PC has not been successful for this purpose since it is difficult to purify the paper support to the same degree as the silica gel support. The steroid derivatives obtained by the method of CLARK and WOTIZ (1963) are more volatile than the steroid chloroacetates, have much higher electron capture affinity (NAKAGAWA et al.,

1966) and should permit the detection of about 10^{-9}—10^{-10} grams of steroid. The use of this technique for the estimation of steroids in biological samples has been difficult from the standpoint of sample purity. Also, if excess reagent is used in the formation of steroid heptafluorobutyrates, enolized Δ^4-3-keto groups may be formed. These groups are extremely unstable and will decompose during PC or TLC (VAN DER MOLEN et al., 1967). Since the sensitivity of detection of steroid heptafluorobutyrates is high, multiple application of aliquots from the same biological sample to GLC should be possible thus increasing the precision of assay.

No discussion of electron capture detection of steroids would be complete without some account of the purity requirements for the samples of biologic origin to be determined by this technique. Extreme purity of all reagents involved is needed and it is the experience of our laboratory that each solvent and each chemical compound involved in a method should be subjected to chloroacetylation or pentafluoro-phenylhydrazone formation. The product(s) should then be exposed to GLC with electron capture detection under exactly the same conditions as for the steroid to be measured. All glassware coming in contact with the sample must be scrupulously clean and a sequence of chromium trioxide—hot water—alkali glass distilled water, and triple-distilled ethanol appears to be a requirement for successful analysis.

Due to the temperature limitations and the sample capacity of the electron capture cell, GLC with electron capture detection of sub-microgram amounts of steroids from biological sources at present utilizes predominately the high detector sensitivity of the technique and not the ability of a GLC column to separate steroids. Thus, prior to GLC, a sample steroid must be free of contaminating compounds. Given the nature of steroid composition in biological samples, it is hardly surprising that prepurification by other chromatographic methods is needed. Prepurification is associated with loss of steroids in the sample. Moreover, during the steps of prepurification the sample can become contaminated with impurities from the systems of PC or TLC used. Such impurities will often give rise to a wide "front" during GLC and it is often not possible to apply the total sample to GLC. Some balance must therefore be struck between steroid loss through processes of purification and width of the "front" during GLC separation of the sample.

4*

The linearity of response of the electron capture detector to steroid concentrations should be established for each compound to be determined. When working with steroid samples of unknown composition, care has to be exercised to keep the sample concentration within the optimal capacity of the electron capture cell. One of the charms and yet one of the dangers of GLC is the ease of compound quantification and the relatively inadequate precision of measurement imposed in electron capture detection by the non-linearity of the detector device at certain compound concentrations.

The instability of the tritium foil electron capture detector deserves the most serious attention in analytical work. At the temperature of operation in the published steroid assays, the sensitivity of the cell will decrease with use due to bleeding of tritium from the radioactive foil (SHOEMAKE et al., 1963). It has been reported that a tritium detector operated at 190 °C will lose 0.5 millicuries per day (KAHN and GOLDBERG, 1965). The tritium activity is between 50—250 millicuries in most of the commercially available detectors. Since the energy of β-radiation is low, any contamination of the tritium foil will decrease the electron current. As a consequence of such decrease, the standing current produced in the cell will be diminished and the sensitivity of the cell at its ordinary operating voltage reduced. In addition to column bleed, application of impure samples and use of impure carrier gas are the most common reasons for cell contamination. The purity of the carrier gas must be checked frequently and one should not rely on stated purity of commercially available carrier gas, but expose it to some repurification process before it enters the column (BROWNIE et al., 1964). The cell itself should be cleaned at frequent intervals. A significant contribution to technology in this field is a recent paper by HOLDEN and WHEATLEY (1967).

RAPP and EIK-NES (1966) observed that synthetic steroids extracted from silica gel thin-layer plates contain impurities which have relatively short retention time (sample "front") on GLC. These impurities decreased the sensitivity of the electron capture cell for steroid quantification. Moreover, this decrease in cell sensitivity at every point in time along the recording was inversely proportional to an increase in baseline caused by material extracted from *purified silica gel*. Since TLC is the usually recommended method for sample purification prior to GLC and since the sensitivity of the electron capture cell decreases at 220°, some means of compensation for spontaneous change in cell sensitivity must be found. In our original method (BROWNIE et al., 1964), we thus introduced the use of an internal standard, i. e., the addition to the purified steroid sample of a known amount of a synthetic steroid chloroacetate just prior to GLC. HORNING and coworkers had introduced the use of an internal standard in GLC work in 1963 (HORNING et al., 1963).

In addition to a check on cell sensitivity at the moment of GLC of the unknown sample, the internal standard will also compensate for compound loss during its transfer to the column which poses a problem when handling nanogram or picogram amounts of steroids (RAPP and EIK-NES, 1966 a). Moreover, the internal standard will compensate for losses occurring during GLC. It is imperative, however, that the sample be free of the internal standard as an endogenous contaminant before GLC, that the internal standard shares many of the physico-chemical characteristics of the sample steroid, and that the sample steroid and the internal standard are eluted from the column closely together and in a position where the baseline does not change rapidly. Finally, the sensitivity of detection of the internal standard should be in the same range as that for the sample steroid. Thus, in our method for the measurement of plasma testosterone, we changed the internal standard from cholesteryl chloroacetate to the chloroacetate of 20β-hydroxypregn-4-ene-3-one. This switch resulted in better precision of assay (RESKO and EIK-NES, 1966). The electron absorbing activity of the chloroacetates of testosterone and 20β-hydroxypregn-4-ene-3-one is approximately the same whereas that of cholesteryl chloro-acetate is much lower (VAN DER MOLEN et al., 1965).

Use of an internal standard improves the precision of assay for submicrogram quantification of steroids (Table 6). The precision of measurement of absolute peak areas is much lower than that obtained by peak ratio estimations. We therefore feel that the use of an internal standard in micromethods for the estimation of steroids by electron capture is not merely important but paramount. This view is not shared by all investigators in this field (VERMEULEN, 1967).

Illustrations of the use of electron capture detection following GLC will be given in subsequent chapters. It is probably not excessive to say that this approach to steroid methodology has already given valuable data on crucial issues like the measurement of specific radio-activity of steroids biosynthetized from labeled steroid precursors. The methodological drawbacks encountered are, however, uncomfortably reminiscent of those of other techniques for the measurement of small amounts of steroids in a biological sample. Sample purity *is a must* and no scientific evidence that has yet been authenticated supplies an irrefutable answer to the problem of microestimation of steroids in samples of "questionable" purity.

Table 6. *Reproducibility of quantification of pure testosterone chloroacetate (T) and of pure 20β-hydroxypregn-4-ene-3-one chloroacetate (P) by electron capture*

Amount chromatographed	Mean peak area (cm²)		
(μg)	T	P	Ratio *
0.005	10.34	12.29	1.19
(n** = 12)	2.29 ***	2.94 ***	0.055 ***

$$* \ \text{Ratio} = \frac{\text{peak area for P}}{\text{peak area for T}}$$

** n — number of samples.

*** One standard deviation.

Mixtures containing equal amounts of both steroids were chromatographed on a 3 ft 1% XE-60 column. The individual data were taken at random from calibration experiments conducted over a period of several months. Attenuation of the detector signal was 1/64 (0.64×10^{-10}) amps for full scale deflection of the recorder pen. The data are from an investigation by VAN DER MOLEN and GROEN (1967).

IX. Structural Analysis by Gas Chromatography-Mass Spectrometry

1. The Gas Chromatograph-Mass Spectrometer as a Combined Instrument

A combination of gas chromatography and mass spectrometry, attained through use of a combined instrument, provides the ability to identify and study individual components of mixtures with or without the prior use of classical separation methods.

The combined instrument represents a major advance in analytical methodology for the study of many biological problems. The technique has been described by RYHAGE (1964) and by LEEMANS and McCLOSKEY (1967). A combined low resolution instrument, designed as a new instrument rather than as a mechanical joining of existing instruments, is now available, and combined high resolution instruments may be available in the future.

There are many ways in which the combined gas chromatograph-mass spectrometer may be used. An illustration of one type of use is demonstrated in Fig. 15 and 16. Companion charts, for OV-17 separations, are shown in Fig. 17 and 18. Fig. 16 and 18 show an analytical separation of human urinary steroids (24 hr collection) after the ingestion of 50 mg of corticosterone. The "steroid profiles" (Fig. 16 and 18) should be compared with the profiles in Fig. 15 and 17. After oral ingestion of corticosterone, a major peak was found with reten-

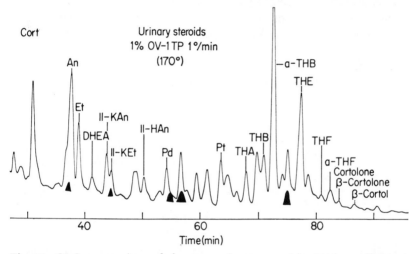

Fig. 16. GLC separation of human urinary steroids (24 hr collection) obtained after ingestion of 50 mg of corticosterone. The steroids were separated as TMSi and MO-TMSi derivatives with a 1% OV-1 column. Enzymic hydrolysis (Glusulase) was employed. The derivatives were prepared by reaction with methoxylamine hydrochloride, followed by reaction with *bis*-trimethylsilylacetamide (BSA) in an uncatalyzed reaction. The steroids which have been identified are the same as those noted in Fig. 15, and also 11β-hydroxyandrosterone (11-HAn) and tetrahydrocorticosterone (THB). *allo*-THF and cortolone are eluted without resolution under these conditions. The "steroid profile" of Fig. 15 is the normal or control pattern, and a major new peak may be observed at the position corresponding to *allo*-tetrahydrocorticosterone (a-THB). Conditions: 12 ft 1% OV-1 (on 100—120 mesh Gas Chrom P) column; temperature programmed at 1°/min from 170°; injector 260°; detector, 300°; nitrogen, 26 psi; flame detector

tion times corresponding to allo-THB (as the MO-TMSi derivative, Fig. 16 and 18) and a peak was also found corresponding to tetra-hydrocorticosterone (THB). Since identification based on GLC data alone can not be regarded as definitive, mass spectra were obtained for the major metabolite and the reference compound (as MO-TMSi derivatives) with a combined instrument. The spectra were identical. In this instance the experimental result was expected because of the earlier work of ENGEL et al. (1955) indicating that the chief metabolite of corticosterone in the human is *allo*tetrahydrocorticosterone. Metabolites of other steroids and steroid drugs may be studied in the same way.

In general, whenever a marked change in a steroid pattern occurs, the compound(s) responsible for new peaks should be studied by mass spectrometry as well as by gas chromatography. A tentative identification may often be made by examination of the mass spectra. Very little data have been published for derivatives of steroids that are used in GLC separations, and the following comments may require modi-

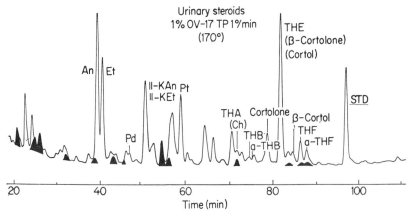

Fig. 17. GLC separation of the TMSi and MO-TMSi derivatives of human urinary steroids (24 hr collection) with a 1% OV-17 column; the sample is the same as that employed for Fig. 15. The solid areas represent contributions from the enzyme preparation (Glusulase). The THA and cholesterol peaks include other unidentified substances. 11-Ketoandrosterone and 11-ketoetiocholanolone are not separated under these conditions. β-Cortolone and cortol are not separated from THE. The internal standard is cholesteryl butyrate (STD). Conditions: 12 ft 1% OV-17 (on 100 to 120 mesh Gas Chrom P) column; temperature programmed from 170° at 1°/min; injector, 260°; detector, 300°; nitrogen, 26 psi; flame detector

fication as a result of greater experience. MO, TMSi and MO-TMSi derivatives show ions at m/e values corresponding to M (molecular weight; the ion is M^+) and M-15 for TMSi and MO-TMSi derivatives, and M and M-31 (M-30 in some cases) for MO and MO-TMSi derivatives. The groups of ion peaks at M and M-15 for TMSi derivatives always show the characteristic silicon isotope distribution. Odd and even values of M correspond to odd and even (including zero) numbers of methoxime functional groups (excluding amino steroids). When the TMSi group is present, a peak is usually also seen at M-90, and if several TMSi groups are present it is usually possible to identify successive loss of fragments corresponding to 90 amu (atomic mass units). The elimination of the C-20, 21 side chain from C_{21} steroids can usually be recognized; the elimination reaction may occur in stepwise fashion.

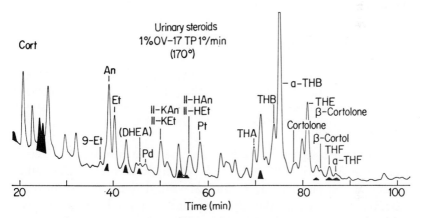

Fig. 18. GLC separation of TMSi and MO-TMSi derivatives of human urinary steroids (24 hr collection) with a 1% OV-17 column; the sample is the same as that employed for Fig. 16 (ingestion of 50 mg of corticosterone). The solid areas represent contributions from the enzyme preparation (Glusulase). The small peak preceding that for androsterone, also seen in Fig. 17, corresponds to Δ^9-etiocholanolone. The DHEA peak contains another (unidentified) compound, and 11β-hydroxyandrosterone and 11β-hydroxyetiocholanolone are not separated. The chief metabolite of corticosterone is *allo*-tetrahydrocorticosterone. A considerable increase in size of a peak corresponding to cholesterol (excreted as cholesteryl sulfate) may be noted; this effect is under investigation. Conditions: 12 ft 1% OV-17 (on 100—120 mesh Gas Chrom P) column; temperature programmed at 1°/min from 170°; injector, 260°; detector, 300°; nitrogen, 26 psi; flame detector

Important diagnostic information may be obtained from a few specific peaks, although all interpretations must be made with care. For example, a peak at m/e 129 is characteristic of TMSi ethers of sterols of the 3β-hydroxy-Δ^5 class. The appearance of a peak at m/e 129, however, does not constitute proof that a 3β-hydroxy-Δ^5 structure is present. This is illustrated in Fig. 19 in the mass spectrum for testosterone as the TMSi ether. The peak at m/e 129 is due to D-ring cleavage to yield a fragment containing the TMSi ether group.

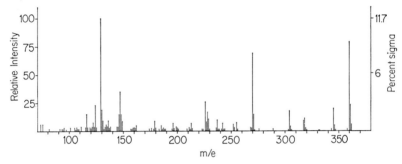

Fig. 19. Mass spectrum of testosterone TMSi ether. The peaks at M and M-15 show the silicon isotope effect. The peak at m/e 129 (base peak) is due to D-ring cleavage to yield an ion containing the TMSi ether group. A peak at M-90 is also present

Another example of a steroid mass spectrum is in Fig. 20. This is from the MO-tri-TMSi ether of tetrahydrocortisone. The ether groups are at positions 3, 17 and 21; the derivative is formed by reaction with *bis*-trimethylsilylacetamide in a catalyzed (trimethylchlorosilane) reaction.

Idealized spectra are usually presented in this way, since the original chart records are on photosensitized paper, and these cannot be reproduced easily.

A detailed study of the mass spectrum for a steroid may involve extensive analysis of electron-impact induced fragmentation reactions. Metastable ions may be involved; the m/e value for a "metastable" signal (m^*) is $m^* = m_2^2/m_1$. The reactions may follow unexpected pathways, although the extensive studies of DJERASSI and his colleagues (1964) have provided much information about relationships between structure and mass spectra for steroids. The current state of knowledge for gas chromatography-mass spectrometry, which usually uses steroid derivatives, is summarized in a recent review (HORNING et al., 1968).

Several precautions should be kept in mind when mass spectra obtained with a combined instrument are interpreted. The experimental record is usually obtained during a period of changing concentration, and the relative intensity of the peaks may vary from one determination to the next if the concentration changes are not similar. A "bias" effect may also occur due to pressure changes in the ion source (LEEMANS and MC-CLOSKEY, 1967). Small changes in the intensity of peaks are not serious, but if M and M-15 peaks are lost for a TMSi derivative the difficulties in interpretation may be formidable until the experimental difficulty is recognized.

Derivatives of epimers do not usually give mass spectra differing by more than normal experimental variation. This experimental limitation is as serious one. A combination of GLC and mass spectrometric data may,

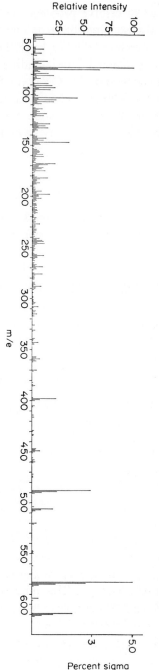

Fig. 20. Mass spectrum of an MO-TMSi derivative of tetrahydrocortisone obtained with a combined instrument (LKB 9000). The derivative was prepared by reaction with BSA-TMCS (catalyzed reaction). Peaks occur at M, M-15, M-31, and M-90, corresponding to loss of the following groups: methyl (15, from a TMSi group), methoxyl (31, from a methoxime group), trimethylsilanol (90). The side chain is eliminated in stepwise fashion, with loss of 103 units (CH_2OTMSi) and 160 units (CH_2OTMSi and $C = NOCH_3$). Major peaks occur at m/e 609 (M), 578 (M-31), 488 (M-31-90) and 398 (M-31-90-90)

however, be used to resolve problems of epimer identification. Positional isomers always give different mass spectra, and TMSi derivatives of steroid epimers always have different GLC properties, as far as is known. Combined data including (1) the mass spectrum, and (2) the GLC retention data for OV-1 (or SE-30) and OV-17 columns should result in a definitive identification for steroids of uncertain structure. If reference compounds are not available, and if the structure is novel, the identification may be more difficult. The availability of reference compounds is of major importance for effective use of these methods.

2. Structural Analytical Methods

The identification of the urinary steroids of the human newborn infant is an example of a current structural analytical problem that may be studied by gas phase analytical procedures. Similar methods may be used for other problems. Fig. 21 shows the "steroid profile" for a newborn infant (age, 5 days; profile from a 24 hr urine collection);

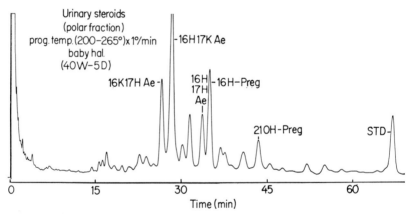

Fig. 21. GLC separation of TMSi derivatives of urinary steroids (24 hr collection) from a newborn infant (age, 5 days). The steroids were obtained by enzymic hydrolysis (Glusulase). The compounds which have been identified are $3\beta,16\alpha$-dihydroxyandrost-5-ene-17-one (16H 17K Ae), 3β, 17β-dihydroxyandrost-5-ene-16-one (16K 17H Ae), $3\beta,16\alpha,17\beta$-trihydroxyandrost-5-ene (16H 17H Ae), $3\beta,16\alpha$-dihydroxypregn-5-ene-20-one (16H-PREG) and $3\beta,21$-dihydroxypregn-5-ene-20-one (21OH-PREG). The internal standard is cholesterylbutyrate (STD). Conditions: 12 ft. 1% SE-30 (on 100—120 mesh Gas Chrom P) column; temperature programmed at $1°$/min from $200°$; injector, $260°$; detector, $300°$; nitrogen, 26 psi; flame detector

the steroids were separated as TMSi ethers. A preliminary CC silicic acid separation of difunctional steroids of the androsterone-etio-cholanolone type was carried out, but this step can be omitted for infant steroid samples. Mass spectra were obtained for all major GLC peaks shown in the illustration. The steroid mixture (free steroids) was subjected to TLC separation (silicic acid) and zones of increasing R_f value were eluted. A GLC analysis of each zone was carried out after conversion of the steroids to TMSi or MO-TMSi derivatives. Fig. 22 shows a typical GLC analytical record (MO-TMSi derivatives) for a TLC zone obtained in an investigation of this kind. At the same time that an enrichment of the sample occurred for major components, the minor components of similar polarity were brought into the same fraction. Mass spectra and GLC retention behavior provided sufficient information for the identification of the compounds noted in Fig. 21. A preliminary description of the method has been published (GARDINER et al., 1966).

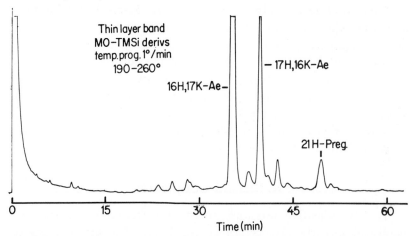

Fig. 22. GLC analysis of steroids in a TLC zone, from a sample of human infant urinary steroids. The TLC separation (silicic acid) yielded several zones; this zone contained keto-diols. The eluted steroids were converted to MO-TMSi derivatives, and the analytical separation was carried out with a 1% OV-1 column. The major steroids were found to be 3β,16α-di-hydroxyandrost-5-ene-17-one (16H, 17K-Ae), 3β,17β-dihydroxyandrost-5-ene-17-one (17H, 16K-Ae) and 3β,21-dihydroxypregn-5-ene-20-one (21H-PREG) by mass spectrometric studies with a combined instrument. Conditions for the GLC separation: 12 ft 1% OV-1 (on 100—120 mesh Gas Chrom P) column; temperature programmed at 1°/min from 190°; injector, 260°; detector, 300°; nitrogen, 26 psi; flame detector

Evidence relating to the presence or absence of functional groups may be obtained by the use of reactions leading to derivative formation. Keto groups at the 3, 16, 17 and 20 positions react to form methoxime derivatives under the usual conditions for derivative formation. Hydroxyl groups at the 21, 3, 16, 20, sec 17, 11, tert 17 may be converted to TMSi ether groups, usually in that order; polyfunctional steroids often give multiple products if the reaction conditions are not selected to yield single products. Oxidation and reduction conditions may often be used to establish structure; the formation of mixed products is not always undesirable since individual components of reaction mixtures (usually including unreacted starting material) may be studied by GLC-mass spectrometric methods.

A few special methods may also be useful. The conversion of 3β-ol-Δ^5 steroid sulfates to i-steroids, and back to 3β-ol-Δ^5 steroids, may be carried out according to FOTHERBY (1959). The conversion of methane (or toluene) sulfonic acid esters of 3β-ol-Δ^5 steroids to i-steroids by thermal elimination of the ester group may also be used to study compounds with this structure, according to VANDENHEUVEL et al. (1965 b). The thermal elimination of the side chain is typical for compounds with a 17α,21-diol-20-one structure (VANDENHEUVEL and HORNING, 1960). The pyro-isopyro thermal conversion is useful in studying compounds of the Vitamins D group (ZIFFER et al., 1960). Periodate oxidation and bismuthate oxidation may be used for side chain oxidations for C-21 steroids.

X. Steroid Conjugates

A comprehensive literature survey for steroid conjugates was published recently (BERNSTEIN et al., 1966). The major types of mammalian conjugates, β-D-glucosiduronic acids and sulfates, present different analytical problems for gas phase work. Glucosiduronic acids may be converted to derivatives without undue difficulty. The derivatives are thermally stable and the chief problems involve technological difficulties arising from the fact that elevated temperatures (above 250°) must be used for the analytical separations. Most of these difficulties have been surmounted. Gas phase analytical studies of sulfates are more difficult, since the thermal elimination of the sulfate group occurs relatively easily.

The following summary of current knowledge relates only to simple glucosiduronic acids and sulfates; double conjugates and other types of conjugates are not included in this brief discussion of the analytical problem.

1. β-D-Glucosiduronic Acids

The most satisfactory derivatives for glucosiduronic acids (glucuronides) are the methyl ester-trimethylsilyl ether (ME-TMSi) derivatives and the trimethylsilyl ester-trimethylsilyl ether (TMSi) derivatives. An experimental procedure for the preparation of ME-TMSi derivatives was given by JAAKONMAKI et al. (1967 a). TMSi derivatives are best prepared by direct reaction of glucosiduronic acids with *bis*-trimethylsilylacetamide (BSA). An example of an analytical separation (ME-TMSi derivatives) of the conjugates of androsterone and etiocholanolone is shown in Fig. 23. The conjugates were isolated from urine by the pyridinium salt extraction procedure of McKENNA and NORYMBERSKI (1960), and the separation was carried out with a 12 ft 1% SE-30 column. The ME-TMSi derivatives were prepared by reaction with diazomethane to form methyl esters, followed by reaction with HMDS-TMCS or BSA-TMCS to form the

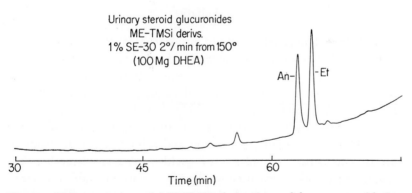

Fig. 23. GLC separation of ME-TMSi derivatives of human steroid β-D-glucosiduronic acids. The sample was obtained by the extraction procedure of McKENNA and NORYMBERSKI (1960) from a 24 hr collection of urine after the ingestion of 100 mg of dehydroepiandrosterone. Preliminary purification was effected by TLC separation of the ME derivatives. Conditions: 12 ft 1% SE-30 (on 80—100 mesh Gas Chrom P) column; temperature programmed at 2°/min from 150°; injector, 260°; detector, 300°; nitrogen, 15 psi; flame detector

TMSi ethers. The usual recommendation of a short column for high temperature work is not necessary if the support has been deactivated and if the phase is thermally stable (OV-1, SE-30, OV-17).

No evidence of adsorption or decomposition has been noted in studies of glucuronides of C_{19} steroids. The acetal structure is thermally stable. The TMSi esters are not entirely satisfactory derivatives when prepared by the HMDS-TMCS method, but BSA-TMCS reaction conditions may be used to prepare TMSi ester-ethers.

The glucuronide of pregnanediol may also be studied in this way (JAAKONMAKI et al., 1967 b), but studies of adrenocortical steroid conjugates may prove to be more difficult.

As has been pointed out by VANDENHEUVEL (1967 a), the separation of a steroid β-D-glucosiduronic acid as the ME-TMSi derivative is not a formidable problem. At the present time the major difficulties with respect to gas phase work lie in extensions to metabolites of the adrenocortical hormones.

Further progress is likely to be slow until better methods for the isolation of glucosiduronic acids from tissue are developed. The existing procedures are satisfactory for steroids of relatively simple structure, but not for those of the adrenocortical series.

2. Sulfates

Sulfate and sulfonate esters of primary alcohols usually may be studied by GLC methods. When esters of secondary alicyclic alcohols are heated, the usual result is an elimination reaction with the formation of one or more products, depending upon the structure of the alcohol. It therefore seems unlikely that the direct separation of steroid sulfates by GLC methods will prove to be practicable, but two indirect approaches (elimination and solvolysis) to the study of sulfate conjugates are likely to yield satisfactory results. The elimination reaction has been studied in detail for sulfonate esters (VANDENHEUVEL et al., 1965 b; VANDENHEUVEL, 1967 b). The product from cholestanol was 2-cholestene (only one product was observed), but cholesterol gave three products. A study of the latter reaction indicated that the i-steroid rearrangement occurred; the products were 3,5-cyclo-6-cholestene, 2,4 or 2,5-cholestadiene (a minor product) and 3,5-cholestadiene. The i-steroid rearrangement did not occur for 5-cholesten-3α-ol (epicholesterol), indicating that the reaction probably proceeded through the homoallylic cation. Sulfate eliminations would be likely to give the same products.

The LIEBERMAN solvolysis procedure may be used to yield a steroid fraction derived entirely from sulfate conjugates. After liberation of the steroids, the usual analytical procedures may be used. Another hydrolysis method of considerable interest is that of FOTHERBY (1959). When aqueous solutions of 3β-ol-$\varDelta^5$ sulfates are heated (95—100°), the sulfate group is eliminated and the steroid undergoes the i-steroid rearrangement. Under slightly acid conditions the reverse rearrangement occurs and the original steroids may be recovered. This procedure, while not widely used, is an excellent one for studies of 3β-ol-$\varDelta^5$ sulfates in urine. The usual GLC procedures may be used after isolation of the steroid fraction.

References

AAKVAAG, A., and K. B. EIK-NES: Metabolism *in vivo* of steroids in the canine ovary. Biochim. biophys. Acta (Amst.) **111**, 273 (1965).
— Gas chromatographic determination of aldosterone in urine with electron capture detection. Acta. Endocr., Suppl. **119**, 96 (1967).
ATTAL, J., S. M. HENDELES, and K. B. EIK-NES: Determination of free estrone in blood plasma by gas phase chromatography with electron capture detection. Anal. Biochem. **20**, 394 (1967).
BARDIN, C. W., and M. B. LIPSETT: Estimation of testosterone and androstenedione in human plasma. Steroids **9**, 71 (1967).
BEERTHUIS, R. K., and J. H. RECOURT: Sterol analysis by gas chromatography. Nature **186**, 372 (1960).
BERNSTEIN, S., E. W. CANTRALL, J. P. DUSZA, and J. P. JOSEPH: Steroid conjugates. Chemical Abstracts Service, American Chemical Society, Washington, D. C., 1966.
BIEMANN, K., P. BOMMER, and D. M. DESIDERIO: Element-mapping, a new approach to the interpretation of high resolution mass sprectra. Tetrahedron Letters **26**, 1725 (1964).
BRODIE, A. H., N. SHIMIZU, S. A. S. TAIT, and J. F. TAIT: A method for the measurement of aldosterone in peripheral plasma using ^{3}H-acetic anhydride. J. clin. Endocr. **27**, 997 (1967).
BROOKS, C. J. W., E. M. CHAMBAZ, and E. C. HORNING: Thin-layer and column chromatographic group separations of steroids as trimethylsilyl ethers. Isolation for GLC analysis of pregnanediol and estriol in pregnancy urine. Anal. Biochem. **19**, 234 (1967).
BROWNIE, A. C., H. J. VAN DER MOLEN, E. E. NISHIZAWA, and K. B. EIK-NES: Determination of testosterone in human peripheral blood using

gas-liquid chromatography with electron capture detection. J. clin. Endocr. **24**, 1091 (1964).

CEJKA, V., E. M. VENNEMAN, and N. BEL-VANDEN BOSCH: Enhancement and modification of isotope fractionation during the partition chromatography of ^{3}H and ^{14}C labeled steroids. J. Chromatog. **22**, 308 (1966).

CHARRANSOL, G., and H. H. WOTIZ: Ultra-micro analysis of plasma estrogens with the electron capture detector. Excerpta Medica Found. Int. Congress Series **111**, 117 (1966) (Abstract).

CLAESSON, S.: A theory for frontal adsorption analysis. Arkiv Kemi, Mineral Geol. **20 A** (1), 1 (1946).

CLARK, S. J., and H. H. WOTIZ: Separation and detection of nanogram amounts of steroids. Steroids **2**, 535 (1963).

COLLINS, W. P., and J. A. SOMMERVILLE: Quantitative determination of progesterone in human plasma by thin-layer and gas-liquid radiochromatography. Nature **203**, 836 (1964).

DJERASSI, C.: In: Structure elucidation of natural products by mass spectrometry. Vols. I and II. H. BUDZIKIEWICZ, C. DJERASSI, and D. H. WILLIAMS (Eds.). San Francisco: Holden-Day, Inc. 1964.

EABORN, C., D. R. M. WALTON, and B. S. THOMAS: Preparation and gas chromatography of steroid bromomethyl dimethylsilyl ethers. Chemistry and Industry (Lond.) 827 (1967).

EGLINTON, G., R. J. HAMILTON, R. HODGES, and R. A. RAPHAEL: Gas-liquid chromatography of natural products and their derivatives. Chemistry and Industry (Lond.) 955 (1959).

ENGEL, L. L., P. CARTER, and L. L. FIELDING: Urinary metabolites of administered corticosterone. I. Steroids liberated by glucuronidase hydrolysis. J. Biol. Chem. **213**, 99 (1955).

EXLEY, D.: The ultramicro determination of testosterone using gas-liquid chromatography with electron capture detection. In: Androgens in normal and pathological conditions. A. VERMEULEN and D. EXLEY (Eds.). Excerpta Medica Found. Int. Congress Series **101**, 11 (1966).

FALES, H. M., and T. LUUKKAINEN: O-Methyloximes as carbonyl derivatives in gas chromatography, mass spectrometry and nuclear magnetic resonance. Anal. Chem. **37**, 955 (1965).

FOTHERBY, K.: A method for the estimation of dehydroepiandrosterone in urine. Biochem. J. **73**, 339 (1959); The isolation of pregn-5-ene-3β, 16α,20α-triol from the urine of normal males. Biochem. J. **71**, 209 (1959). See also: The isolation of 3β-hydroxy-Δ^5-steroids from the urine of normal man. Biochem. J. **69**, 596 (1958).

GARDINER, W. L., and E. C. HORNING: Gas-liquid chromatographic separation of C$_{19}$ and C$_{21}$ human urinary steroids by a new procedure. Biochim. biophys. Acta (Amst.) **115**, 524 (1966).

—, C. J. W. BROOKS, E. C. HORNING, and R. M. HILL: Urinary steroid pattern of the human newborn infant. Biochim. biophys. Acta (Amst.) **130**, 278 (1966).

GLUECKAUF, E.: Theory of chromatography. Part. 9. The "theoretical plate" concept in column separations. Trans. Faraday Soc. 51, 34 (1955).

GOLD, N., and J. F. CRIGLER: Effect of tritium labeling of cortisol on its physico-chemical properties and its metabolism in man. J. clin. Endocr. 26, 133 (1966).

HAMILTON, R. J., W. J. A. VANDENHEUVEL, and E. C. HORNING: An extension of the "steroid number" concept to relationships between the structure of steroids and their gas chromatographic retention times observed with selective phases. Biochim. biophys. Acta. (Amst.) 70, 679 (1963).

HOLDEN, A. V., and G. A. WHEATLEY: Cleaning of tritium foil electron capture detectors. J. Gas Chromatog. 5, 373 (1967).

HORNING, E. C., K. C. MADDOCK, K. V. ANTHONY, and W. J. A. VANDENHEUVEL: Quantitative aspects of gas chromatographic separations in biological studies. Anal. Chem. 35, 526 (1963).

—, C. J. W. BROOKS, L. JOHNSON, and W. L. GARDINER: Separation, identification and estimation of human steroid hormones and their metabolites. Applications to adrenocortical steroids. Separ. Sci. 1, 555 (1966).

—, M. G. HORNING, N. IKEKAWA, E. M. CHAMBAZ, P. I. JAAKONMAKI, and C. J. W. BROOKS: Studies of analytical separations of human steroids and steroid glucuronides. J. Gas Chromatog. 5, 283 (1967).

—, C. J. W. BROOKS, and W. J. A. VANDENHEUVEL: In: Advances in lipid research. R. PAOLETTI and D. KRITCHEVSKY (Eds.). New York: Academic Press 1968.

HORNING, M. G., K. L. KNOX, C. E. DALGLIESH, and E. C. HORNING: Gas-liquid chromatographic study and estimation of several urinary aromatic acids. Anal. Biochem. 17, 244 (1966).

—, A. M. MOSS, and E. C. HORNING: Formation and gas-liquid chromatographic behavior of isomeric steroid ketone methoxime derivatives. Anal. Biochem. in press.

JAAKONMAKI, P. I., K. L. KNOX, E. C. HORNING, and M. G. HORNING: The characterization by gas-liquid chromatography of ethyl β-D-glucosiduronic acid as a metabolite of ethanol in rat and man. European J. Pharmacol. 1, 63 (1967 a).

—, K. A. YARGER, and E. C. HORNING: Gas-liquid chromatographic separation of human urinary steroid glucuronides. Biochim. biophys. Acta (Amst.) 137, 216 (1967 b).

JAMES, A. T., and A. J. P. MARTIN: Gas-liquid partition chromatography: the separation and micro-estimation of volatile fatty acids from formic to dodecanoic acid. Biochem. J. 50, 679 (1952).

KAHN, L., and M. C. GOLDBERG: The emanation of tritium gas from two electron capture detectors. J. Gas Chromatog. 3, 287 (1965).

KARMEN, A., and H. R. TRITCH: Radioassay by gas chromatography of compounds labelled with carbon-14. Nature 186, 150 (1960).

—, I. McCaffrey, and R. L. Bowman: Radioassay by gas-liquid chromatography of lipids with carbon-14. J. Lipid Res. **3,** 4 (1962).

— —, J. W. Winkelman, and R. L. Bowman: Measurement of tritium in the effluent of a gas chromatography column. Anal. Chem. **35,** 536 (1963 a).

— —, and B. Kliman: Derivative ratio analysis: A new method for isotope measurement of acetylable steroids by gas liquid chromatography. Anal. Biochem. **6,** 31 (1963 b).

— Calibration of flow-through detectors of ^{14}C in gas-liquid chromatographic effluents. J. Lipid Res. **8,** 61 (1967).

Kirschner, M. A., and M. B. Lipsett: Isotope effects in gas-liquid chromatography of steroids. J. Lipid Res. **6,** 7 (1965).

Klein, P. D., D. W. Simborg, and P. A. Szczepanik: Detection and composition of isotope fractionation in the adsorption chromatography of dual labelled compounds. Pure appl. Chem. **8,** 357 (1964).

— In: Advances in chromatography, Vol. III. J. C. Giddings and R. A. Keller (Eds.). New York: Marcel Dekker 1966.

Kliman, B.: Analysis of aldosterone in urine by double isotope dilution and gas-liquid chromatography. In: Gas chromatography of steroids in biological fluids. M. B. Lipsett (Ed.). New York: Plenum Press 1965.

—, and C. Briefer: Collection of carbon-14 and tritium labelled steroids in gas-liquid chromatography with application to the analysis of testosterone in human plasma. In: Steroid gas chromatography. J. K. Grant (Ed.). Endocrin. Soc. Memoir No. 16. London: Cambridge University Press 1967.

Kovats, E.: Gas-chromatographische Charakterisierung organischer Verbindungen. Teil 1: Retentionsindices aliphatischer Halogenide, Alkohole, Aldehyde und Ketone. Helv. chim. Acta **41,** 1915 (1958).

Landowne, R. A., and S. R. Lipsky: The electron capture of haloacetates: a means of detecting ultramicro quantities of sterols by gas chromatography. Anal. Chem. **35,** 532 (1963).

Leemans, F. A. J. M., and J. A. McCloskey: Combination gas chromatography-mass spectrometry. J. Amer. Oil Chem. Soc. **44,** 11 (1967).

Lloyd, B. J., G. C. Haltmeyer, and K. B. Eik-Nes: Measurement of cortisol (F_k) and corticosterone (B_k) by electron capture following gas phase chromatography. Fed. Proc. **26,** 483 (1967) (Abstract).

Lovelock, J. E.: A sensitive detector for gas chromatography. J. Chromatog. **1,** 35 (1958). See also: The "argon" detector. In: Gas chromatography 1958. D. H. Desty (Ed.). New York: Academic Press 1958.

—, and S. R. Lipsky: Electron affinity spectroscopy. A new method for the identification of functional groups in chemical compounds separated by gas chromatography. J. Amer. Chem. Soc. **82,** 431 (1960).

— Affinity of organic compounds for free electrons with thermal energy: Its possible significance in biology. Nature **189,** 729 (1961).

—, P. G. Simmonds, and W. J. A. Vandenheuvel: Affinity of steroids for electrons with thermal energies. Nature **197,** 249 (1963).

MAKITA, M., and W. W. WELLS: Quantitative analysis of fecal bile acids by gas-liquid chromatography. Anal. Biochem. 5, 523 (1963).

MARTIN, A. J. P., and R. L. M. SYNGE: A new form of chromatogram employing two liquid phases. 1. A theory of chromatography. 2. Application to the micro-determination of the higher monoamino acids in proteins. Biochem. J. 35, 1358 (1941).

—, and A. T. JAMES: Gas-liquid chromatography: the gas-density meter, a new apparatus for the detection of vapours in flowing gas streams. Biochem. J. 63, 138 (1956).

MASON, L. H., H. J. DUTTON, and L. R. BAIR: Ionization chamber for high temperature gas chromatography. J. Chromatog. 2, 322 (1959).

McKENNA, J., and J. K. NORYMBERSKI: The extraction and measurement of urinary 17-oxo steroid hydrogen sulphates. Biochem. J. 76, 60 P (1960).

MENINI, E., and J. K. NORYMBERSKI: An approach to the systematic analysis of urinary steroids. Biochem. J. 95, 1 (1965).

NAKAGAWA, K., N. L. McNIVEN, E. FORCHIELLI, A. VERMEULEN, and R. I. DORFMAN: Determination of testosterone by gas-liquid chromatography using an electron capture detector. I. Responses of haloalkyl derivatives. Steroids 7, 329 (1966).

OAKS, D. M., H. HARTMAN, and K. P. DIMICK: Analysis of sulphur compounds with electron capture/hydrogen flame dual channel gas chromatography. Anal. Chem. 36, 1560 (1964).

RAISINGHANI, K. H., R. I. DORFMAN, and E. FORCHIELLI: A gas chromatographic method for the estimation of nanogram quantities of progesterone using electron capture detection. Abstr. meeting on gas chromatographic determination of hormonal steroids. Rome, September, 1966.

RAPP, J. P., and K. B. EIK-NES: Gas chromatography with electron capture detection of some corticosteroid derivatives. J. Gas Chromatog. 3, 235 (1965).

— — Determination of deoxycorticosterone and aldosterone in biological samples by gas chromatography with electron capture detection. Anal. Biochem. 15, 383 (1966 a).

— — The effect of front size on electron capture detector sensitivity. J. Gas Chromatog. 4, 376 (1966 b).

RAY, N. H.: Gas chromatography. I. The separation and estimation of volatile organic compounds by gas-liquid partition chromatography. J. appl. Chem. (Lond.) 4, 21 (1954); II. The separation and analysis of gas mixtures by chromatographic methods. J. appl. Chem. (Lond.) 4, 82 (1954).

RESKO, J. A., and K. B. EIK-NES: Diurnal testosterone levels in peripheral plasma of human male subjects. J. clin. Endocr. 26, 573 (1966).

RYHAGE, R.: Use of a mass spectrometer as a detector and analyzer for effluents emerging from high temperature gas-liquid chromatography columns. Anal. Chem. 36, 759 (1964).

SHOEMAKE, G. R., J. E. LOVELOCK, and A. ZLATKIS: The effect of temperature and carrier gas on rate of loss of tritium from radioactive foils. J. Chromatog. 12, 314 (1963).

STEINBERG, D.: Radioassay of aqueous solutions mixed with solid crystalline fluors. Nature 183, 1253 (1959).

SUPINA, W. R., R. S. HENLY, and R. F. KRUPPA: Silane treatment of solid supports for gas chromatography. J. Amer. Oil Chem. Soc. 43, 202 A (1966).

SWEELEY, C. C., and E. C. HORNING: Microanalytical separation of steroids by gas chromatography. Nature 187, 114 (1960).

THOMAS, B. S., C. EABORN, and D. R. M. WALTON: Preparation and gas chromatography of steroid chloromethyldimethylsilyl ethers. Chem. Comm. 2, 408 (1966).

VANDENHEUVEL, W. J. A.: Gas-liquid chromatography of steroid glucuronosides. J. Chromatog. 28, 406 (1967 a).

— The gas-liquid chromatographic behavior of sterol sulfonates. Effect of structure upon the nature of their elimination reaction. J. Chromatog. 26, 396 (1967 b).

—, and E. C. HORNING: Gas chromatography of adrenal cortical steroid hormones. Biochem. biophys. Comm. 3, 356 (1960).

—, C. C. SWEELEY, and E. C. HORNING: Separation of steroids by gas chromatography. J. Amer. chem. Soc. 82, 3481 (1960).

—, and E. C. HORNING: Study of retention time relationships in gas chromatography in terms of the structure of steroids. Biochim. biophys. Acta (Amst.) 64, 416 (1962).

—, W. L. GARDINER, and E. C. HORNING: Substituted hydrazones as derivatives of ketones in gas chromatography. J. Chromatog. 18, 391 (1965 a).

—, R. N. STILLWELL, W. L. GARDINER, S. WIKSTRÖM, and E. C. HORNING: Gas chromatographic behavior of methanesulfonates and p-toluenesulfonates of sterols. J. Chromatog. 19, 22 (1965 b).

—, W. L. GARDINER, and E. C. HORNING: The influence of the treatment of the support upon properties of thin-film gas chromatography column packings. J. Chromatog. 25, 242 (1966).

— — — A comparison of the behavior of the hydrocarbons used as reference standards in the determination of "steroid numbers" and "methylene units". Selective retention of steroid hydrocarbons by polar stationary phases. J. Chromatog. 26, 387 (1967).

VAN DER MOLEN, H. J.: Personal communication (1967).

—, D. GROEN, and J. H. VAN DER MAAS: Steroid monochloroacetates: physical-chemical characteristics and their use in gas-liquid chromatography. Steroids 6, 195 (1965).

—, and D. GROEN: Determination of progesterone in human peripheral blood using gas-liquid chromatography with electron capture detection. J. clin. Endocr. 25, 1625 (1965).

VAN DER MOLEN, H. J., J. H. VAN DER MAAS, and D. GROEN: Preparation and properties of steroid heptafluorobutyrates. In press (1967).

—, and D. GROEN: Quantitative determination of submicrogram amounts of steroids in blood using electron capture and flame ionization detection following gas-liquid chromatography. In: Steroid gas chromatography. J. K. GRANT (Ed.). Endocrin. Soc. Memoir No. 16. London: Cambridge University Press 1967.

VERMEULEN, A.: Personal communication (1967).

WASSERMANN, G. F., and K. B. EIK-NES: Unpublished (1967).

WENTWORTH, W. E., and R. S. BECKER: Potential method for the determination of electron affinities of molecules: application to some aromatic hydrocarbons. J. Amer. chem. Soc. 84, 4263 (1962).

WOODFORD, F. P., and C. M. VAN GENT: Gas-liquid chromatography of fatty acid methyl esters: the "carbon number" as a parameter for comparison of columns. J. Lipid Res. 1, 188 (1960).

WOLFGANG, R., and F. S. ROWLAND: Radioassay by gas chromatography of tritium and carbon-14 labelled compounds. Anal. Chem. 30, 903 (1958).

ZIFFER, H., W. J. A. VANDENHEUVEL, E. O. A. HAAHTI, and E. C. HORNING: Gas chromatographic behavior of vitamins D_2 and D_3. J. Amer. chem. Soc. 82, 6311 (1960).

Chapter 2

Gas Phase Chromatographic Methods for Estrogens in Biological Fluids

H. Adlercreutz and T. Luukkainen

I. Introduction

During the past two decades interest in studying the biological significance, metabolism and excretion of the estrogens has increased considerably and a great variety of methods have been developed for the estimation of this class of steroids. Among the latest developments in the field of estrogen methodology are gas phase chromatographic procedures.

For details of the chemical properties, biological and clinical significance, biogenesis and metabolism of the estrogens as well as the different methods, other than GLC, available in this field, the reader is referred to publications by Breuer (1960), Brown (1960), Diczfalusy and Lauritzen (1961), O'Donnell and Preedy (1961), Preedy (1962), Adlercreutz (1962), Loraine and Bell (1966) and a book edited by Paulsen (1965).

This survey deals with the problems of GLC estimation of estrogens and presents some of the recent methods developed for the quantitation of these steroids in biological fluids and tissues.

II. General Considerations

1. Hydrolysis

Virtually all estrogens in the human are present in conjugated form, and free estrogens have been found only in blood and some tissues (ovary, placenta). Since the estimation of estrogen glucosiduronates is at a preliminary stage of development and sulfates have not been determined successfully by GLC, it is neccessary to include a hydrolysis step in all methods which are intended to measure the total amount of estrogens present in a biological sample.

Two types of hydrolytic procedures, acid and enzyme hydrolysis, are commonly used and the choice between them is mainly dependent on how many and which estrogens are to be estimated and whether the estimations are for clinical or research purposes. In addition, the nature of the biological extract determines the type of hydrolysis to be employed.

A thorough study of the optimal conditions for acid hydrolysis of urinary estrogens has been carried out by Brown and Blair (1958). Maximum yields are obtained when 15 volumes of concentrated hydrochloric acid are boiled under reflux with 100 volumes of urine for one hour, or when 20 volumes of hydrochloric acid are boiled with 100 volumes of urine under reflux for 30 minutes. These results were confirmed by Preedy (1962). The hydrolytic procedure involving autoclaving of the urine samples with 3% sulfuric acid suggested by Frandsen (1965) seems also to be satisfactory.

For clinical purposes and provided only estrone, 17β-estradiol and/or estriol are to be estimated, acid hydrolysis of urinary estrogens may be used when these steroids are to be estimated with GLC. In glucose-containing urine samples, however, acid hydrolysis can not be used, since glucose has a destructive effect on estrogens during hot acid hydrolysis. If urine specimens are diluted with water before acid hydrolysis, this destructive effect can be avoided (Brown and Blair, 1958; Hobkirk et al., 1959). Dilution with 10 volumes of water makes the sample size so large that for urine obtained from nonpregnant women processing is often inconvenient. For such urine samples, therefore, enzymic hydrolysis is preferable or the glucose can be completely eliminated by gel filtration (Beling, 1963) of the conjugated estrogens before acid hydrolysis. All glucose present in the urine of diabetic patients will be removed prior to the conjugated estrogens during gel filtration of urine on Sephadex G 25 (Adlercreutz and Luukkainen, 1964; Adlercreutz et al., 1967 a; Adlercreutz, 1968). In fact, for estrone, estradiol and estriol conjugates in urine from pregnant women the combination of gel filtration and acid hydrolysis gives results comparable to those obtained by a combination of gel filtration and enzyme hydrolysis (Table 1), if GLC is used as the final step.

Enzymic hydrolysis of urinary estrogen conjugates is more time-consuming and expensive than acid hydrolysis, but appears to give the best yield in most cases (KATZMAN et al., 1954; BEER and GALLAGHER, 1955; BROWN and BLAIR, 1958; BLOCH and GIBREE, 1959; BUGGE et al., 1961). Of the different enzymes used, that prepared from the mollusc *Helix pomatia* seems to be preferable (BLOCH and GIBREE, 1959; SLAUNWHITE and SANDBERG, 1960; BUGGE et al., 1961). The estrogen sulfates may be hydrolyzed over a wide pH range (ADLERCREUTZ, 1962) but for the estrogen glucosiduronates there is an optimal pH at 4.1—4.2 (WAKABAYASHI and FISHMAN, 1961; ADLERCREUTZ, 1962; BELING, 1963). If this low pH is used for the enzyme hydrolysis of urinary estrogen conjugates, a strong inhibition of the enzymes may occur due to partial conversion of the D-glucosaccharic acid present in the urine to its 1:4 lactone (MARSH, 1962). It seems likely that this phenomenon has influenced the results obtained by different workers, and in fact the hydrolysis of estrogen conjugates in untreated urine with *Helix pomatia* extract has been found to be optimal at a pH of 5.0—5.2 (BLOCH and GIBREE, 1959; BUGGE et al., 1961).

More adequate conditions for enzymic hydrolysis of conjugated estrogens in urine can be obtained by combining gel filtration and enzyme hydrolysis under optimal conditions for hydrolysis of the conjugates, since it has been shown that gel filtration of the urine eliminates most of the enzyme inhibitors present (BELING, 1963; ADLERCREUTZ and LUUKKAINEN, 1964; KUSHINSKY and OTTERNESS, 1964; ADLERCREUTZ et al., 1967 a; ADLERCREUTZ, 1968). In this laboratory a comparative investigation has been made of three different types of hydrolytic procedures using estrogen estimation by GLC as the final step. Fifty ml urine samples of pooled urine from 5 different pregnant women were treated with A) 15 vol. % hydrochloric acid and boiling for 1 hour, B) gel filtration with Sephadex and boiling for 1 hour with 15 vol. % hydrochloric acid and C) gel filtration with Sephadex and enzymic hydrolysis with *Helix pomatia* extract. Duplicate estimations were carried out on all samples, and the concentrations of estrone, 17β-estradiol and estriol determined after GLC on two different columns. The mean relative values for the three estrogens found by each method can be seen in Table 1. Acid and enzymic hydrolysis following gel filtration gave essentially the same values for the three classical estrogens and the differences found were not signif-

Table 1. *Comparison of different hydrolytic procedures for cleavage of conjugated estrogens in late pregnancy urine. The experiments were carried out with 50-ml samples from a pool of five urine specimens from different women. The method used for estrogen estimation is presented in Flowsheet 6. Quantitative data were obtained from two different liquid phases and all analyses were carried out in duplicate*

Method of hydrolysis	Relative amounts		
	estrone	estradiol	estriol
Acid hydrolysis	85	74	59
Gel filtration + acid hydrolysis	93	100	100
Gel filtration + enzyme hydrolysis	100	95	95

icant. Acid hydrolysis carried out directly on the urine without gel filtration caused significant losses of the estrogens. These findings agree well with those of BROWN and BLAIR (1958), showing that dilution of pregnancy urine before acid hydrolysis increased the recovery of estrogens. These workers were of the opinion that the combined effect of a normal constituent of urine and boiling with acid caused the destruction of estrogens. It seems that gel filtration eliminates this or these constituents from urine, and therefore acid and enzymic hydrolyses give equal values for the three classical estrogens if gel filtration precedes hydrolysis and GLC is used as final step. Gel filtration also eliminates glucose and many drugs which may interfere with steroid estimation.

Most methods used for the estimation of estrogens in blood or plasma involve acid hydrolysis, and it has been found that the recoveries are rather low if free estrogens are added to blood before hydrolysis. ROY and BROWN (1960) recorded recoveries between 47 and 56% of estrogens added to blood from pregnant women. ADLERCREUTZ (1964 a) found a somewhat higher recovery in such experiments if enzymic hydrolysis was carried out on extracts of blood, but in some blood samples inhibition of the enzyme was strong. Later it was found that a combination of gel filtration of extracts of blood and enzymic hydrolysis gives the most satisfactory results for estrogen estimation in blood or plasma (unpublished observations). For bile specimens acid hydrolysis should not be used (ADLERCREUTZ, 1962) and enzymic hydrolysis must be carried out following some purification of the bile samples. This can be done by precipitation of fatty material in cold methanol and purification of the glucosiduronate fraction by solvent partition (ADLERCREUTZ, 1962). Gel filtration on Sephadex G 25 can be substituted for the solvent partition (ADLER- CREUTZ and LUUKKAINEN, 1966; ADLERCREUTZ et al., 1967 a). These procedures give very satisfactory results.

2. Extraction

Following hydrolysis of the conjugated estrogens the liberated steroids are usually extracted with ethyl ether. Chloroform, used by some workers in this field, is not suitable because the partition coefficients of estriol and other polar estrogens between water and chloroform are not favorable. It is of great importance to have per- oxide-free ether. Washing of the ether with $FeSO_4$ or $AgNO_3$ solution and redistillation should be carried out even on commercially available "peroxide-free" ether. New batches of ether must be prepared twice a week and stored at $+4\,^{\circ}C$. If polar estrogens other than estriol are estimated, the aqueous phase must be saturated with sodium chloride before ether extraction. In all phases of the extraction procedure alkalinity must be avoided if the labile ring D α-ketolic or 2- hydroxylated estrogens are to be estimated. In such cases, the extract can only be rapidly washed with saturated sodium bicarbonate solution, freshly made up, and then rinsed with distilled water.

3. Purification

The purification procedures used in GLC methods do not differ from those used in other procedures for the estimation of estrogens. Since the detection system in GLC is not specific, the samples usually require more thorough purification than is needed for other methods based on colorimetry or fluorimetry. On the other hand, with increas- ing numbers of steroids to be estimated the purification procedures are less laborious if the method involves GLC, since separation and estimation of closely related compounds can often be carried out simultaneously.

a) Solvent Partition

Two of the most useful solvent partitions are those described by ENGEL et al. (1950) and by BROWN (1955). Both separate phenolic estrogens from neutral steroids. The first is a partition between toluene and sodium hydroxide solution. It seems to be especially valuable in work with bile and blood extracts (ADLERCREUTZ, 1962, 1964 a) and it has been used in combination with GLC for bile estrogens by LUUKKAINEN and ADLERCREUTZ (1963), for blood estrogens by ADLERCREUTZ (1964 a), EIK-NES et al. (1965) and TOUCHSTONE and MURAWEC (1965), and for urinary estrogens by YOUSEM (1964). The partition between benzene-petroleum ether and 2 per cent ethanol in water and/or sodium hydroxide solution employed in the method of BROWN has been used in a great number of GLC methods for estrogens (ADLERCREUTZ and LUUKKAINEN, 1963, 1965 a, b; WOTIZ and CHATTORAJ, 1964, 1965; COX and BEDFORD, 1964). The only disadvantage of using the benzene-petroleum ether mixture for the separation of phenolic from neutral steroids is the great amount of impurities present in commercially available benzene. Such impurities interfere in GLC. With appropriate redistillation this drawback can be overcome.

b) Column Chromatography

Chromatography of the estrogens as their methyl ethers (LUUKKAINEN and ADLERCREUTZ, 1963; MENINI, 1965 a, b; ADLERCREUTZ and LUUKAINEN, 1965 a, b; ADLERCREUTZ et al. 1967 a) or acetates (WOTIZ and CHATTORAJ, 1965; WOTIZ and CLARK, 1966) or as free steroids (TOUCHSTONE and MURAWEC, 1965) on alumina has been included in several methods. Methylation of the estrogens may be carried out as described by BROWN (1955). By this technique only estrone, estradiol and estriol can be estimated since the coditions are not optimal for monomethylation of the other estrogens, and as a result formation of a number of derivatives of other estrogens will occur (NOCKE, 1961). When working with methyl ethers of the estrogens other hydroxyl groups on the steroid structure can be used for the formation of double derivatives. Such derivatives show considerably improved GLC properties (LUUKKAINEN and ADLERCREUTZ, 1963; COX and BEDFORD, 1964; ADLERCREUTZ and LUUKKAINEN, 1965 a, b; MENINI, 1965 a, b; EIK-NES et al., 1965; ADLERCREUTZ et al., 1967 a).

In contrast to the wide experience gained for chromatography of the estrogen methyl ethers, data on chromatography of estrogen acetates on alumina are rather meager (WOTIZ and CHATTORAJ, 1965; WOTIZ and CLARK, 1966) and the usefulness of the method has yet to be evaluated. Purification of the acetylated monomethyl ethers of estrogens on alumina (MENINI, 1965 a, b) is another interesting approach to the problem. Chromatography of free estrogens on alumina in combination with GLC (TOUCHSTONE and MURAWEC, 1965) appears not to be superior to the above-mentioned procedures, but it seems that a modification of this technique, adopting the already well known method of ITTRICH (1960), might be worthwhile, since by this procedure all three classical estrogens can be separated on the same column.

Partition chromatography on Celite columns in combination with GLC has, to the best of our knowledge, not been used for estrogen purification. Hence, no statement as to the usefulness of Celite columns in combination with GLC of estrogens can be made. Nor is there any report of the combination of ion exchange chromatography of estrogens and GLC.

c) Thin-layer Chromatography

Thin-layer chromatography (TLC) has until recently found rather limited use for estrogen estimation in combination with GLC. This might be due to the fact that silica gel contains impurities which interfere considerably with the GLC estimation of steroids. However, by washing the plates with methanol or ether-methanol and reactivating the plates after such washing this difficulty can be avoided.

The capacity for estrogen separation by TLC is good, but the procedure is comparatively laborious for routine assay. In addition, extracts of more than 10% of 24-hour urine samples can frequently not be handled satisfactorily by TLC (WOTIZ and CLARK, 1966).

A quantitative GLC method involving TLC for 7 different estrogens in urine samples from pregnant and nonpregnant women has been published by WOTIZ and CHATTORAJ (1964). Upon re-examination of this technique it was discovered that the method was not suitable for urine samples from nonpregnant women (WOTIZ and CLARK, 1966) since the thin-layer chromatograms were occasionally overloaded when working with such samples. Other methods including TLC are those of EIK-NES et al. (1965) for the estimation of radioactive estradiol in plasma and homogenates and of ATTAL et al. (1967) for determination of estrone in plasma.

For qualitative work TLC is one of the best chromatographic procedures for estrogen separation (LISBOA and DICZFALUSY, 1962;

Lisboa, 1966 a). It has been used in combination with GLC for bile and urinary estrogens (Adlercreutz and Luukkainen, 1965 a; Luukkainen and Adlercreutz, 1965). By combining TLC and GLC and using several different derivatives of the estrogens a high degree of method specificity is achieved.

d) Paper Chromatography

The main advantage in using paper chromatography in combination with GLC is that eluates from paper do not contain compounds interfering with GLC in methods for estrogens. Another advantage is that paper chromatography is less laborious than TLC for routine assays. But paper chromatograms are easily overloaded and it is therefore desirable to purify extracts containing estrogens to some degree prior to paper chromatography.

In work with polar estrogens it is found that their elution from paper is somewhat difficult. Using methanol and a rather large elution volume even estrogens containing up to 4 hydroxyl groups can be quantitatively eluted. The separatory capacity of paper chromatography for estrogens is good and a great number of well investigated solvent systems are available (Preedy, 1962; Neher, 1964).

A quantitative method for determination of urinary estrogens involving paper chromatography and GLC has been presented by Adlercreutz et al. (1967 a). Paper systems are used for the separation of the ketonic estrogens and for some polar estrogens. The same procedure, with slight modifications, was also used for bile estrogens (Adlercreutz and Luukainen, 1966; Adlercreutz et al., 1967 a). In addition, Eik-Nes et al. (1965) included paper chromatography in a GLC method for blood estrogens. It seems likely that paper chromatography, in combination with GLC, will continue to be one of the most useful tools for the quantitative estimation of the estrogens present in small amounts in biological fluids.

e) Gel Chromatography

If during gel filtration the buffer or distilled water is replaced by a two-phase system consisting of a stationary nonorganic phase and a mobile organic phase, this procedure could be called gel chromatography. Such chromatography has been used by Beling (1963) for the separation of estrogen conjugates, by Adlercreutz (1965) and by

ADLERCREUTZ et al. (1967 b) for the quantitative estimation of estrogen sulfates in urine from pregnant women. In combination with GLC, gel chromatography has been used for purification of polar estrogens (ADLERCREUTZ et al., 1967 a). In addition such a step using an ammonia: n-butanol: tert. butanol system has been included in a method for the estimation of estrogens in normal urine (presented in this chapter). The procedure gives considerable purification of the sample, and all estrogens obtained after gel filtration and enzymic hydrolysis of an extract of 500 ml of nonpregnancy urine can be readily obtained in a 13-ml fraction when eluted from a 50-cm × 1-cm gel column.

III. Use of Estrogen Derivatives

Adequate GLC of estrogens as free compounds is possible for those containing only one or two hydroxyl groups. GLC of other estrogens results in irreversible adsorption and/or thermal decomposition on the column and submicrogram analysis of "free" estrone and estradiol does not give satisfactory quantitative results because of adsorption. However, analysis of larger amounts of these steroids on the same column can give quantitative results.

In many of the methods derivatives are formed at an early stage of sample purification. The Girard reaction is used to divide estrogens into ketones and nonketones. This step enhances the specificity of a method and also increases sample purification. Since the original method of BROWN (1955) methylation of the phenolic hydroxyl group has been used to change the polarity of estrogens thereby achieving increased purification as a result of altered chromatographic and partition properties of the sample.

1. Girard Separation

The procedure described by GIVNER et al. (1960 a) may be used with some small changes. Instead of reagent P the Girard reagent T is used and the procedure is not repeated, since on careful investigation it was found in this laboratory that after a single procedure 94% of estrone, 16α-hydroxyestrone and 16-keto-estradiol could be recovered as judged from GLC analysis of the hydrolyzed and extracted Girard complex. Complex formation is effected at room temperature and extraction of the nonketonic estrogens is carried out with ether from a NaCl-saturated solution. Following hydrolysis of the Girard complex with acid at room temperature, the ketonic estrogens are extracted with ether. The hydrazones of the ketones can be purified by subjecting these derivatives to TLC (LISBOA, 1966 b).

2. Methyl Ethers

The phenolic hydroxyl can be converted to its 3-methyl ether as described by BROWN (1955). Epimeric estriols are converted to multiple compounds by this method (NOCKE, 1961). Methyl ethers of estrogens have fair GLC properties and their retention times are shorter than those of the corresponding acetates (LUUKKAINEN and ADLERCREUTZ, 1963). Methyl ethers of estrogens can be converted to double derivatives in order to improve their GLC properties. Acetates of methylated estrogens may be used for the determination of the classical estrogens (Cox and BEDFORD, 1964; MENINI, 1965 a, b) and TMSi ethers of methylated estradiol and estriol may be used for the identification and determination of estrogens in biological samples (LUUKKAINEN and ADLERCREUTZ, 1963, 1965; ADLERCREUTZ and LUUKKAINEN, 1965 a, b, 1967 a).

3. Acetates

Acetates are usually prepared by dissolving the steroid in a mixture of equal parts of acetic anhydride and dry pyridine. This mixture is placed in the dark for 17 to 24 hours at room temperature. Excess reagents are then evaporated under reduced pressure or in a nitrogen stream at 45 °C and the residue is dissolved in ethyl acetate or hexane.

According to WOTIZ and CHATTORAJ (1965), estrogens are acetylated by dissolving them in a mixture of five parts of acetic anhydride and one part of pyridine and keeping the mixture at 68 °C for one hour. To the acetylated mixture 10 ml of distilled water is added, while stirring thoroughly with a glass rod. The sample is then transferred to a small separatory funnel and extracted twice with 10 ml and once with 5 ml of light petroleum ether. The vessel used for acetylation is also rinsed with petroleum ether and the washings added to the separatory funnel. The combined petroleum ether fractions are washed with 8% $NaHCO_3$ solution (5 ml) followed by 2-ml portions of water until the wash fraction is neutral.

The procedure of WOTIZ and CHATTORAJ (1965) is complicated and the high temperature recommended for the reaction is a cause for concern. The extraction procedure used in this method separates almost completely the acetylated products from the partly acetylated ones. Conversion to the acetates is usually between 92—100%. Acetates are stable and form excellent derivatives for purification or for work with preparative GLC.

4. Trimethylsilyl Ethers (TMSi Ethers)

TMSi ethers of estrogens are easy to prepare and their gas chromatographic properties are good because they are highly volatile and are not adsorbed on the column. During GLC of such derivatives the stereochemical differences between the epimers are accentuated, an effect which is of importance in the separation of estrogens.

The steroid sample can be further purified and divided into subgroups after the sample has been converted to trimethylsilyl ethers by TLC (ADLERCREUTZ and LUUKKAINEN, 1965 a; BROOKS et al., 1966). After elution from the TLC plates a second conversion of the sample to TMSi derivatives is necessary to circumvent the problem of partial hydrolysis occurring during elution from the TLC plate. An interesting method of purification of a sample converted to TMSi derivatives is by microsublimation (BROOKS et al., 1966) before GLC analysis.

Trimethylsilyl ethers can be prepared by the original procedure of LUUKKAINEN et al. (1961) by dissolving the estrogens in 1 ml of anhydrous tetrahydrofuran or chloroform, then adding 100 µl of hexamethyldisilazane and 5 µl of trimethylchlorosilane and allowing the well stoppered glass tubes to stand overnight at room temperature. After evaporation of the solvent and reagents the residue is dissolved in 1 ml of n-hexane and centrifuged and the clear supernatant is pipetted into another tube. The precipitate is washed with 0.5 ml of n-hexane. The combined hexane extracts are then evaporated to the desired volume. Chloroform or tetrahydrofuran can be replaced by pyridine in this procedure.

A very useful modification for TMSi ether formation has been reported by GRUNDY et al. (1965). These workers used a mixture consisting of dry pyridine, hexamethyldisilazane and trimethylchlorosilane (9:3:1). If protected from contamination from water vapor this mixture remains effective for at least 6 months. For one mg of steroid 100 μl of mixture is used and the stoppered vial is left at room temperature for 1 hr. The sample can then be analyzed directly, or alternatively it may be evaporated to dryness and the residue dissolved in n-hexane. (See Chapter 1 for a discussion of TMSi derivatives in GLC.)

5. O-Methoximes

Ketones are converted to O-methoximes by reaction of methoxylamine hydrochloride in pyridine with steroids containing a keto group (overnight at room temperature). After evaporation of the excess pyridine the residue is extracted with benzene and the pyridine hydrochloride removed by centrifugation (FALES and LUUKKAINEN, 1965).

Methoximes of the estrogens can be subjected to TLC or other chromatographic separations; the changes in the chromatographic mobility of such derivatives will often give better sample purification. For analysis by GLC methods the methoximes of estrogens are converted to double derivatives by the formation of TMSi ethers of the hydroxyl group(s) or by methyl ether formation of the phenolic hydroxyl group(s).

6. Acetonides

BREUER and PANGELS (1961) separated cis-glycolic estriol epimers from estriol and 16,17-epiestriol by forming the acetonide of the cis-glycolic steroids, dissolved in acetone, using hydrogen chloride as catalyst. It was found by ADLERCREUTZ et al. (1966) that the reaction was quantitative if trimethylchlorosilane was used as an acid catalyst and that the GLC properties of the mono TMSi ethers of the acetonides were good. It was also observed that specific determination of urinary 17-epi- and 16-epiestriol was possible by making use of the acetonide derivative.

Acetonides are prepared by dissolving estrogens in 10 ml of freshly distilled acetone and adding 100 μl of trimethylchlorosilane. The reaction mixture is shaken for 2 hours at room temperature, 1 ml of 1 N sodium hydroxide solution is added and the solvent is evaporated under reduced pressure below 40 °C. The residue is dissolved in 25 ml of 1 N sodium hydroxide solution which is extracted twice with half the volume of chloroform. The combined chloroform extract, which contains the cis-glycolic estriols, 16-epiestriol and 17-epiestriol, is evaporated to the desired volume and analyzed directly or after conversion of the remaining hydroxyl groups to TMSi ethers. The alkaline water residue is acidified and saturated with sodium chloride. The non-cis-glycolic estrogens present in this fraction are extracted with ether (3 × 1/1 vol.).

7. Derivatives of Estrogens for Electron Capture Detection

a) Chloroacetates

Chloroacetylation is carried out according to BROWNIE et al. (1964): To the dried residue is added 0.5 ml of a solution of mono-chloroacetic anhydride in tetrahydrofuran (10 mg per ml) and 0.1 ml of pyridine. The reaction is carried out overnight in a desiccator. After addition of 1 ml of distilled water the chloroacetates are extracted 3 times with 1 ml of ethyl acetate. The combined ethyl acetate extracts are washed once with 1 ml of 6N HCl, and twice with 1 ml of distilled water, and evaporated to dryness. The dry residue is dissolved in the desired volume of benzene or tetrahydrofuran.

Only samples of high purity containing one or two estrogens can be used, because short columns are employed to elute the estrogen derivatives in a reasonable time and at a reasonable temperature during GLC (EIK-NES et al., 1965).

b) Heptafluorobutyrates

Heptafluorobutyrates are prepared according to CLARK and WOTIZ (1963) by dissolving the steroid in tetrahydrofuran. A large excess of heptafluorobutyric anhydride is then added. The solution is heated at 60 °C for 30 min and evaporated to dryness in a stream of dry nitrogen; the residue is dissolved in acetone. The derivative formation is, according to WOTIZ et al. (1966), quantitative (93 to 100%), a view not shared by EXLEY and CHAMBERLAIN (1966) who found that the conversion of estrogens to heptafluorobutyrates is not quantitative.

c) Monochloroalkylsilyl Ethers

Monochloroalkylsilyl ether derivative formation was reported by THOMAS et al. (1966) for use in GLC. Good separation was obtained with both selective and nonselective phases. These steroid derivatives were stable in TLC.

In a more recent report, THOMAS and WALTON (1966) demonstrated that the substitution of bromine for the chlorine atom in the trimethylsilyl ether radical produced more promising results with regard to sensitivity of detection. Monobromomethyldimethylsilyl ethers could be analyzed on long GLC columns without undue increases in retention times. In the preliminary trial 0.1 nanogram of these derivatives of steroids was detectable. Further progress in the preparation of these derivatives may make it possible to carry out ultramicroanalysis of the estrogens.

d) Pentafluorophenylhydrazones

Pentafluorophenylhydrazones are prepared by the method of ATTAL et al. (1967). The steroid is dissolved in 0.2 ml methanol and 0.2 ml of a solution containing 10 mg pentafluorophenylhydrazine in 9 ml methanol and 1 ml acetic acid is added. The sample is left overnight at room temperature. The next morning 1 ml of water is added and the mixture is extracted three times with 2 ml hexane each time. The hexane extract is washed once with 2 ml 1 N sulphuric acid and then with water (2 ml portions) to neutrality. The washed hexane is evaporated to dryness under nitrogen and the residue purified by TLC. Commercially available pentafluorophenylhydrazine has to be purified extensively before it can be used as a reagent.

IV. Quantification and Identification of Gas Chromatographic Peaks of Estrogens

The quantification of estrogens by GLC presents many difficulties. Because of the wide variation in the concentrations of different estrogens in biological samples it is frequently impossible to use internal standards. In our laboratory we employ calibration curves obtained with reference standards. Estradiol-17β is used for all diols and estriol for all triols (not when acetonide derivatives of *cis*-glycolic triols are estimated, in which case the corresponding reference standard is used). New calibration curves for all compounds are prepared for each series of analyses and for all columns. Often the reference compounds need purification by TLC and recrystallization, because otherwise they give rise to several peaks during GLC. Quantification is done by calculating the peak area from the product of the height of the peak and its width at half height. This calculation is valid if the shape of the peak is almost ideal (as with trimethylsilyl ether derivatives). In methods where compounds are determined as free steroids, planimetric estimation of the peak area gives the best results.

The instrumentation and the sensitive detection system of GLC will often provoke the inexperienced worker to extend GLC techniques beyond the limits at which reliability and specificity can be evaluated. It should be realized that the estimation of some urinary estrogens is already at the level of one part of estrogen to 10^8 parts of extract and that most commercially available solvents used for extraction and purification of the sample may contain interfering impurities at that level. The result is therefore that all glassware and all solvents used must be tested almost daily for interfering impurities. Moreover, when using GLC for the estimation of steroids in biological samples every effort must be made to study the specificity of the estimation. There are many problems in which GLC estimation of estrogens can provide interesting new knowledge and valuable clinical information without working at the borderline of established specificity and assumed identification.

The standard requirement of this laboratory when estimating estrogens in biological samples by GLC is that a retention time identical with that of a given reference standard should be achieved on the same instrument and on the same day as the analysis. This retention time must show the same relationship to a marker compound, like cholestane, throughout the course of the study. It should be remembered that relative retention times given in the literature can not be used for steroid identification. Moreover, we have found that the retention effect of a given functional group at a given carbon atom can not be used for calculation of the retention time of a missing reference standard. In the estrogen series of steroids the interaction between different functional groups frequently changes the specific retention effect of a functional group (Table 2).

Table 2. *Relative retention times (to cholestane) of the trimethylsilyl ether derivatives (TMSi) of some estrogens. Gas inlet pressure 2.0 kg/cm²*

TMSi of	1% XE-60 195°C	3% F-60 213°C	1% Z 184°C	2% QF-1 198°C	0.8% JXR 210°C	1% NGS 195°C	JXR-XE-60 205°C
E_1 *	1.15	0.62	2.33	1.51	0.52	3.25	—
2metE$_1$	2.06	0.91	4.27	2.29	0.79	—	—
2OHE$_1$	1.84	0.97	2.83	2.03	0.89	3.28	1.43
6βOHE$_1$	1.47	0.82	2.46	1.91	0.73	3.14	1.23
7αOHE$_1$	1.39	0.73	1.89	1.81	0.68	2.54	1.14
11βOHE$_1$	—	0.95	1.99	2.81	—	2.70	1.21
16αOHE$_1$	1.74	1.03	2.84	1.75	—	3.76	1.39
6ketoE$_1$	3.52	1.18	8.53	5.16	0.93	14.50	3.06
16ketoE$_1$	2.24	1.22	3.86	2.32	—	—	—
6ketoE$_2$	2.45	1.33	3.18	2.94	—	—	1.91
11ketoE$_2$	—	1.12	—	1.67	—	—	—
16ketoE$_2$	2.11	1.14	3.08	2.21	1.09	4.68	1.64
E$_2$	0.83	0.70	1.01	0.81	0.66	—	0.79
17αE$_2$	0.70	0.63	0.87	0.71	—	—	0.70
11Δ17αE$_2$	0.62	0.53	0.84	—	—	—	—
2metE$_2$	1.34	1.05	1.78	1.21	—	—	1.22
3met11Δ17αE$_2$	—	0.45	—	—	—	—	—
3metE$_2$	—	0.58	—	—	—	—	—
2OHE$_2$	1.10	1.05	1.28	1.08	1.13	1.21	1.18
6αOHE$_2$	1.24	1.04	1.34	1.19	1.16	1.44	1.19
6βOHE$_2$	1.01	0.92	1.15	1.04	1.00	1.12	1.04
7αOHE$_2$	—	0.71	0.81	0.89	0.79	—	—
11βOHE$_2$	0.87	0.77	2.42	0.91	—	—	0.87
15αOHE$_2$	1.21	1.06	1.23	1.24	—	—	1.20
E$_3$	1.41	1.29	1.73	1.43	1.44	1.77	1.43
16epiE$_3$	1.67	1.39	1.78	1.63	1.52	1.96	1.60
17epiE$_3$	1.39	1.23	1.63	1.39	1.29	1.63	1.42
16,17epiE$_3$	1.18	1.11	1.37	1.20	1.25	1.32	1.27
2metE$_3$	2.25	1.91	3.06	2.04	—	—	2.23
2OHE$_3$	1.91	1.94	2.45	1.82	—	2.12	—
6αOHE$_3$	1.56	1.70	2.18	1.85	—	2.08	—
15αOHE$_3$	3.02	2.37	—	2.56	—	5.96	—

* E_1 = estrone (3-hydroxyestra-1,3,5(10)-trien-17-one), E_2 = estradiol (estra-1,3,5(10)-triene-3,17β-diol), E_3 = estriol (estra-1,3,5(10)-triene-3,16α, 17β-triol). The following abbreviations are used: met = methoxy, OH = hydroxy, keto = keto, Δ = double bond, epi = steric epimer of the parent compound.

The final sample produced through purification by methods of unknown specificity should be studied by GLC, after first making a suitable derivative and using a nonselective liquid phase. Through this preliminary work valuable information can be obtained, since the absence of steroids from the sample at the level of detection sensitivity used can be established by the absence from the chromatogram of peaks with the same retention times as the corresponding derivatives of the reference standards.

A retention time on the chromatogram identical with that of a reference standard could signify that the peak may be identical with the reference standard or with another compound, perhaps even non-steroidal in nature, but with similar molecular weight and polarity. The quantity of the expected steroid should be calculated and the sample should then be analyzed on at least two selective phases. If a peak fails to appear on these chromatograms at the expected position, it is proof that this particular steroid is not present in the sample. If the quantity decreases during repeated GLC, it demonstrates that the peak on the first chromatogram was not due to a single substance and the sample needs additional purification. The presence of a peak on one nonselective and on two selective phases and with the same retention time as a reference standard suggests the possible identity of the compound with the reference standard.

Such tentative identification warrants further experiments. A part of the sample can be converted to different derivatives and analyzed with the corresponding derivative of the reference steroid on different liquid phases. Thereafter, the sample can be subjected to paper or thin-layer chromatographic analysis and the areas with mobilities similar to the corresponding reference standard can be analyzed by GLC on different liquid phases. It has been reported that the estrogens can be chromatographed on TLC plates as TMSi ethers (ADLERCREUTZ and LUUKKAINEN, 1965 a). The value of gas chromatographic identification can be further enhanced by reduction or oxidation of the sample and demonstration that the product of the chemical reaction has the same GLC mobilities as the reference compounds treated with the same reagent. Further, certain estrogens, such as *cis*-glycolic estriols, can be selectively converted to acetonides, extracted from the other estriols and analyzed as acetonides or after conversion of the phenolic hydroxyl to TMSi ether derivatives and then carried through GLC on different liquid phases. This stereoselective derivative formation results in a very specific determination of 16- and 17-*epi*estriols (ADLERCREUTZ et al., 1966).

If gas chromatography is the only tool used for compound identification, the identity of the compound (provided microgram or submicrogram amounts are available) can be established by determining the partition values of the compound in a binary solvent system of equal volumes of two immiscible phases, where the partition coefficient for authentic material has already been determined (BEROZA and BOWMAN, 1965). It is our experience that if a compound is present in microgram and submicrogram amounts in the sample, identification can best be achieved by recording the mass spectrum of the compound as it emerges from the gas chromatographic column with a gas chromatograph — mass spectrometer combination instrument (LUUKKAINEN and ADLERCREUTZ, 1965, 1967; ADLERCREUTZ et al., 1967 a; ADLERCREUTZ and LUUKKAINEN, 1967). The sensitivity limit of this method is at 50 nanograms of a compound and with this instrument isomeric and epimeric estrogens can be identified by using different ionization energy or better by combining the retention data and mass spectra. By recording multiple spectra from the different parts of the same peak it can be decided whether the peak is homogeneous or contaminated with some other material.

The second method which can be used even if only a small amount of the steroid is present in the sample is crystallization to constant specific activity. This method is useful only if the sample has been obtained after administration of labeled steroid and if the appropriate carrier is available in reasonable amounts and at reasonable price. Because of the difficulties of this technique with stereoisomers which tend to co-crystallize and in absence of a sufficient amount of a non-radioactive carrier standard, crystallization to constant specific activity is of limited value in the identification of estrogens other than estrone, estradiol and estriol.

Collection of the eluted steroids from the GLC column in glass U-tubes chilled in liquid nitrogen can be used (FALES et al., 1962), because the argon carrier gas is condensed along with the steroids. The fraction collected can be studied with different techniques depending on the amount of material present.

If the amount of the sample is less than 100 μg but over 5 μg, ultraviolet adsorption spectrometry gives valid information and the sample can be recovered after the analysis. The formation of a sulfuric acid chromogen is not recommended.

In our experience the analysis of an estrogen sample below 100 μg with infrared spectrophotometry using KBr pellets is difficult and the spectrum is too diffuse to permit confident identification. More valuable information can be obtained if the estrogen sample is dissolved in carbon tetrachloride and the characteristic bonds of the functional groups determined by infrared spectrophotometry. The bond at 2853 cm^{-1}, due to the aromatic methoxyl (BRIGGS et al., 1957) strongly suggests that the methyl ether derivative of an isolated compound is an estrogen bearing a methyl ether group at the phenolic hydroxyl.

After recovery from carbon tetrachloride, the sample can be converted to a suitable derivative and a part of it studied with a low- or high-resolution mass spectrometer, using a probe introduced into the ion source, or with a gas chromatographic inlet system. The correct use of the last-mentioned method provides currently the best identification method for estrogens found in biological samples, but these techniques are not available in every laboratory at the present time. Therefore parts of the collected sample may require analysis by other methods. Microchemical reactions on paper or thin-layer chromatograms can be carried out in every laboratory and the reader is referred to some of the recent monographs or reports in the field (LISBOA and DICZFALUSY, 1963; NEHER, 1964; ADLERCREUTZ and LUUKKAINEN, 1965 a). If the collected sample is crystalline and the structure unknown, it can be studied by X-ray crystallography (KENNARD, 1966).

With samples of more than 100 μg, rather conclusive identification can be made by using KBr pellets and infrared spectroscopy. Moreover, if the sample is larger than 1 mg, melting-point determinations and nuclear magnetic resonance spectrometry can be added to the arsenal of identification methods.

V. Methods for the Estimation of Estrogens in Biological Extracts

Estimations of urinary estrogens by GLC have been carried out for samples of urine from pregnant and nonpregnant women. For the former samples, methods are available for the estimation of estriol, for all three "classical" estrogens and finally for a number of estrogen metabolites. In addition, GLC methods have been reported for the estimation of estrogens in bile, plasma, tissue extracts and incubation media.

1. Methods for Estriol in Urine of Pregnant Women

Method of Wotiz *and* Martin *(1961, 1962)*

The procedure has been described three times with small variations in the extraction or in the acetylation techniques. In Flow-sheet 1 the method is outlined according to the text of a recent monograph by Wotiz and Clark (1966, p. 259). The only difference from the method originally suggested is that a wash with 8% $NaHCO_3$ solution has been included and acetylation is carried out in a slightly different way.

Flow-sheet 1. *Method of* Wotiz *and* Martin *(1961, 1962) for estriol in pregnancy urine*

Acid hydrolysis of 100 ml urine with 15 vol. % HCl and reflux at 100° C.

Ether extraction with $1 \times 1/1$ vol. $+ 2 \times 1/2$ vol.
Ether extract washed with 1/4 vol. of 8% $NaHCO_3$ solution.
Ether evaporated to dryness.

Dry residue dissolved in acetone and transferred to a screw-cap vial. Acetone dried in a stream of N_2 or air.

Acetylation with 0.1 ml of pyridine and 0.5 ml of acetic anhydride for 1 hr at 60—70° C. Mixture evaporated to dryness and dissolved in 0.1 ml of acetone.

GLC: 6 ft $\times$ 4 mm 4% SE-30 column at 250° C.

Comment: This method was first suggested for the estimation of all three classical estrogens in pregnancy urine (Wotiz and Martin, 1961). Only one gas chromatogram obtained by this procedure, showing the results for a third-trimester urine sample, has been presented (Wotiz and Martin, 1962). Later, the method was thought to be useful only for estrone and estriol in pregnancy urine (Wotiz and Chattoraj, 1965) and finally Wotiz and Clark (1966, p. 232) claim that "this method was found to be quite useful for the rapid determination of estriol in the second half of pregnancy".

In Fig. 1 one gas chromatogram obtained from one late-pregnancy urine sample by the method of Wotiz and Martin (1962) is shown and compared with gas chromatograms obtained by two other procedures (Yousem, 1964; Adlercreutz and Luukkainen, 1965 b). All these gas chromatograms were obtained from the same urine, using different methods for sample purification and for GLC. Employing the method of WOTIZ and MARTIN (1962), the peak shape is not ideal and some impurity is still present in the sample with slightly longer retention time than estriol triacetate (Fig. 1).

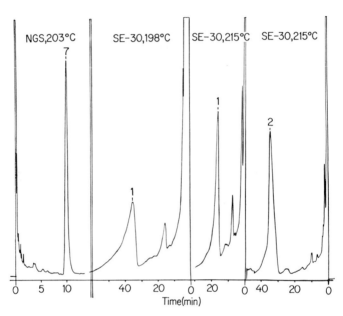

Fig. 1. GLC determination of estriol from the same 24-h urine specimen with different methods. Method of ADLERCREUTZ and LUUKKAINEN (1965 b): 7 = 3-methyl ether of estriol 16,17diTMSi; Method of YOUSEM (1964): 1 = free estriol (two gas chromatograms); Method of WOTIZ and MARTIN (1962): 2 = estriol-3,16,17-triacetate. Estriol excretion 12.4 mg/ 24 h. Injected amounts correspond to 0.5 ml of 24-h urine sample. Columns: U-shaped 6-ft×4-mm glass tubes, stationary phases 1⁰/₀ on 100—120 mesh Gas-chrom P. All gas chromatograms presented in this chapter were obtained with F & M Model 400 or 402 with hydrogen flame ionization detector

Method of YOUSEM (1964)

The method of YOUSEM (1964) is presented in Flow-sheet 2. As can be seen, the main difference from the procedure of WOTIZ and MARTIN (1962) is that free estriol is chromatographed on a QF-1 stationary liquid phase at 180—200 °C.

Flow-sheet 2. *Method of* YOUSEM *(1964) for the estimation of estriol in pregnancy urine*

Acid hydrolysis (ENGEL et al., 1950) of 200 ml of urine.

Extraction with ether $(1 \times 1/1$ vol. $+2 \times 1/2$ vol.).
Ether extract washed with 1/10 vol. of saturated $NaHCO_3$ solution and 3/100 vol. of water. Ether evaporated to dryness.

Dry residue dissolved in 200 ml of toluene, extracted with $4 \times 1/4$ vol. of 1 N NaOH and washed twice with 1/20 vol. of water. Aqueous extracts combined and washed with 1/10 vol. of hexane.

The aqueous solution acidified to pH 9.0 with 6 N H_2SO_4 and extracted with $4 \times 1/4$ vol. of water, dried with sodium sulfate and evaporated to dryness.

Dry residue dissolved in 1 ml of triple distilled alcohol and GLC on a 2% QF-1 column at 180—200° C.

Comment: Hitherto no GLC record of a urine sample subjected to YOUSEM's method has been presented. We therefore decided to try the method, and our experience with this technique is shown in Fig. 1. The stationary liquid phase was SE-30, in order to make comparisons with the method of WOTIZ and MARTIN (1962). The peak is broad and nonsymmetric, but the specificity is probably not less than for rapid chemical methods involving colorimetric estimation of estrogens in crude extracts of pregnancy urine. Owing to adsorption on the column, which is seen in Fig. 1, the calibration curves will not be linear. By increasing the temperature a somewhat better peak shape is obtained (Fig. 1).

The recovery of estriol added before hydrolysis was $78.6 \pm 11.8\%$ (YOUSEM, 1964). Nothing is known about the sensitivity of the procedure but estimations seem to have been carried out starting from the 6th week of pregnancy (YOUSEM, 1964).

Method of ADLERCREUTZ and LUUKKAINEN (1965 b)

This GLC procedure is based mainly on the work by LUUKKAINEN and ADLERCREUTZ (1963) studying GLC properties of TMSi derivatives of methylated estrogens. In this method a double derivative of the estriol is formed, namely the $16\alpha,17\beta$-ditrimethylsilyl ether of estriol 3-methyl ether. The methylation procedure, including a phase-change purification step, enhances the specificity of the method considerably. In addition, the gel filtration procedure of BELING (1963) was adopted, which means a high purification of the samples before hydrolysis and also an improvement of the yield of estrogens during both acid and enzyme hydrolysis. The procedure is presented in Flow-sheet 3.

Flow-sheet 3. *Method of* ADLERCREUTZ *and* LUUKKAINEN *(1965 b) for the estimation of estriol in pregnancy urine*

Gel filtration of 10 ml of urine on Sephadex G_{25} medium (pearl form). Peak I and peak II containing conjugated estrogens collected separately.

|

Peak I and peak II hydrolyzed separately for 16 hr at 37° C in 0.15 M acetate buffer, pH 4.1—4.2, with 600 Fishman units of β-glucuronidase and 6000 units of phenol sulfatase *(Helix pomatia* extract) per ml of reaction mixture. Alternatively acid hydrolysis according to BROWN (1955).

|

Hydrolysate of peak I and peak II combined. Carbonate buffer pH 10.5 added (BROWN, 1955). Extracted with $3 \times 1/1$ vol. of ethyl ether.

|

Ether evaporated to 4 ml under a stream of nitrogen and then extracted with $3 \times 1/2$ vol. of 1 N NaOH.

|

NaOH extract diluted to 15 ml with distilled water. 0.3 g boric acid added. Methylation (BROWN, 1955) in the same tube, using 0.3 ml dimethyl sulfate.

|

Methylated estrogens extracted once with 8 ml of benzene. Benzene washed with 1 ml of distilled water. Benzene evaporated to dryness.

|

Formation of TMSi ether derivatives of the methylated compounds.

|

Gas chromatography on Z, NGS and/or SE-30 liquid phases. [Alternatively, Kober reaction according to NOCKE (1961).]

Comment: The extraction procedure used in this method is not so rapid as in the two previous methods but all steps can be carried out in test-tubes, which is an advantage. Gel filtration takes about 2 hr, acid hydrolysis 1 hr (if enzymic hydrolysis is carried out, 16 hr are required), and finally the methylation procedure consumes 1 hr. The GLC estimation is rapid and the conditions can be regulated so that the retention time of the estriol peak is short. The formation of the TMSi ethers can be carried out in 1 hr; however, we prefer to do this overnight.

This is the only method that has been tested by adding conjugated estriol to the urine samples before processing the sample. A mean recovery of estriol-16(17?)-glucosiduronate of 85.5% was found (5 estimations). The small number of recovery experiments performed is due to the fact that the different steps of the procedure have previously been investigated very thoroughly, using the Kober reaction (KOBER, 1931) as the final step. The gel filtration method in combination with enzyme hydrolysis of the estrogens was investigated by BELING (1963) and most of the results were confirmed in a large study

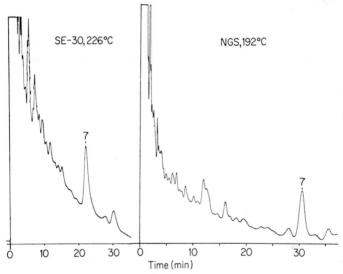

Fig. 2. GLC determination of estriol from the same 24-h urine specimen, using acid and enzyme hydrolysis by the method of ADLERCREUTZ and LUUKKAINEN (1965 b). 7 = 3-methyl ether of estriol-16,17diTMSi. The daily excretion of estriol 92 μg. 1% SE-30 (acid hydrolysis) and 1% NGS (enzymic hydrolysis) on 100—120 mesh Gas-chrom P in 6-ft×4-mm glass U-tubes

in this laboratory (ADLERCREUTZ, 1968). The losses during the gel filtration procedure are negligible for estriol; hydrolysis also gives losses of only a few percent and methylation gives a 95% yield (BROWN, 1955; ADLERCREUTZ, 1962). TMSi formation is complete as judged from IR spectrophotometric data (LUUKKAINEN et al., 1961).

The precision and sensitivity of the method have been investigated by duplicate estimation on urine obtained at different stages of pregnancy (Table 3). At low levels the precision decreases, and the method is not intended to be used for samples containing less than about 100—200 μg estriol/24-hr urine sample. This level must be regarded as the sensitivity limit of the procedure, which means that estimations can be carried out starting from about the 6th week of pregnancy (Fig. 2).

It is obvious that the specificity of the method is rather good, owing to the phase-change purification step involving methylation of the phenolic hydroxyl. Minor quantities of an unknown compound (probably 16-*epi*estriol) occurring at the shoulder of the peak (Fig. 1, ADLERCREUTZ and LUUKKAINEN, 1965 b) can not be regarded as influencing the specificity of the estimation, since its quantity is very small. As judged from mass spectrometric investigations with a gas chromatograph-mass spectrometer, the peak is homogeneous and the spectrum is identical with that of a reference standard. Even at low steroid concentration the gas chromatographic-mass spectrometric data suggest that the specificity of the method is satisfactory (LUUK-KAINEN and ADLERCREUTZ, 1967).

Results Obtained with the Methods for the Estimation of Estriol in Pregnancy Urine

As far as we know, the methods described seem not to have been used except in the laboratories where they were developed. WOTIZ and MARTIN (1962) have presented results obtained with urine from women nine months pregnant, and YOUSEM (1964) gives a figure showing the distribution of estriol throughout normal pregnancy. In addition, some few values for three patients with pathological pregnancies were presented by YOUSEM. Recently, SCOMMEGNA and CHATTORAJ (1966) published results of estriol determinations during the two last trimesters of pregnancy, using a further modification of the method of WOTIZ and MARTIN (1962). The estriol excretion was found to be similar to that reported by BELING (1963). Estriol determinations were also made during pathological pregnancies in order to monitor the fetal well-being in utero after intrauterine blood transfusions. It thus seems that the modified method may give valuable clinical information.

In Table 3 the results of estriol determination in urine obtained during both normal and pathological pregnancies are shown, using the method of ADLERCREUTZ and LUUKKAINEN (1965 b). For hormone estimation comparisons have also been carried out with a similar

Table 3. *Data on duplicate estimation of estriol in pregnancy urine by the
method of* ADLERCREUTZ *and* LUUKKAINEN *(1965 b)*

Month of pregnancy	Estriol mg/24 h	Condition	Month of pregnancy	Estriol mg/24 h	Condition
II	0.22 0.33	Normal	VI	8.10 7.57	Normal
II	0.24 0.24	Normal	VI	8.12 7.88	Hypertension
III	0.62 0.84	Normal	VII	18.6 18.7	Normal
III	0.72 0.54	Normal	VII	4.96 4.85	Hypertension
III	0.82 0.79	Normal	VII	5.72 5.52	Normal
IV	3.84 4.03	Normal	VIII	16.9 17.0	Gestanon treatment
IV	1.69 1.53	Normal	VIII	2.24 2.38	Toxemia
IV	2.20 2.14	Normal	VIII	13.9 12.7	Normal
IV	4.96 4.73	Normal	IX	10.3 10.2	Toxemia
IV	3.22 3.22	Normal	IX	13.7 13.5	Normal
IV	6.20 5.85	Normal	X	30.8 31.6	Normal
IV	4.96 4.85	Normal	X	20.0 19.3	Normal
V	6.30 6.11	Normal	X	25.3 26.5	Normal
V	9.64 9.62	Normal	X	56.8 54.7	Normal
V	4.94 4.85	Normal			

method using colorimetric estimation of estriol (BELING, 1963) and
for most urines the agreement was good. However, in some cases
great discrepancies between the two methods were seen when the
urine came from subjects not receiving drugs or other compounds
known to influence the Kober reaction. This "unknown material"

which must give rise to a positive Kober reaction could be separated from estriol by gas chromatography. In one case a compound with GLC retention behavior like that of 16-*epi*estriol but not identical with this compound was present in the urine (LUUKKAINEN and ADLERCREUTZ, 1966).

For scientific purposes, therefore, a gas chromatographic procedure seems superior to a colorimetric one, but only if the specificity of the former method has been well established. A direct gas chromatographic-mass spectrometric check on the identity of the compound under investigation is very valuable but not possible in routine clinical work, owing to the expensive instruments needed.

Conclusion

Compared to the procedure of ADLERCREUTZ and LUUKKAINEN (1965 b), it seems that the method of WOTIZ and MARTIN (1962) and YOUSEM (1964) are less practicable due to the large urine volume needed but more rapid at the expense of accuracy and specificity. If however, the answer to the clinician has to be given the same day, our laboratory still prefers to use acid hydrolysis and a colorimetric final estimation for estriol. For nonroutine work a GLC procedure is to be recommended. Especially for drug-contaminated or bile-stained urine a specific gas chromatographic method seems better than a colorimetric one since estimation by GLC is not subject to interference, as in the Kober reaction, by drugs (BROWN et al., 1957 a, b) or biliary compounds (ADLERCREUTZ, 1962; ADLERCREUTZ and SCHAUMAN, 1964).

2. Methods for the Estimation of Estrone, Estradiol-17β and Estriol in Pregnancy Urine

Method of WOTIZ and CHATTORAJ *(1965)*

This method (WOTIZ and CHATTORAJ, 1965) includes alumina chromatography of the estrogen acetates (Flow-sheet 4) and is a further development of the method of WOTIZ and MARTIN (1962), which apparently did not have the required specificity for the estimation of all three estrogens, as first suggested.

Comment: Chromatography of the estrogen acetates on alumina separates estrone acetate and estriol triacetate from estradiol di-

Flow-sheet 4. *Method of* WOTIZ *and* CHATTORAJ *(1965) for the estimation of estrone, estradiol-17β and estriol in pregnancy and nonpregnancy urine*

Acid hydrolysis, ether extraction, washing of the ether extract and evaporation of ether to dryness (BROWN, 1955).

|

Separation of phenolic and neutral fractions by partition between benzene-petroleum ether and 1 N NaOH.

|

NaHCO$_3$ solution added to the aqueous extract until pH 9.5—10. Extraction with ether. Ether extract washed with 8% NaHCO$_3$ and evaporated to dryness.

|

Acetylation with 0.1 ml pyridine and 0.5 ml acetic anhydride for 1 hr at 68° C.

|

Solvent partition (see section on acetylation).

|

Alumina chromatography:
    (a) 25% benzene in petroleum ether, 10 ml (discarded)
    (b) 50% benzene in petroleum ether, 15 ml (discarded)
    (c) 75% benzene in petroleum ether, 20 ml: first 5 ml
        (discarded), next 10 ml collected (estradiol diacetate),
        last few ml (discarded)
    (d) benzene, 20 ml: first 15 ml collected (estrone acetate
        + estriol triacetate).
GLC: 6 ft by 4 mm, 3% QF-1 column (3000 plates or better).

acetate and seems to be a considerable advance as compared with the original procedure of WOTIZ and MARTIN (1962). The mean recoveries of free estrogens added after (?) acid hydrolysis to one male urine were found to be 72.4, 75.6 and 82.8% for estrone, estradiol and estriol, respectively. The mean losses during alumina chromatography were found to be 6.2—7.5%. It is not clearly indicated whether the standard estrogens were added to the urine before or after hydrolysis; but from the results published it is most probable that the standards were added after hydrolysis. The acid hydrolysis procedure used (BROWN, 1955) destroys about 20% of the three estrogens (BROWN and BLAIR, 1958; ADLERCREUTZ, 1962). The sensitivity of the procedure appears good; the method has also been used for urine samples from nonpregnant women and the duplicate assays presented from such samples agree well (see later). The specificity of the method was investigated for pregnancy urine and the chromatographic as well as spectrophotometric data obtained suggest that this aspect of the method is satisfactory. The authors claim that one technician can carry out 25 estimates a week.

Method of FISHMAN and BROWN (1962)

These authors made one of the first attempts to estimate estrogens by GLC. The method is practically identical with that of WOTIZ and MARTIN (1962), but enzymic hydrolysis is used.

Comment: The authors evidently made no real attempt to develop a GLC procedure for urinary estrogens; the experiments were carried out more with the aim of making comparisons with the original procedure of BROWN (1955) in order to obtain further information regarding the specificity of the colorimetric method. The results obtained suggest that for estrone and estriol the agreement between the two procedures is good, but for some urines discrepancies were found with regard to estradiol concentration. There are two reasons for these discrepancies: 1) the GLC method was obviously not very specific for estradiol, 2) the estradiol fraction contains another Kober-positive estrogen, 11-dehydroestradiol-17α, in an amount comparable with that of estradiol-17β (Table 4, LUUKKAINEN and ADLERCREUTZ, 1965).

GLC was carried out on a SE-30 column, and it was shown that the calibration curves for the estrogen acetates were not linear.

Method of ADLERCREUTZ and LUUKKAINEN (1965 b)

The method is presented in Flow-sheet 5. Purification steps from the procedure of BROWN (1955) have been combined with gel filtration of the conjugated estrogens and enzymic hydrolysis. Estrone is estimated as its methyl ether, estradiol as its 17β-TMSi ether derivative of the 3-methyl ether, and estriol as its 3,16α,17β-tri TMSi ether derivative. It is possible to use several different GLC columns for the final estimation and those mentioned are only examples of columns which have been used. As shown in a previous study (ADLERCREUTZ and LUUKKAINEN, 1965 b), a great number of other polar estrogens can be detected in the estriol fraction. The recovery of these substances, however, is not quantitative and it is necessary to use at least four different columns in order to obtain a reasonable degree of specificity. Therefore this procedure has been considerably modified to allow more satisfactory estimation of the other estrogens (see later).

Flow-sheet 5. *Method of* ADLERCREUTZ *and* LUUKKAINEN *(1965 b) for the estimation of estrone, estradiol-17β, and estriol in urine of pregnant women*

Gel filtration of 10—20 ml of urine on Sephadex G_{25} medium. Peak I and peak II containing conjugated estrogens collected separately and hydrolyzed for 16 hr at 37° C in 0.15 M acetate buffer, pH 4.1, with 600 Fishman units of β-glucuronidase and 6000 units of phenol sulfatase (*Helix pomatia* extract) per ml of reaction mixture.

|

Hydrolysate of peak I and peak II combined. Carbonate buffer, pH 10.5 added (BROWN, 1955).

|

Extracted with 3×1/1 vol. of ethyl ether. Ether evaporated to dryness.

|

Dry residue dissolved in 0.1 ml of ethyl alcohol. 3 ml of benzene and 3 ml of petroleum ether added.

|

1.

Benzene-petroleum ether extracted with 2×1/2 vol. of distilled water.

|

Water extracted with 3×1/1 vol. of ether. Ether washed with 1/20 vol. of 8⁰/₀ $NaHCO_3$ solution. Ether washed with 1/40 vol. of distilled water.

|

Ether evaporated to dryness.

|

Formation of TMSi derivatives.

|

GLC of the estriol fraction: XE-60 and/or Z and/or SE-30 liquid phases.

2.

Benzene-petroleum ether extracted with 2×1/2 vol. of 0.4 N NaOH

|

NaOH extract diluted to 15 ml with 0.4 N NaOH, 0.3 g boric acid added. Methylation according to BROWN (1955).

|

Methylated estrogens extracted with 8 ml of hexane. Hexane washed with 1 ml of distilled water.

|

Hexane evaporated to dryness.

|

Formation of TMSi derivatives of the methylated estrone-estradiol fraction.

|

GLC: XE-60 and/or Z liquid phases.

Comment: The method presented in Flow-sheet 5 has been tested with conjugated estrogens added to the urine samples before enzymic hydrolysis. Since reference standards of naturally occurring glucosiduronates of estrone and estradiol are not available, the method was tested with estrone and estradiol 3-sulfate added to gel-filtered urine samples. This was done since small amounts of the sulfates, especially estradiol sulfate, are adsorbed on the gel column during gel filtration. Since the concentration of these sulfates, especially estradiol sulfate, is rather low (ADLERCREUTZ, 1965; ADLERCREUTZ et al., 1967 b), the amounts of urinary estrogen sulfates lost during gel filtration are negligible. The mean recovery of estrone sulfate was 86.5% (5 determinations) and that of estradiol 3-sulfate was 78.0% (5 determinations). The corresponding value for estriol-16(17?)-glucosiduronate was 96.5% (5 determinations).

This method is recommended only for urines containing at least 1 mg estriol/24-h specimen. It is possible to use this method for estriol concentrations of ≥ 200 µg/24-h urine specimen, but it is suggested that in such cases the method of ADLERCREUTZ et al. (1967 a) (see later) should be used, since the concentration of estradiol is usually too low for adequate quantification.

When the final fractions (from a late pregnancy urine sample) were subjected to TMSi ether formation and injected into a gas chromatograph-mass spectrometer, it was found that mass spectra of the compounds estimated were identical with those of the corresponding reference standards. In addition, the retention times were identical with those of the reference compounds on five different GLC columns.

Method of ADLERCREUTZ et al. (1967 a)

The method is presented in Flow-sheet 6. With this method a fourth estrogen can also be quantitated, e. g. 11-dehydro-estradiol-17α (LUUKKAINEN and ADLERCREUTZ, 1965). The method is recommended for urine samples containing less than 1 mg estriol/24-h urine specimen. Since an additional estrogen can be estimated with this procedure, we usually prefer to use this technique for the study of estrogen excretion during pregnancy.

Comment: Gas chromatograms showing results obtained from samples from the second month of pregnancy are presented in Fig. 3 and 4. The peak occurring before the TMSi derivative of estradiol-17β 3-methyl ether has an identical retention time with that of the TMSi derivative of estradiol-17α 3-methyl ether. This compound is probably the TMSi derivative of 11-dehydro-estradiol-17α 3-methyl ether, but since the NGS column gives a high background at the temperatures necessary for investigating this problem by gas chro-

Flow-sheet 6. *Method of* ADLERCREUTZ *et al. (1967 a) for the estimation of
estrone, estradiol-17β, 11-dehydroestradiol-17α and estriol in urine*

Gel filtration of 50—200 ml of urine on Sephadex G_{25} medium (pearl form).
Peak I and peak II containing conjugated estrogens collected separately
and hydrolyzed for 16 hr at 37° C in 0.15 M acetate buffer, pH 4.1, with
1000 Fishman units of β-glucuronidase and 1,000,000 units of phenol sulfatase (*Helix pomatia* extract) units per ml of reaction mixture.

Hydrolysate of peak I and peak II combined and extracted with 1×1/1 vol.
+ 2×1/2 vol. of ethyl ether. Ether washed with 1/5 vol. of carbonate buffer
(BROWN, 1955), with 1/30 vol. of 8% $NaHCO_3$ solution and 1/40 vol. of
distilled water. Ether evaporated to dryness.

Dry residue dissolved in 1 ml of ethyl alcohol. 25 ml of benzene and 25 ml
of petroleum ether added.

1.	2.
Benzene-petroleum ether extracted with 2×1/2 vol. of distilled water.	Benzene-petroleum ether extracted with 2×1/2 vol. of 0.4 N NaOH.
Methylation (BROWN, 1955)	Methylation (BROWN, 1955).
Extraction of the methylated estrogens with 15 ml of benzene. Washing of the extracts twice with 3.0 ml of distilled water.	Extraction of the methylated estrogens with 15 ml of hexane. Washing of the extract twice with 3.0 ml of distilled water.
Chromatography according to BROWN (1955).	Chromatography according to BROWN (1955).
Formation of TMSi derivatives of the methylated estriol fraction.	Formation of TMSi derivatives of the methylated estradiol fraction.
GLC of the estriol fraction: F-60 and/or JXR and/or NGS liquid phases. (Alternatively, Kober reaction according to NOCKE [1961].)	GLC of the methylated estrone and estradiol fractions: Z and/or XE-60 and/or F-60 liquid phases. (Alternatively, Kober reaction according to NOCKE [1961].)

matography-mass spectrometry, we have not been able to definitely
establish that this peak on an NGS column is identical with the
TMSi derivative of 11-dehydro-estradiol-17α 3-methyl ether. In
addition, the peak sometimes contains contaminating material, as
seen in Fig. 4. As demonstrated previously, on the Z column the

retention times of the TMSi derivatives of 3-methyl ether of estradiol-17α and 11-dehydro-estradiol-17α are identical. Since NGS and Z are both selective columns, it seems likely that the same phenomenon

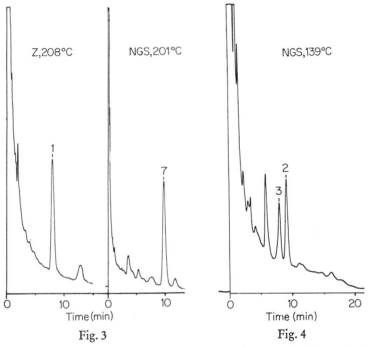

Fig. 3   Fig. 4

Fig. 3. GLC of methylated estrone and estriol fraction by the method of ADLERCREUTZ et al. (1967 a). Urine sample from the second month of pregnancy. Excretion of estrone 110 μg/24 h and estriol 720 μg/24 h. Injected amounts 0.22 μg and 0.61 μg, respectively. 1 = methyl ether of estrone, 7 = 3-methyl ether of estriol-16,17diTMSi. Both liquid phases 1% on 100—120 mesh Gas-chrom P in 6-ft×4-mm glass U-tubes

Fig. 4. GLC of methylated diol fraction as TMSi ethers obtained from the same urine sample as in Fig. 3. Daily excretion of estradiol 27 μg/24 h. 2 = estradiol-17β, 3 = 11-dehydro-estradiol-17α(?). 1% NGS on 100 to 120 mesh Gas-chrom P in a 6-ft×4-mm glass U-tube

occurs when an NGS column is used. In Fig. 5 another gas chromatogram of the estradiol fraction from pregnancy urine is depicted, showing the position of the TMSi derivative of 11-dehydro-estradiol-17α 3-methyl ether on an SE-30 column.

This method differs from the methods of ADLERCREUTZ and LUUK-KAINEN (1965 b) only with regard to chromatography of the methylated estrogens and the amounts of solvents used. Therefore, additional recovery experiments were not considered necessary, since the losses entailed by the chromatography step are known to be no greater than 5% at most (ADLERCREUTZ, 1962). Assuming a 5% loss during chromatography, the recovery of estrone sulfate would be about 82%, estradiol 3-sulfate about 73% and estriol-16(17?)-glucosiduronate about 89%, if a 10-ml urine sample is used. Moreover, an extensive investigation has been made of this method, where the Kober reaction was used as the final step. The average recovery of the three estrogen conjugates (10 analyses) processed from 50-ml nonpregnancy urine was 84.5, 73.2 and 71.6% for estrone sulfate, estradiol-3-sulfate and estriol-16(17?)-glucosiduronate, respectively. The value somewhat lower than expected for estriol-16(17?)-glucosiduronate is probably due to interference from urinary "impurities" with the colorimetric estimation of estriol. Since the procedure of WOTIZ and CHATTORAJ (1965) has not been tested with conjugated estrogens added before hydrolysis, no comparisons of the recovery values of the two methods can be made.

The precision of the method has been investigated by duplicate estimates (Table 4) and the results of this study are satisfactory. It is not possible, however, to achieve the same level of precision with the GLC method as with the colorimetric method. The precision of the latter method, (expressed as the standard deviation of the differences between duplicate estimates at low levels) working with 50-ml nonpregnancy urine samples, is 0.19, 0.20 and 0.71 µg/24-h for estrone, estradiol-17β and estriol, respectively. The sensitivity of the method involving GLC is also less adequate than that of the method using colorimetric estimation of the estrogens. The amounts, which

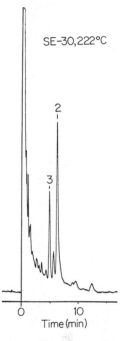

Fig. 5. GLC of methylated diol fraction obtained from pregnancy urine by the method of ADLERCREUTZ et al. (1967 a) on 1% SE-30. Stationary phase on Anakrom ABS 100 to 120 mesh in a 6-ft ×4 mm glass U-tube. 2 = 3-methyl ether of estradiol-17βTMSi and 3 = 3-methyl ether of 11-dehydroestradiol-17αTMSi

Table 4. *Estimation of estrone, estradiol-17β, 11-dehydroestradiol-17α and estriol in pregnancy urine by the method of* Adlercreutz *et al. (1967 a). Some duplicate estimations are included*

Month of pregnancy	Estrone mg/24 h	Estradiol-17β mg/24 h	11-Dehydro-estradiol-17α mg/24 h	Estriol mg/24 h	Condition
II	0.17	0.015	0.019	0.72	Normal
	0.15	0.014	0.017	0.53	(Duplicate)
III	0.10	0.020	0.003	0.4	Normal
III	0.33	0.083	0.012	1.2	Normal
	0.22	0.061	0.006	1.2	(Duplicate)
IV	0.041	0.028	0.007	1.6	Normal
IV	0.46	0.015	— *	2.1	Normal
	0.49	— **	— **	2.3	(Duplicate)
V	— *	0.016	0.006	— *	Normal
VI	— *	0.25	0.04	— *	Normal
VI	— *	0.024	0.008	— *	Normal
VI	0.45	0.092	0.015	6.3	Normal
VI	0.18	0.064	0.026	7.8	Normal
VI	0.58	0.18	0.022	9.5	Normal
	0.34	0.14	0.015	8.7	(Duplicate)
VI	— *	0.66	0.15	21.1	Normal
VI	0.35	0.084	0.034	7.8	Normal
VII	0.71	0.45	0.028	12.6	Normal
	0.56	0.40	0.029	15.9	(Duplicate)
VII	— *	0.46	0.14	29.8	Normal
VIII	0.037	0.008	0.010	4.1	Bleedings
	0.046	0.007	0.008	4.1	(Duplicate)
VIII	— *	0.53	0.20	41.5	Normal
IX	1.10	0.078	— *	27.8	Normal
IX	— *	0.43	0.19	45.8	Normal
IX	1.18	0.037	— *	74.0	Normal
X	0.54	0.23	— *	3.0	Edema
	0.40	— **	— **	3.0	(Duplicate)
X	0.29	0.18	0.05	12.9	Toxemia
	0.30	0.21	0.07	12.5	(Duplicate)
X	1.24	0.39	0.037	16.9	Normal
X	— *	0.13	0.08	— *	Normal
X	— *	0.24	0.09	— *	Twin pregnancy
	— *	0.28	0.13	— *	(Duplicate)
X	2.16	0.38	0.11	30.1	Normal
X	— *	0.58	0.32	36.5	Normal
X	— *	0.68	0.42	— *	Normal
X	— *	0.74	0.33	53.0	Normal
X	0.72	— *	— *	75.1	Recurrent jaundice of pregnancy

      * not estimated   ** sample lost

differ significantly from zero (P = 0.01), were 0.4, 0.4 and 1.5 µg/24 h for estrone, estradiol-17β and estriol, respectively, if colorimetry is used. With the GLC method values in this range can be estimated, but interfering peaks sometimes occur and therefore a modification of the method is recommended for use at estrogen levels below 2—5 µg/24 h (see later). However, the GLC procedure has the distinct advantage that it shows greater specificity, especially at low levels when at least one nonselective and two selective GLC columns are used. Only in this respect is the colorimetric method unable to compete with the GLC procedure.

The specificity of the GLC method has been investigated for pregnancy urine samples with a gas chromatograph-mass spectrometer. It was found that even at low levels the peaks used for estrogen estimation were identical with those of the reference standards.

Results Obtained with the Methods for the Estimation of Estrone, Estradiol and Estriol in Pregnancy Urine

Using the original procedure, WOTIZ (1963) estimated the three classical estrogens throughout one pregnancy. The results obtained did not agree with those reported by other investigators; especially the values for estradiol were peculiar, being higher in the beginning of pregnancy. It thus seems likely that some other compound must have been estimated in addition to estradiol. To overcome these difficulties (see WOTIZ and CLARK, 1966), WOTIZ and CHATTORAJ (1965) incorporated alumina chromatography of the estrogen acetates. This step seems to have been a great help. Estrogen excretion values during pregnancy have not been published using the modified method. WOTIZ and CLARK (1966) have presented two gas chromatograms showing the results of analysis from a late (?) pregnancy urine sample.

Results obtained with the method of ADLERCREUTZ et al. (1967 a) are shown in Table 4. With this method it seems possible to obtain a reliable estimate of the estradiol-17β content in the urine of pregnant women. It is interesting to note the comparatively low value for this estrogen in many subjects. This could indicate that the values obtained by colorimetric procedures are too high. A few comparisons between the GLC method and the corresponding colorimetric procedure (ADLERCREUTZ, unpublished) have also been carried out in our laboratory and the estradiol values were always higher with the colorimetric method (approximately corresponding to the amount of estradiol-17β + 11-dehydroestradiol-17α) provided that no drugs interfered with the latter estimation. For the first time quantitative values for 11-dehydro-estradiol-17α are presented (Table 4), showing that the amount of this estrogen excreted during pregnancy is mostly lower, but often rather near the estradiol values. The physiological significance of this estrogen is still not known.

Conclusions

The method of Wotiz and Chattoraj (1965) is somewhat easier to carry out than that of Adlercreutz and Luukkainen (1965 b). In the latter method the hydrolysis step used is obviously more adequate and the accuracy may be somewhat better (Table 1). The sensitivity of the procedures is likely to be about the same. The specificity of the two procedures is difficult to compare, since in the method of Wotiz and Chattoraj (1965) only GLC data and fluorescence spectra are available. The mass spectrometric data obtained for urinary estrogens purified by the method of Adlercreutz et al. (1967 a) will be presented elsewhere. Mass spectra of some estrogens obtained from urine have already been presented (Luukkainen and Adlercreutz, 1965, 1967; Adlercreutz et al., 1967 a).

It seems, therefore, that the choice of method is a matter of deciding which derivative of the estrogens should be used for GLC.

3. Methods for the Estimation of Estrone, Estradiol and Estriol in Nonpregnancy Urine

Several methods are available for the estimation of the three classical estrogens in nonpregnancy urine. Most of these methods include derivative formation and chromatography on alumina, which seems to be an absolutely necessary step in GLC methods for low-titer urines.

Method of Wotiz *and* Chattoraj *(1964)*

The method involves acid hydrolysis, a TLC step and GLC of the acetylated extract. The authors claim that "in some instances further purification was necessary prior to GLC". In that event the extract was subjected to another TLC. It seems scarcely credible that such crude extracts could be chromatographed in a satisfactory way by

TLC and the authors seem to have drawn the same conclusion in a later publication (WOTIZ and CHATTORAJ, 1965).

Method of WOTIZ and CHATTORAJ (1965)

This method is a further development of the above-mentioned procedure. The TLC steps were excluded and chromatography of the estrogen acetates on alumina was included. Some other slight modifications were also made. The method has already been discussed rather extensively under the section on methods for pregnancy urine samples. Some additional comments, however, seem indicated.

Comment: It is not reported how much urine must be used per assay. Nor is it stated how much of the urine from one male subject was used for the few recovery experiments carried out. As mentioned already, it is not known whether the estrogens were added to the urine samples for recovery experiments before or after acid hydrolysis. The duplicate estimates using 9 nonpregnancy urine samples indicate good reproducibility and some chromatographic tracings have been presented, without, however, any indication of the concentration of estrogens in the sample. Somewhat more is known about the specificity of the method, which has been established using different GLC columns and both acetates and TMSi ether derivatives for identification. Fluorescence spectra suggesting that the compounds eluted from the alumina column are identical with the reference standards have also been presented.

Method of COX and BEDFORD (1964)

Almost simultaneously, several authors suggested the use of TMSi ether or acetate derivatives of estrogen methyl ethers for GLC of estrogens (LUUKKAINEN and ADLERCREUTZ, 1963; COX and BEDFORD, 1964; ADLERCREUTZ and LUUKKAINEN, 1964; 1965 a; MENINI, 1965 a, b). These derivatives were found to be very suitable for GLC work and have been incorporated into several methods. COX and BEDFORD (1964) combined the procedure of BROWN (1955) for estimation of urinary estrogens with GLC of these estrogens as double derivatives. In their preliminary report they showed that TMSi ether and acetate derivatives gave equally good results, but seemed to have preferred the acetates on account of easier preparation and better stability. No definite method was presented but it has been found that the combination of BROWN's (1955) procedure with

GLC of the TMSi derivatives of the estrogen 3-methyl ethers works rather well (ADLERCREUTZ and LUUKKAINEN, 1964; 1965 b).

Method of MENINI (1965 a, b) for the estimation of estriol and estrone + estradiol

A similar approach to the problem of the estimation of estrogens in nonpregnancy urine has been presented by MENINI (1965 a, b). The method starts with a borohydride reduction in order to convert estrone conjugates to estradiol conjugates. This step is followed by acid hydrolysis (BROWN, 1955), saponification of the estrogens (BROWN et al., 1957 b), partition between benzene, light petroleum, ethanol and aqueous alkali for the separation of estradiol from estriol, methylation and chromatography according to BROWN (1955). Following acetylation, the estrogens are rechromatographed on alumina and then submitted to GLC as the same double derivatives, as suggested by COX and BEDFORD (1964).

Comment: The gas chromatograms published indicate a high degree of purity of the samples. Pure estradiol and estriol added to water and processed by the method were recovered in the range of 68—77%. Nothing is known about the recovery from urine samples. It seems that the author has not taken into consideration the possibility of the conversion of many other compounds to estriol and estradiol by borohydride. Both 16α-hydroxyestrone and 16-ketoestradiol will be converted to estriol and perhaps also other estrogens. Hence it is somewhat difficult to say which estrogens are estimated and therefore also difficult to evaluate the significance of the results. Further studies with this method are therefore awaited with interest, but it is possible that estimation of the total estrogens substituted at carbon 17 and at carbons 17 and 16 might be as useful as the specific estimation of the "classical" estrogens.

Method of ADLERCREUTZ et al. (1967 a)

Investigations on the combination of the method of BROWN (1955) with GLC for nonpregnancy urine samples (ADLERCREUTZ and LUUKKAINEN, 1964; 1965 b) demonstrated that the GLC technique was not suitable for routine clinical assays. In order to enhance recovery during hydrolysis, gel filtration (BELING, 1963) was included in the method, but still it was found that at very low concentrations of estrogens difficulties were encountered in quantitative estimation (see section on methods for pregnancy urine, where this method has been presented in detail). As indicated previously, amounts less than 2—5 µg/24-h urine specimen can not be satisfactorily estimated with this method and we therefore used the original procedure, which involves a colorimetric estimation of the estrogens (ADLERCREUTZ, to be published), for routine clinical assays. There is, however, a need for a specific method for measurement of estradiol concentrations down to about 0.1 µg/24-h specimen.

Modification of the method ADLERCREUTZ et al. (1967 a) for the estimation of estrone, estradiol-17β and estriol in nonpregnancy urine

Analysis is performed on 500 ml of urine or $^1/_3$ of the 24-hour urine sample, which is filtered through a 50-cm × 5-cm Sephadex G 25 (pearl form) column. This treatment will concentrate the estrogen conjugates to be analysed to a volume of 200—250 ml, depending on the rate of column flow. Enzymic hydrolysis is carried out as described previously. Following ether extraction, washing of the extract and evaporation of the ether to dryness, the free estrogens, dissolved in 1 ml of the butanolic phase are chromatographed on a Sephadex G 25 (pearl form) column (50 cm × 1 cm in the solvent system n-butanol:tertiary butanol:conc. ammonia:water (300:100:60:340 v/v) and the fractions (5 × 2.6 ml) are collected with a fraction collector. This procedure has been used previously for the purification of estrogen sulfates in pregnancy urine (ADLERCREUTZ, 1965; ADLERCREUTZ et al., 1967 b). Starting from the first drops of the butanolic phase, which can easily be recognized, the first fractions are collected and evaporated to dryness and the original procedure described in Flow-sheet 6 is then followed. The purification obtained is considerable.

The column is prepared in aqueous ammonia and if the Sephadex is removed from the column after chromatography and washed thoroughly with water, the same support medium can be used for several years.

Comment: In Fig. 6 are recorded three steroid fractions obtained from the urine of a nonpregnant woman. The exact concentration of each estrogen is indicated in the legend. The estradiol-TMSi peak represents 0.03 µg estradiol and gives a 5-cm-high peak at an attenuation of 8 with a range of 10 (F & M, model 400, gas chromatograph equipped with a hydrogen flame ionization detector). The concentration of estradiol in this urine was 0.8 µg/24 h and it seems possible to estimate estrogens down to about the 0.1 µg/24 h level. So far we have not analyzed any urine containing less than 0.8 µg/24 h for any of these estrogens. The additional step included had been thoroughly investigated previously during development of the method for estrogen sulfates in pregnancy urine, and it was found to be quantitative; no significant losses were noted. The amount of urine used is large in this procedure and further recovery studies are necessary.

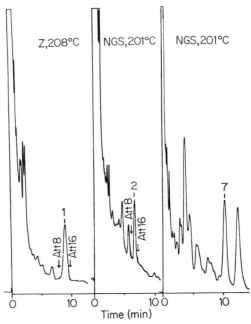

Fig. 6. GLC-analysis of a nonpregnancy urine sample by the method of ADLERCREUTZ and LUUKKAINEN, a modification reported in this chapter. Figures from left to right. 1 = methylated estrone (2.2 µg/24 h); methylated diol fraction as TMSi ether derivatives. 2 = estradiol-17β (0.8 µg/24 h); methylated triol fraction as TMSi ether derivatives, 7 = estriol (20 µg/24 h). 1% Z on 100—120 mesh Gas-chrom P in a 6-ft×4-mm glass U-tube. 1% NGS on 100—120 mesh Gas-chrom P in a 6-ft×4-mm glass U-tube. Att = attenuation

The estriol peak in Fig. 6 has been analyzed with a gas chromatograph-mass spectrometer recording several spectra from this peak. It was found that the compound was pure and identical with the diTMSi ether derivative of estriol 3-methyl ether (LUUKKAINEN and ADLERCREUTZ, 1967).

Conclusions

The hope expressed by some authors that GLC methods would yield versatile and more practicable methods for the estimation of estrogens in urine is still far from being realized. As shown above, the methods are as complicated as the colorimetric or fluorometric procedures and our laboratory still prefers to use colorimetric methods for routine clinical assays. However, there is an increasing need for specific and highly sensitive methods for the estimation of estrogens in urine. With current improvements in the construction of gas chromatographs, it seems possible to develop such methods. The successful application of a suitable method will hinge on scrupulous purification of the solvents and glassware, and for a new laboratory much work may be required before all interfering factors have been excluded. It is therefore not likely that highly sensitive and specific GLC methods will be used for routine work in the near future.

4. Methods for the Estimation of Estrone, Estradiol, Estriol and other Estrogens in Pregnancy Urine

Very few chemical methods for the estimation of estrogens other than the classical ones have hitherto been presented (GIVNER et al., 1960 b; KUSHINSKY et al., 1960; BREUER, 1964; KUSHINSKY and DEMETRIOU, 1963). In this field, however, it seems that GLC methods may have some advantages, owing to the high separation capacity of the GLC columns. The first attempt to estimate estrogens other than the classical ones was made by WOTIZ and CHATTORAJ (1964). This method has since been slightly modified by the same authors (WOTIZ and CHATTORAJ, 1965).

Method of WOTIZ *and* CHATTORAJ *(1964, 1965) for the estimation of estrone, estradiol-17β, estriol, 2- methoxyestrone, 16α-hydroxyestrone, 16-ketoestradiol and 16-epiestriol in pregnancy urine*

In the original procedure the two ring D α-ketolic estrogens could not be separated. In the modified procedure this was possible using a combination column of 0.5% EGA (stabilized) and 2.5% SE-30. The method is presented in Flow-sheet 7. As can be seen, this method includes two TLC steps and five different GLC estimations.

Flow-sheet 7. *Method of* WOTIZ *and* CHATTORAJ *(1964, 1965) for the estimation of estrone, 2-methoxyestrone, estradiol-17β, 16α-hydroxyestrone, 16-ketoestradiol, 16-epiestriol and estriol in pregnancy urine*

Enzymic hydrolysis (GIVNER et al., 1960 a).
|
Ether extractions ($1 \times 1/1$ vol. $+ 2 \times 1/2$ vol.). Ether washed with $1 \times 1/10$ vol. of 8% $NaHCO_3$ solution and with $2 \times 1/20$ vol. of water. Extract dried over Na_2SO_4. Ether extract evaporated to dryness.
|
TLC in system benzene : ethyl acetate (1 : 1) (incompletely saturated)
      Fraction A: estrone, 2-methoxyestrone
      Fraction B: estradiol, ring D-α-ketols
      Fraction C: 16-*epi*estriol
      Fraction D: estriol
Fractions eluted with ethanol.
|
TLC of fraction B in system petroleum ether : dichlormethane : ethanol (10 : 9 : 1) (completely saturated). Fractions (estradiol + ring D-α-ketols) eluted with ethanol.
|
All fractions evaporated to dryness.
|
Acetylation with 0.1 ml pyridine and 0.5 ml acetic anhydride for 1 hr at 68° C. Addition of 5 ml of water and extraction with 1×10 ml and 2×5 ml of petroleum ether. Petroleum ether evaporated to dryness.
|
Dry residue dissolved in 50 or 100 μl of acetone.
|
GLC: 3% SE-30 on 80—100 mesh alcohol washed Diatoport S, 4 ft by 4 mm column. Fractions A and B: column temperature 228° C, 20 psi N_2; Fraction C and D: column temperature 238° C, 20 psi N_2.

Comment: The recovery values reported by the authors vary from 72 to 91%, the highest value being found for 16α-hydroxyestrone. The latter value is astonishingly high, since two TLC chromatograms are used for the purification of the α-ketolic fraction. Losses may also be incurred during acetylation of the labile α-ketolic estrogens in pyridine.

No values for precision have been presented, but this is understandable, since the enormous amount of work involved in such procedures makes it practically impossible to establish dependable precision values until the method has been in use for several years. The specificity of the method has been investigated using multiple TLC, different color reactions, borohydride reduction followed by TLC and GLC (WOTIZ and CLARK, 1966).

From the data published using this method (WOTIZ and CHATTORAJ, 1964) difficulties must have been encountered during processing of some of the urines. No measurable estradiol values could be found in one patient whose urine was assayed for this hormone at different stages of pregnancy. In later work it was suggested that storage of the samples caused changes in the estradiol values (WOTIZ and CLARK, 1966). One wonders whether storage may also have influenced the concentration of the other estrogens assayed. Another difficulty seems to have been spreading of a large estriol peak to the area of 16-*epi*estriol during GLC, making the quantitation of the latter compound impossible. It is our opinion that TLC of crude urinary extracts is very difficult; the recovery of the compounds is poor. It is moreover not known how much urine was used in the recovery experiments of WOTIZ and CHATTORAJ (1965). The gas chromatograms presented from this method will not give any notion of the reliability of the method, since many compounds occur near the solvent front. Finally no gas chromatogram showing the separation of the two diacetates of the ring D α-ketolic estrogens has been published. It seems, therefore, that further work on the procedure is necessary before it can be accepted as a definite improvement in this area of estrogen research.

Method of ADLERCREUTZ *et al. (1967 a) for the estimation of estrone, estradiol-17β, 11-dehydroestradiol-17α, 16α-hydroxyestrone, 16-keto-estradiol, 2-methoxyestrone, estriol, 16-epiestriol and 17-epiestriol in pregnancy urine*

The method is presented in Flow-sheet 8. It should be pointed out that this method is still being explored and should not be regarded as final. The method has been modified for use on bile and plasma. The method is rather complicated but its specificity has been enhanced through a modification including acetonide formation of estrogen *cis*-glycols. The *cis*-glycols are separated from the other polar estrogens by solvent partition and the TMSi ether derivatives of the acetonides are subjected to GLC. In this way, one of the paper chromatograms is eliminated and it seems that 17-*epi*estriol can more easily be quantitated (see Flow-sheet 8, 1 b. Modified procedure).

Flow-sheet 8. *Method of* ADLERCREUTZ *et al. (1967 a) for the estimation of estrone, estradiol-17β, 11-dehydroestradiol-17α, 16α-hydroxyestrone, 16-ketoestradiol-17β, 2-methoxyestrone, estriol, 16-epiestriol and 17-epiestriol in pregnancy urine*

Gel filtration of 50—500 ml of urine on Sephadex G_{25} medium (pearl form). Peak I and peak II containing conjugated estrogens collected separately and hydrolyzed for 16 hr at 37° C in 0.15 M acetate buffer, pH 4.1, with 1000 Fishman units of β-glucuronidase and 1,000,000 units of phenol sulfatase (*Helix pomatia* extract) per ml of reaction mixture.

|

Hydrolysate of peak I and peak II combined, saturated with NaCl and extracted with $3 \times 1/1$ vol. of ethyl ether. Ether washed with 1/20 vol. of 8% $NaHCO_3$, saturated with NaCl and 1/40 vol. of distilled water. Ether evaporated to dryness.

|

Girard separation of ketonic steroids from nonketonic steroids with Girard reagent T in a single procedure using the amounts of reagents suggested by GIVNER et al. (1960 a, b). The nonketonic estrogens extracted from the NaCl-saturated solution with $3 \times 1/1$ vol. of ether and the ketonic estrogens, following hydrolysis, are extracted with $1 \times 1/1$ vol. and $2 \times 1/2$ vol. of ether.

Processing of ketonic fraction

Ether extract containing the ketonic estrogens washed with 1/20 vol. of 8% $NaHCO_3$ and 1/40 vol. of distilled water and evaporated to dryness.

|

Paper chromatography in the solvent system cyclohexane : toluene (1 : 1 v/v)/formamide separating the estrogens into 3 fractions:

Fraction A: 2-methoxyestrone + some 17-ketosteroids

Fraction B: estrone

Fraction C: 16α-hydroxyestrone and 16-ketoestradiol

All fractions eluted from the paper with 50 ml of methanol.

|

Fraction C rechromatographed further on paper in the solvent system chloroform/formamide and both α-ketolic estrogens eluted in the same fraction with 50 ml of methanol.

|

Formation of TMSi derivatives of the compounds following evaporation of the methanolic extracts.

|

GLC of estrone fraction: 1% Z.

GLC of 2-methoxyestrone fraction: 1% NGS.

GLC of fraction containing α-ketolic estrogens: 1% NGS or 1% QF-1

Processing of nonketonic fraction

Ether extract, following Girard separation, washed with 1/40 vol. of NaCl-saturated 8% NaHCO₃ solution and a very small amount of distilled water and evaporated to dryness.

Dry residue dissolved in 1 ml of ethyl alcohol. 25 ml of benzene and 25 ml of petroleum ether added.

1.

Benzene-petroleum ether extracted with 3×1/2 vol. of distilled water (1).

2.

Benzene-petroleum ether extracted with 2×1/2 vol. of 0.4 N NaOH (2).

1. Processing of water extract

1 a. Original procedure:

Aqueous extract saturated with NaCl, extracted with 3×1/1 vol. of ether and washed with 1/20 vol. of NaCl-saturated carbonate buffer, pH 10.5 (BROWN, 1955), NaCl-saturated 8% NaHCO₃ solution (1/40 vol.) and a very small amount of distilled water. Ether evaporated to dryness.

Gel chromatography on a 1 cm×15 cm Sephadex G₂₅ column in the solvent system n-butanol : toluene : 25% (conc.) ammonia : distilled water (150 : 50 : 20 : 180 v/v). Sample applied to the top of the column in 1 ml of the organic phase and an 8 ml fraction, starting from the front of the mobile phase, is collected and evaporated to dryness.

Paper chromatography in the solvent system toluene : ethyl acetate (9 : 1 v/v)/ 50% aqueous methanol, which separates the estrogens into two main fractions:

      Fraction D: 16-*epi*estriol and 17-*epi*estriol (+ some 2-methoxy-
              estriol).
      Fraction E: estriol, 16,17-*epi*estriol, 6α-hydroxyestradiol-17β,
              6β-hydroxyestradiol-17β, 15α-hydroxyestriol.

Both fractions eluted with 50 ml methanol. Methanolic extract evaporated to dryness.

Formation of TMSi derivatives of the compounds.

GLC of both fractions on at least one selective and one nonselective liquid phase (NGS, JXR, F-60).

1 b. Modified procedure:

Ether extraction and washing of the ether extract as described for the original procedure. Ether evaporated to dryness.

Dry residue dissolved in 25 ml of 1 N NaOH and extracted with 7×25 ml of chloroform which is discarded.

Aqueous phase acidified with 3 N HCl and saturated with NaCl. Extracted with 3×25 ml of ether, ether dried over Na₂SO₄. Ether extract filtered and evaporated to dryness under a stream of nitrogen.

Residue dissolved in 10 ml of dry acetone and 0.1 ml of trimethylchlorsilane and shaken at room temperature 2 h. The acid neutralized with 1 ml of 1 N NaOH and the acetone evaporated in a rotating evaporator at temperature below 40° C. 25 ml of 1 N NaOH added to the residue and mixture extracted with 2×12,5 ml of chloroform, which is dried over Na₂SO₄. The chloroform extract is filtered and evaporated to dryness.

I

TMSi ether derivative formation of the *cis*-glycols (16-*epi*- and 17-*epi*estriol).

GLC: SE-30 and NGS.

II

Aqueous extract neutralized with 3 N HCl, saturated with NaCl and extracted with 3×25 ml of ether. Ether evaporated to dryness.

Formation of TMSi ether derivatives of the compounds in the estriol fraction.

GLC: several different phases (NGS, JXR, XE-60, SE-30 or F-60).

2. Processing of the NaOH extract (diol fraction)

NaOH extract following partition between benzene-petroleum ether and 0.4 N NaOH is methylated according to Brown (1955).

To the methylated extract 10 ml of 5 N NaOH is added and the mixture extracted with 15 ml of hexane. Hexane extract washed with 2×3 ml of distilled water.

Chromatography of hexane extract on partially deactivated alumina according to Brown (1955). Estradiol-3-methyl ether fraction collected and evaporated to dryness.

Formation of TMSi ether derivatives of methylated diols.

GLC of the derivatives of estradiol-17β and 11-dehydroestradiol-17α on F-60 or SE-30 liquid phases.

Comment: At least 50 ml urine should be processed. It is possible to use up to 500 ml of urine, but for paper chromatographic separation of the ketones, extracts of more than 50 ml urine should not be chromatographed on one paper. This step is the weakest one in the

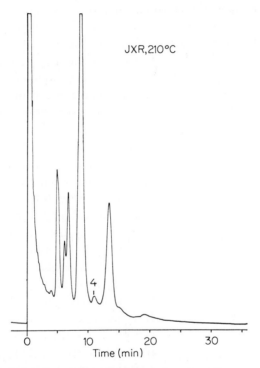

Fig. 7. GLC of the 2-methoxyestrone fraction from late pregnancy urine by the method of ADLERCREUTZ et al. (1967 a) (Flow-sheet 8). 4 = 2-methoxyestrone. Other compounds mainly 17-ketosteroids. 0.8% JXR on 100 to 120 mesh Anakrom AB in a 6-ft × 4-mm glass U-tube

procedure and work is now in progress to find a more suitable technique for the separation of the ketones contained in extracts of more than 50 ml of urine.

GIVNER et al. (1960 a, b) suggested that the Girard separation for ketonic estrogens should be carried out twice, using reagent P in order to obtain quantitative results. But a single procedure, with Girard reagent T, was found to give quantitative results (ADLERCREUTZ et al., 1967 a). Before extraction of the nonketonic estrogens from the aqueous phase containing the Girard complex the aqueous phase must be saturated with NaCl in order to get quantitative results for the highly polar estrogens. It was also found that during the ether extraction procedures involved in the Girard separation the ketolic estrogens are especially sensitive to peroxides in the ether. Saturated sodium bicarbonate solution can be used for washing the ether extract containing the ketonic estrogens following hydrolysis of the Girard complex and extraction of the liberated ketones. The recovery of estrone, 16α-hydroxyestrone and 16-ketoestradiol was found to be 91—99% for the whole procedure involved in the Girard separation described in Flow-sheet 8.

In Figs. 7, 8 and 9 gas chromatograms of the ketones obtained from pregnancy urine samples are presented. From these tracings the effect of one or two paper chromatographic systems on the purity of the fraction containing the ring D α-ketolic compounds is clearly demonstrated. The 2-methoxy-estrone fraction is rather impure owing to contamination with 17-ketosteroids. It is possible to separate 2-methoxy-estrone from these compounds by a phenolic partition, but during such partition some losses of the estrogen must be expected. We have not so far found this step necessary.

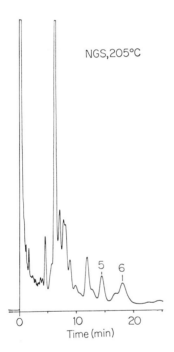

Fig. 8. GLC of the polar ketonic fraction as TMSi obtained from late pregnancy urine by the method of ADLERCREUTZ et al. (1967 a) (Flow-sheet 8). Gas chromatogram was obtained following one paper chromatographic purification. 5 = 16α-hydroxy-estrone, 6 = 16-ketoestradiol. 1% NGS on 100—120 mesh Gas-chrom P in a 6-ft×4-mm glass U-tube

Fig. 10 shows a gas chromatogram of the diol fraction obtained by this method. Sometimes difficulties are encountered with GLC of this fraction and several different columns should be used for the separation and estimation of estradiol-17β and 11-de-hydroestradiol-17α. The best liquid phases for this fraction are F-60 and SE-30.

In Fig. 11 the TMS derivatives of 16- and 17-*epi*estriol acetonides obtained from late pregnancy urine are shown. Gas chromatograms indicating the presence of 17-*epi*estriol in pregnancy urine have not been presented previously. Unless this compound is separated from

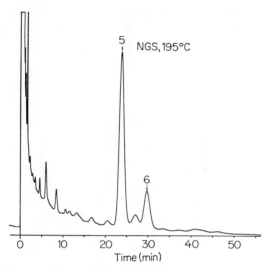

Fig. 9. GLC of the polar ketonic fraction obtained from late pregnancy urine by the method of ADLERCREUTZ et al. (1967 a) (Flow-sheet 8). Gas chromatogram following two paper chromatographic purifications. Conditions as in Fig. 8. Daily excretion of 16α-hydroxyestrone (5) = 1.49 mg/24 h and 16-ketoestradiol (6) = 0.27 mg/24 h. Conditions as in Fig. 4

estriol prior to GLC no liquid phase will separate the 17-*epi*estriol from a large estriol peak.

Chloroform extraction of the polar estrogen fraction before acetonide formation leads to considerable purification. Following acetonide formation additional purification is achieved by a second chloroform extraction. The fraction obtained is fairly pure, but a good column is still needed for separation of the large amount of different polar triols and tetrols present in the urine. In order to illustrate the difficulties involved in the estimation of polar estrogens by GLC some gas chromatograms are presented in Figs. 12, 13 and 14. In Fig. 15 a gas chromatogram of the estriol fraction obtained by the original method (ADLERCREUTZ et al., 1967 a) is shown. There is some evidence suggesting the presence of 6α-hydroxyestradiol, 6β-hydroxyestradiol,

11β-hydroxyestradiol and 16,17-*epi*estriol, in addition to estriol in the gas chromatograms in Figs. 12—15.

Most work on the reliability of this procedure has been concerned with the specificity of estimation. Recovery at each of the different

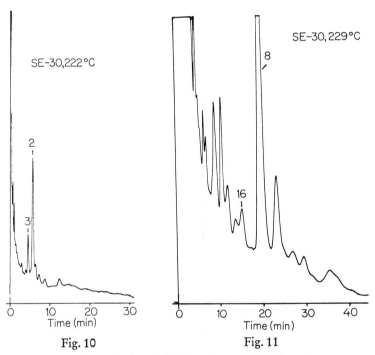

Fig. 10   Fig. 11

Fig. 10. GLC of the methylated diol fraction as TMSi from late pregnancy urine by the method of ADLERCREUTZ et al. (1967 a) (Flow-sheet 8). acetonide. 16 = 3-monoTMSi of 17-*epi*estriol-16α,17α acetonide. 1% SE-30 on 100—120 mesh Gas-chrom P in a 6-ft×4-mm glass U-tube

Fig. 11. GLC of the cis-glycolic triol fraction from late pregnancy urine obtained by the method of ADLERCREUTZ et al. (1967 a) (Flow-sheet 8), a modification presented in this chapter. 16-*epi*estriol excretion 290 μg/24 h, 17-*epi*estriol excretion 8 μg/24 h. 8 = 3 monoTMSi of 16-*epi*estriol-16β,17β acetonide. 16 = 3-monoTMSi of 17-*epi*estriol-16α,17α acetonide. 1% SE-30 on 100—120 mesh Gas-chrom P in a 6-ft×4-mm glass U-tube

steps added to the original method has been carefully investigated. The loss during paper chromatography is about 5%; occasionally, however, losses up to 10% have been incurred. As mentioned, the Girard separation is quantitative, as is also the formation of acetonides. The recovery of estriol in the different steps involved in the formation of acetonides is about 89%. 6α- and 6β-Hydroxyestradiol are partly destroyed during this step and therefore this modification cannot be used for the evaluation of their quantity. Compound re-

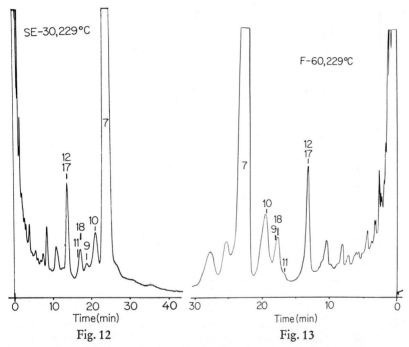

Fig. 12   Fig. 13

Fig. 12. GLC of the polar noncis-glycolic fraction from late pregnancy urine obtained by the method of ADLERCREUTZ et al. (1967 a) (Flow-sheet 8), a modification presented in this chapter. 7 = estriol-3,16,17triTMSi, 9 = 6α-hydroxyestradiol-3,6,17triTMSi, 10 = 16,17-*epi*estriol-3,16,17-tri TMSi, 11 = 6β-hydroxyestradiol-3,6,17triTMSi, 12 = 11β-hydroxyestradiol-3,11,17triTMSi, 17 and 18 = unknown compounds. 3% F-60 on 100 to 120 mesh Anakrom ABS in a 6-ft×4-mm glass U-tube

Fig. 13. Same urine sample as in Fig. 12 on 1% SE-30. Numbers correspond to the same steroids as in Fig. 12

covery is therefore lowest for the ring D α-ketolic compounds (60 to 65%) if two paper chromatography steps are included, as is necessary for urine samples. For estradiol and estriol the recovery is about 70 to 80%. The estimated values for estrone, 16α-hydroxyestrone, 16-keto-estradiol, 2-methoxyestrone, estradiol-17β, 11-dehydroestradiol-17α, estriol-16-*epi*estriol and 17-*epi*estriol have not been corrected for losses during processing.

No estimate of precision for this method can be given at present since a rather limited number of samples has been assayed. The sensi-

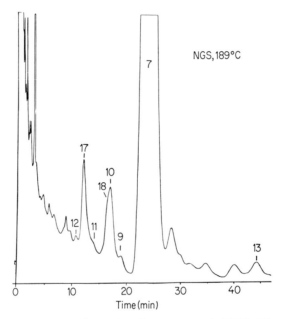

Fig. 14. Same urine sample as in Fig. 12 on 1% NGS. Numbers correspond to the same steroids as in Fig. 12. 13 = 2-methoxyestriol-3,16,17 triTMSi

tivity limit for the different compounds is, moreover, not known at present.

For investigation of the specificity, GLC on at least five different stationary liquid phases has been used, in addition to conventional methods such as paper chromatography, TLC and color reactions. Using direct gas chromatography — mass spectrometry, the following compounds, estimated as TMSi derivatives in this method are identical with the reference standards: estrone, estradiol-17β, 11-dehydro-estradiol-17α, 16α-hydroxyestrone, 16-ketoestradiol, estriol and 16-*epi*estriol. 16-*Epi*estriol and 17-*epi*estriol have also been identified in the same way as the TMSi ether derivatives of their acetonides (ADLERCREUTZ et al., 1966). In addition, after TLC separation of material in the 6α-hydroxyestradiol-17β peak obtained with the original procedure, steroid identity was established by GLC followed by mass-spectrometry (ADLERCREUTZ, HEIKKILÄ, LUUKKAINEN, to be published).

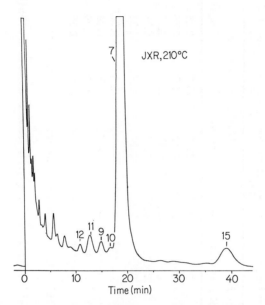

Fig. 15. GLC of the polar triol fraction as TMSi obtained from late pregnancy urine (twin pregnancy), by the original method of ADLERCREUTZ et al. (1967 a) (Flow-sheet 8). 7 = estriol, 9 = 6α-hydroxyestradiol, 10 = 16,17-*epi*estriol, 11 = 6β-hydroxyestradiol, 12 = 11β-hydroxyestradiol, 15 = 15α-hydroxyestriol. 0.8% JXR on 100—120 mesh Anakrom AB in a 6-ft×4-mm glass U-tube

Results Obtained with GLC Methods for the Estimation of Newer Estrogen Metabolites in Pregnancy Urine

WOTIZ and CHATTORAJ (1964) estimated estrone, estradiol-17β, 2-methoxyestrone, Ring D α-ketols, estriol and 16-*epi*estriol in the urine of a pregnant woman at 6 different stages of pregnancy. Their failure to detect any estradiol in this urine was later (WOTIZ and CLARK, 1966) suggested to be due to prolonged storage. The other estrogen values recorded seem to be in agreement with the values obtained by other workers using colorimetry for final estimation.

Table 5. *Estimation of some estrogens (mg/24 h) in pregnancy urine by the method of* ADLERCREUTZ *et al.* (1966 a)

Case no.	Month of pregnancy	Ketonic fraction *					$\Delta_{11}17\alpha E_2$	Nonketonic fraction *		
		$2metE_1$	E_1	$16\alpha OHE_1$	$16ketoE_2$	$17\beta E_2$		E_3	$16epiE_3$	$17epiE_3$
1.	VII	0.11	1.04	1.49	0.27	0.18	0.10	15.7	0.25	—**
2.	VII	0.04	0.21	1.09	0.63	0.15	0.12	13.0	0.33	—**
3.	VIII	0.05	1.89	2.28	0.42	0.24	0.17	22.0	0.25	—**
4.	IX	0.15	0.41	5.95	0.42	0.27	0.18	24.4	0.39	—**
5.	X	0.10	0.82	9.89	0.83	0.49	0.27	29.2	1.21	—**
6.	VII ***	—****	—****	—****	—****	—****	—****	2.3	0.067	0.019
7.	IX ***	—****	—****	—****	—****	—****	—****	7.5	0.24	0.050
8.	X ***	—****	—****	—****	—****	—****	—****	9.0	0.29	0.008
9.	X ***	—****	—****	—****	—****	—****	—****	11.8	0.25	0.017

* E_1 = estrone, E_2 = estradiol, E_3 = estriol, OH = hydroxy, met. = methoxy, Δ = double bond

** Not detectable

*** Modification of the method including acetonide formation of *cis*-glycols (ADLERCREUTZ et al., 1966)

**** Not estimated

Preliminary results obtained with the method of ADLERCREUTZ et al. (1967 a) are shown in Table 5. The first five estimations were carried out with the original procedure (ADLERCREUTZ et al., 1967 a) and no 17-*epi*estriol could be detected.

In Table 5, some values for 11-dehydroestradiol-17α are also recorded. This steroid seems to be of quantitative importance, since it appears to be present in amounts corresponding to those of 2-methoxyestrone.

Using the new modification (Flow-sheet 8) of the procedure of ADLERCREUTZ et al. (1967 a), the proportions of estriol, 16-*epi*estriol and 17-*epi*estriol were estimated in four urine samples. The results are shown in Table 5. This estimation is very specific, since the mass spectra obtained from the TMSi derivatives of the acetonides of both 16- and 17-*epi*estriol were identical with those of the corresponding derivatives of the reference standards (see also Fig. 11).

Conclusions

It is not possible to draw definitive conclusions with regard to the reliablity of the two above-mentioned procedures. When attempts are made to separate closely related compounds, the TMSi ether derivatives appear to give more accurate results and in addition they are excellent compounds for the gas chromatography-mass spectrometric investigations intended for the establishment of their identity. These facts seem to suggest that the TMSi ether derivatives are of more value than acetates in research work on metabolites of estrogens present in low concentrations in biological fluids.

5. Methods for the Estimation of Estrogens in Blood

Only a few applications of GLC methods for the estimation of blood or plasma estrogens have been presented. This is due to the small amounts of estrogens present in this biological fluid.

Method of ADLERCREUTZ *(1964 a) for the estimation of estrone, estradiol-17β and estriol in the "sulfate" and "glucosiduronate" fractions of pregnancy blood*

The method, which is described in Flow-sheet 9, was at first used only in combination with colorimetric estimation of the purified methylated estrogens. GLC was primarily used for investigation of

Flow-sheet 9. *Method of* ADLERCREUTZ *(1964 a) for the estimation of estrone, estradiol-17β and estriol in the "sulfate" and "glucosiduronate" fractions of pregnancy blood*

Heparinized blood is centrifuged and at least 20 ml of plasma is used for each analysis. The plasma is added dropwise to methanol to a final concentration of 30 : 70 (plasma : methanol). The precipitate is removed by centrifugation and washed with 70% aqueous methanol. The combined methanolic extract is kept in a freezer at —17° C for at least 24 h, then centrifuged at —17° C (1500 rpm) for 45 min.

Methanol phase evaporated to dryness. Residue dissolved in 50 ml of 0.1 N NaOH saturated with NaCl and extracted with 3×1/1 vol. of n-butanol-petroleum ether (70 : 30 v/v) saturated with H₂O and NaCl.

"Sulfate" fraction
Butanol-petroleum ether combined and washed with 1/10 vol. of 0.1 N NaOH saturated with NaCl

Washing combined with "glucosiduronate" fraction

Butanol-petroleum ether phase evaporated to dryness

Residue dissolved in 50 ml of 0.15 M acetate buffer, pH 5.0

Extracted with 4×1/2 vol. of ether (= free estrogens). For estimation ether can be processed as described in section on processing of the ether extracts

Ether evaporated from aqueous phase containing estrogen sulfates in a rotating evaporator.

Enzymic hydrolysis for 12—16 h with 1,000,000 phenol sulfatase units/ml of *Helix pomatia* extract at 37° C

Extracted with 4×1/2 vol. of ether

"Glucosiduronate" fraction
Aqueous phase acidified with 2 N HCl to pH 2—3. Extracted with 4×1/2 vol. of n-butanol saturated with H₂O and NaCl

Butanol phase neutralized with N NaOH and evaporated to dryness

Residue dissolved in 50 ml of 0.15 M acetate buffer, pH 4.1

Enzymic hydrolysis with 1000 Fishman units/ml of *Helix pomatia* extract at 37° C for 36—48 h

Extracted with 4×1/2 vol. of ether

Processing of the ether extracts

(All three ether extracts containing free estrogens, estrogen "sulfates" and estrogen "glucosiduronates" processed separately but in the same way)

|

Ether extract washed with 1/5 vol. of BROWN's (1955) carbonate buffer, pH 10.5, with 1/20 vol. of 8⁰/₀ NaHCO₃ solution and with 1/40 vol. of distilled water. Ether evaporated almost to dryness.

|

Moist residue dissolved in 30 ml of toluene. Toluene extracted with 4×1/2 vol. of 1 N NaOH.

|

pH of aqueous phase adjusted to 10 with ammonium sulfate and extracted with 4×1/2 vol. ether. Ether extract washed with 1/8 vol. of 8⁰/₀ NaHCO₃ solution and with 1/25 vol. of distilled water. Ether evaporated to dryness.

|

To the residue 1 ml of ethanol is added and the extract is transferred to a separatory funnel with 25 ml of benzene and 25 ml of petroleum ether. Following this step the procedure is exactly the same as described in Flowsheet 6.

the specificity of the procedure. Later, when gas chromatographs with a hydrogen flame ionization detector and more sensitive electrometers became available, this method was found to be useful, especially when problems concerning "sulfate" or "glucosiduronate" conjugation had to be solved. The same derivatives were used as in the method for the estimation of the three classical estrogens in urine.

Comment: The reliability of the method has been tested using colorimetry as the final step. The recovery of conjugated estrogens added to methanolic extracts of 25-ml blood samples was found to be as follows: estrone sulfate = 82.6⁰/₀, estradiol-3-sulfate = 82.9⁰/₀, estriol-3-sulfate 81.2⁰/₀ and estriol-16(17?)-glucosiduronate 49.5⁰/₀. The precision of the method was found to be for estrone = 0.020 µg/ 25 ml, for estradiol = 0.021 µg/25 ml and for estriol = 0.044 µg/25 ml. The sensitivity of the method for a single determination (P = 0.01) was found to be for estrone = 0.06 µg/25 ml, for estradiol = 0.08 µg/ 25 ml and for estriol 0.14 µg/25 ml. The specificity of the procedure has been evaluated using five different GLC columns (SE-30, F-60, QF-1, XE-60 and NGS). The specificity of the same method for bile estrogens (ADLERCREUTZ, 1962) has been extensively investigated using TLC, counter-current distribution and different color reactions and with infrared spectrophotometry for the estriol fraction, which provides further support for the view that the blood method is specific for estrone, estradiol and estriol. The specificity of the separation of estrogen "sulfates" from estrogen "glucosiduronates" has been evaluated by counter-current distribution studies of eight different estrogen conjugates (ADLERCREUTZ, 1964 a).

The method has only been used on blood samples obtained from late pregnancy. Electron capture detection methods are needed for investigation of the small amounts of these steroids present in blood during early pregnancy.

Method of KROMAN *et al. (1964) for the estimation of estrone, estradiol-17β and estriol in normal human plasma*

The authors used a ^{90}Sr ionization detector and report a sensitivity permitting the detection of as little as 0.002 µg of estradiol-17β, an equivalent amount of estrone and 0.025 µg of estriol. Even with hydrogen flame detectors values of 2 nanogram of estrogens in biological fluids are most difficult to determine with any degree of accuracy and the sensitivity reported by KROMAN et al. (1964) has never been obtained by other investigators working with ^{90}Sr or other argon ionization detectors. The gas chromatograms presented show peaks which can hardly be due to estrogens, and they occur too close to the solvent front, which means that the peaks can not be quantitated. The authors are of the opinion that the GLC of free estrogens, including estriol, gives satisfactory results, an opinion shared by few investigators in this field. No data regarding the specificity of the peaks are presented.

Method of EIK-NES *et al. (1965) for the estimation of 17β-estradiol-^{14}C or -^{3}H in plasma and tissue homogenates*

The method is a further development of a method published by AAKVAG and EIK-NES (1964) and has been used by the same authors (AAKVAG and EIK-NES, 1965 a, b) for studies on steroid biosynthesis in the canine ovary. They make use of the monochloroacetate derivative of the methylated radioactive estradiol-17β and an electron capture detector. The method is presented in Flow-sheet 10.

Comment: This double derivative has not been used previously and is an interesting new method. The sensitivity of the method is very high, — about 0.005 µg of the double derivative can be estimated quantitatively. The gas chromatograms show base-line separation of

Flow-sheet 10. *Method of* Eik-Nes *et al. (1965) for the estimation of specific radioactivity of estradiol-17β-¹⁴C or -³H in plasma and tissue homogenates*

Extraction according to Eik-Nes et al. (see Eik-Nes et al., 1965).

Toluene-sodium hydroxide partition.

Aqueous extract neutralized and extracted with methylene dichloride. Methylene dichloride evaporated to dryness.

Dry residue chromatographed on paper in the solvent system benzene/formamide. Zone corresponding to estradiol-17β eluted.

Extract chromatographed in the solvent system chloroform/formamide. Elution of the estradiol fraction.

Methylation according to Brown (1955).

Methylated estrogen extracted with hexane and the hexane extract washed with water. Evaporated to dryness.

TLC in the solvent system benzene : ethyl acetate (4 : 1 v/v). Estradiol methyl ether fraction scraped off the plate, dissolved in water and extracted with benzene. Benzene evaporated to dryness.

Formation of monochloroacetate derivative of the methylated estradiol fraction (Brownie et al., 1965).

TLC in benzene. Fraction containing estradiol derivative eluted, evaporated to dryness and dissolved in benzene containing 0.4 μg cholesterol chloroacetate. 1/10 of the sample is used for calculation of radioactivity, the rest is evaporated and dissolved in 15 μl of toluene.

GLC: 3 ft glass column with XE-60 phase. An electron capture detector is used.

the peaks which can readily be quantitated. The recovery through the whole procedure is 27—46⁰/o, which is rather low, but it may be improved with experience. The specificity of the method has been evaluated by crystallization to constant specific activity of the radioactive estradiol in biological material purified as described in Flow-sheet 10. The procedure is rather laborious but is the only one described for the estimation of specific radioactivity of estradiol synthesized from radioactive estradiol precursors. When working with an electron capture detector a very high degree of purification is needed in order to obtain specific results, which also means high quality control of solvents (BROWNIE et al., 1964).

Method of WOTIZ et al. (1966) for the estimation of estrone, estradiol-17β and estriol in human plasma

A preliminary report has been presented (WOTIZ et al., 1966). These workers used an electron capture detector and heptafluoro-butyrate derivatives of the estrogens (CLARK and WOTIZ, 1963). The recovery through the method is checked by adding radioactive reference standards before the plasma is subjected to the method. The method includes protein precipitation, enzymic hydrolysis and extraction, followed by liquid-liquid partitioning into a weak and a strong phenol fraction. The weak phenols are separated into estrone and estradiol on an alumina column and the three fractions are each chromatographed on impregnated glass-fiber paper. After development, the radioactive zones are eluted and chromatographed once more on glass fiber paper. Following derivative formation with heptafluorobutyric anhydride in tetrahydrofuran-hexane, the derivatives are chromatographed independently on a 3% QF-1 column at 200 °C.

Comments: The losses during the procedure can be corrected and this results in good precision, averaging about ± 5%. Since hepta-fluorobutyrate derivatives of estrogens are not very stable in material from biological samples, the total amount of ^{14}C-activity of the internal standards estimated before GLC may not be directly proportional to the amount of heptafluorobutyrate derivative estimated by GLC. In the chromatograms the peaks corresponding to the derivatives of the estrogens seem to be free from interfering impurities.

Modification of the method of ADLERCREUTZ et al. (1967 a) for the estimation of estrogens in pregnancy blood

The same method as was suggested for bile (see later) has been used in preliminary experiments for plasma samples obtained from pregnant women. The purification of the triol fraction can be made either by the original procedure for urine (ADLERCREUTZ et al., 1967 a) or by extracting the *cis*-glycols from the *trans*-glycols following aceton-ide formation (ADLERCREUTZ et al., 1966). In order to recover all estrogen sulfates, which are to some degree adsorbed on the Sephadex column, the column is re-eluted with 10% ethanol in water (volume $= 3 \times V_i$), and the ethanolic solution is added to the estrogen fraction (peak II) (BELING, 1963), which is evaporated to dryness. This procedure is necessary for samples of plasma and bile, because of the relatively large amount of estrone sulfate in plasma from pregnant women and in samples of bile (ADLERCREUTZ, 1962; 1964 a, b). The dry residue is dissolved in water and hydrolyzed with enzyme as described in Flow-sheet 12 for bile estrogens.

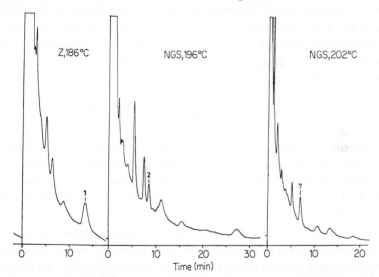

Fig. 16. GLC of late pregnancy plasma estrogens by the modification of the method of ADLERCREUTZ et al. (1967 a) for plasma, as presented in this chapter. Estrone-3-TMSi (1) = 2.0 μg/100 ml, injected 0.14 μg, 3-methyl ether of estradiol-17β-TMSi (2) = 0.4 μg/100 ml, injected 0.03 μg, estriol-3,16,17triTMSi (7) = 3.3 μg/100 ml, injected 0.09 μg. Values not corrected for losses during the procedure. Conditions as in Fig. 6

Comment: The recovery of estrone sulfate, added to a methanolic extract of 50 ml of plasma and carried through the whole procedure (with the exception of the paper chromatographic step) has been found to be 91.0%. The corresponding values for estradiol-3-sulfate and estriol-16(17?)-glucosiduronate were 86.3% and 81.1% respectively. No other conjugates of estrogens have been available for investigation. No figures can be given for the precision of the method or for its sensitivity. If only estrone, estradiol and estriol are to be estimated, the plasma samples can be processed as described for urine following precipitation of fatty material in cold methanol and gel filtration (see

Flow-sheet 6). In order to give an idea of the purity of the fractions, three gas chromatograms of the estrone, estradiol and estriol fractions obtained from late pregancy plasma and processed by the extended procedure involving Girard separation of the ketones from the non-ketones and paper chromatography of the ketones are shown in Fig. 16. Since the method is practically the same as that used for urine, it is possible that the specificity is approximately the same. However, work is in progress to definitely establish the specificity of the peaks, using an LKB 9000 gas chromatograph-mass spectrometer. Some other estrogens have also been detected in pregnancy blood and the results obtained to date suggest that it will be possible to identify these plasma steroids.

Method of ATTAL *et al. (1967) for the determination of free estrone in human plasma*

In this method the derivative for the GLC using electron capture detection is the 3-methyl-ether-17-pentafluorophenylhydrazone of purified plasma estrone. The method is presented in Flow-sheet 11. The GLC is carried out on a 2-ft × 0.4 cm glass U-column filled with 1% XE-60.

Comment: The recovery of radioactive estrone added to plasma samples is 34%, but since the losses can be corrected and the precision of the method is high, the low recovery is of no significance. Estrone concentrations above 0.001 µg/sample can be detected with a satis-factory degree of precision. The specificity of the method was eval-uated by infusing the ovary of a dog given HCG with radioactive androstenedione, processing the radioactive estrone obtained by the method and, following addition of non-radioactive reference stan-dard, crystallizing the estrone as its 3-methyl-ether-17-pentafluoro-phenylhydrazone derivative to constant specific activity.

Results Obtained with the Methods for the Estimation of Estrogens in Blood

The high values for blood estrogens obtained by KROMAN et al. (1964) suggest that their method is not specific for the compounds estimated. They found up to 3.80 µg estrone, 6.11 µg estradiol-17β and 6.53 µg estriol/100 ml of plasma from nonpregnant women. In nonpregnant women WOTIZ et al. (1966) found mean values of 0.241 µg, 0.166 µg and 0.299 µg/100 ml of plasma for estrone, estradiol

Flow-sheet 11. *Method of* ATTAL *et al. (1967) for the estimation of free estrone in human plasma*

A solution of estrone-6,7-H³ (3000 cpm) dried in a glass tube, 10 ml of plasma added, mixture extracted 3×2/1 vol. of ether. Ether extract washed with 1/10 vol. of 8⁰/₀ ammonium bicarbonate solution and 1/10 vol. of water. Ether evaporated to dryness.

|

Dry residue dissolved in 5 ml of toluene, extracted 3× with 2 ml of 1 N NaOH.

|

NaOH extract diluted with 1.5 ml of 1 N NaOH and 5 ml of 4.5⁰/₀ (w/v) boric acid in water. Solution kept for 5 min. at 40° C. 0.5 ml dimethyl-sulfate added, mixture shaken vigorously and left overnight at 40° C. Addition of 2.5 ml of 20⁰/₀ (w/v) NaOH in water. Extraction of the methylated estrone with 12 ml of hexane. Hexane extract washed with 2 ml of distilled water until neutral and evaporated to dryness.

|

Dry residue submitted to TLC in the system benzene : methanol (99 : 1 v/v). Estrone methyl ether fraction eluted with 6 ml of ethyl acetate. Extract evaporated to dryness.

|

Dry residue dissolved in 0.2 ml of methanol and 0.2 ml of pentafluoro-phenylhydrazine solution (10 mg of pentafluorophenylhydrazine in 9 ml of methanol and 1 ml of acetic acid). The mixture left overnight at room temperature. 1 ml of water added and solution extracted with 3×2 ml of hexane. Extract washed with 2 ml of 1 N H_2SO_4 and water. Extract evaporated to dryness.

|

Dry residue submitted to TLC in benzene and estrone methyl ether fraction eluted with 6 ml of ethyl acetate:benzene (5:95 v/v). Eluate washed with 0.5 ml of distilled ether, centrifuged and organic solvent layer removed and evaporated to dryness.

|

Dry residue dissolved in 1 ml of benzene and 1/10 aliquot assayed for radio-activity. The remaining solution transferred to 2 ml conical microcentrifuge tube and 10 μl of a methanolic solution of deoxycorticosterone acetate (3 μg/ml) added to the tube as internal standard. Following mixing and evaporation to dryness the residue is dissolved in 15 μl of toluene. 10 μl of this solution used for GLC on a 2 ft×0.4 cm glass U-tube with 1⁰/₀ XE-60 on 80—100 mesh Gas Chrom Q.

and estriol respectively. These values are much closer to the results obtained with colorimetric procedures, but since the colorimetric procedures are not very specific at low levels the values cannot be compared.

We have not found previous reports of estrogen levels in pregnancy plasma estimated by GLC methods. The results presented in Fig. 16 are thus some of the first ones obtained with this technique for estrogen estimation in plasma of pregnant women.

ATTAL et al. (1967) have estimated the amount of free estrone in the plasma of both men, nonpregnant women and pregnant women. A rather astonishing result is that in some samples of male plasma, the level of free estrone is higher than in women at ovulation time (mean value of such women: 0.046 µg/100 ml). In late pregnancy slightly less than 1 µg free estrone/100 ml of plasma was found.

Conclusions

It seems that GLC methods for plasma and blood estrogens are still in a preliminary stage of development and further progress in this field is awaited with interest. The combination of GLC and mass spectrometry might be able to solve many problems connected with the identity of the peaks used for estimation and it is likely that several new estrogens will be detected in human blood by this technique.

6. Methods for the Estimation of Estrogens in Bile

Investigations involving GLC of estrogens in extracts of bile samples have been reported only from this laboratory. LUUKKAINEN and ADLERCREUTZ (1963) combined the method of ADLERCREUTZ (1962) for the estimation of estrogens in human bile with GLC as the final step. Estrone was estimated as its 3-methyl ether, and for estradiol and estriol the TMSi derivatives of the 3-methyl ethers were employed for the estimation. The gas chromatograms presented are of the estrogens from bile samples obtained from pregnant women and samples after administration of estriol to a female patient with T-tube drainage of the main bile duct. They showed a high degree of purification, since practically no other peaks could be found in the gas chromatograms, which suggests a high specificity of the extraction procedure. At that time only an argon ionization detector was available, which prohibited quantitative estimations in bile samples with lower titers of estrogens.

ADLERCREUTZ and LUUKKAINEN (1965 a) reported the isolation and identification of estradiol-17α in bile of the pregnant cow. In this report the gas chromatographic behavior of the acetylated and methylated estradiols was described, in addition to the TLC behavior of TMSi derivatives of estrogens. The gas chromatograms presented showed a high purity of the final extracts. A quantitative estimation of the estradiol-17α content in the bile of one cow was also carried out.

Further investigation of pregnancy bile samples by ADLERCREUTZ and LUUKKAINEN (1965 c) showed that human bile presumably contains at least 8 different estrogens. The amounts found were too small to permit final identification. In addition to the already identified "classical" estrogens (ADLERCREUTZ, 1962), GLC evidence was obtained for the presence of 16-ketoestradiol, 16α-hydroxyestrone, 16,17-epiestriol, 16-epiestriol, 17-epiestriol and estradiol-17α. The results for 16-ketoestradiol, 16α-hydroxyestrone, 16α-hydroxyestriol and 16-epiestriol have since been confirmed (ADLERCREUTZ and LUUKKAINEN, 1966, 1967) and in addition a number of peaks corresponding to some other estrogens could be detected, but final identification was not possible.

Method of ADLERCREUTZ *et al. (1967 a) for the estimation of estrone, estradiol-17β, estriol, 16α-hydroxyestrone, 16-ketoestradiol, 16-epiestriol and 17-epiestriol in human pregnancy bile and in bile following estrogen administration*

The method which resembles that for the measurement of these estrogens in urine, is shown in Flow-sheet 12. The initial part of this method is similar to the original method of ADLERCREUTZ (1962) but following precipitation of fatty material in cold methanol the extract is evaporated to dryness, dissolved in 0.3 M NaCl solution and filtered on a suitable Sephadex column (the size depends on the amount of bile). If more than 100 ml of bile is processed, precipitation in cold methanol must be repeated. Up to 500 ml of bile has been processed without great difficulty provided that repeated methanol precipitations have been used. Either procedure (Flow-sheet 8) for the purification of the polar estrogens may be used, and for the ketolic estrogens two paper chromatographic steps are included if the amount of these estrogens is believed to be less than 0.5 µg/bile sample.

Flow-sheet 12. *Method of* ADLERCREUTZ *et al.* *(1967 a) for the estimation of estrone, estradiol-17β, estriol, 16α-hydroestrone, 16-ketoestradiol-17β, 16-epiestriol and 17-epiestriol in human pregnancy bile and in bile following estrogen administration*

Bile (10—500 ml) + methanol (30:70 v/v) kept at $-17°$ C for 48 h. Centrifuged at $-17°$ C (1500 rpm) for 45 min. Methanol phase evaporated to dryness. Procedure repeated by adding 70% aqueous methanol (v/v) to the dry residue if more than 100 ml of bile is processed.

|

Dry residue dissolved in 50 ml of 0.3 M NaCl solution and filtered through a Sephadex G_{25} (pearl form) column (2×35 cm). Eluted with distilled water. Peak I and peak II containing conjugated estrogens collected separately. The column is then re-eluted with 10% ethanol in water (150 ml) and this fraction is combined with peak II (fraction contains some free estrogens and estrogen sulfates adsorbed on the column).

|

Ethanolic extract evaporated to dryness and dissolved in 50 ml of 0.15 M sodium acetate buffer, pH 4.1. To the aqueous fraction containing peak I conjugates 1/10 vol. of 1.5 M sodium acetate buffer, pH 4.1, is added.

|

Both fractions hydrolyzed separately with 1000 Fishman units β-glucuronidase and 1,000,000 units of sulfatase *(Helix pomatia* extract) per ml reaction mixture at 37° C for 16—48 h.

|

Bile extracts processed as described in Flow-sheet 8.

Comment: The precipitation in cold methanol has previously been found to give no losses (ADLERCREUTZ, 1962), and the recovery of estrogen conjugates is the same as for the corresponding blood method. No data on the precision and sensitivity of the method can be given, but an idea of the latter is obtained from the data presented in Table 6 and in Figs. 17, 18 and 19. In a slightly modified version of the method the specificity has been investigated by gas chromatography-mass spectrometry (ADLERCREUTZ and LUUKKAINEN, 1967) with satisfactory results. The method is rather laborious but this drawback must be considered in relation to the information obtained.

Results Obtained with the Method for Estimation of Estrogens in Bile

Some preliminary quantitative results have been obtained with this method. Three of the samples analyzed were obtained from patients with recurrent jaundice during pregnancy and, as shown previously (ADLERCREUTZ et al., 1967 b), the values for bile estrogens in such patients were very low. Despite the very low concentration in these bile samples, it was often possible to estimate some of the estrogens not previously quantified in human bile. Following intramuscular administration of estradiol benzoate the estimation of the

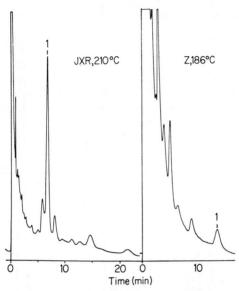

Fig. 17. GLC of two estrone (1) fractions as TMSi ether derivative obtained by the method of ADLERCREUTZ et al. (1967 a) for bile.
Left figure: bile sample from a patient with T-tube in main bile duct following administration of 25 mg of estradiol benzoate intramuscularly. Conditions as in Fig. 7. Right figure: bile sample obtained from a patient with recurrent jaundice of pregnancy in the icteric stage. Estrone (1) concentration 0.67 μg/100 ml of bile. Conditions as in Fig. 6

estrogens in bile was comparatively simple. Surprisingly low values were found for the estrogens in the first 12-hour bile sample obtained during such experiments (Table 6).

The gas chromatograms in Figs. 18 and 19 show peaks corresponding to 16-*epi*estriol, 16α-hydroxyestrone and 16-ketoestradiol. The peaks are rather well separated and can readily be quantified. Since mass spectrometric data of the corresponding peaks from pregnancy urine indicate that the peaks found are identical with the corresponding derivative of the reference standards, it can be con-

cluded that the data obtained confirm and extend the observations of
ADLERCREUTZ and LUUKKAINEN (1965 c) with regard to the presence
of 16α-hydroxyestrone, 16-ketoestradiol and 16-*epi*estriol in human
bile (for some recent results see ADLERCREUTZ and LUUKKAINEN, 1967).

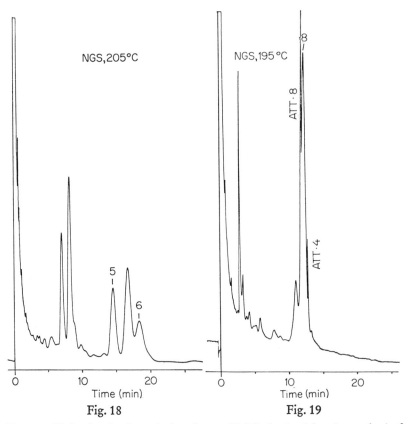

Fig. 18   Fig. 19

Fig. 18. GLC of polar ketonic fraction as TMSi obtained by the method of
ADLERCREUTZ et al. (1967 a) for bile following one paper chromatographic
purification. Bile from a patient with a T-tube in the main bile duct after
administration of 25 mg of estradiol benzoate intramuscularly. 5 = 16α-
hydroxyestrone-3,16diTMSi, 6 = 16-ketoestradiol-3,17triTMSi. Conditions
as in Fig. 8

Fig. 19. GLC of the 16-*epi*estriol (8) fraction obtained from bile following
administration of 25 mg of estradiol benzoate intramuscularly to a patient
with T-tube drainage of the main bile duct. Same method as in Fig. 18.
Conditions as in Fig. 8. The small peak before 16-*epi*estriol-3,16,17tri-
TMSi (8) is a small overlapping of estriol in this fraction

Table 6. *Estimation of estrogens in human bile by the method of* ADLERCREUTZ *et al. (1967 a).* (+) = *Peak obtained too small for quantitation.* (−) = *Not detectable*

Case	Diagnosis	Month of pregnancy	Estrogens μg/100 ml *						
			E_1	E_2	$16\alpha OHE_1$	$16\text{-keto}E_2$	E_3	$16\text{-}epiE_3$	$17\text{-}epiE_3$
1	Patient with T-tube drainage of the main bile duct. First 12-h bile sample following intramuscular administration of 25 mg of estradiol benzoate	Nonpregnant	1.7	0.04	26.2	8.1	3.2	0.8	—
2	As above	Nonpregnant	7.9	5.2	19.9	18.9	78.0	10.4	2.5
3 **	Recurrent jaundice of pregnancy, icteric stage	X	0.33	0.04	0.82	0.49	2.61	0.15	—
4 **	As above	VIII	0.67	—	+	+	0.88	—	—
5 **	As above	X	2.91	+	+	+	4.34	—	—

* E_1 = estrone, E_2 = estradiol-17β, E_3 = estriol, OH = hydroxy, keto = keto
** Preliminary results obtained in a study of recurrent jaundice of pregnancy (ADLERCREUTZ, LUUKKAINEN, SVANBORG and ÅNBERG)

7. Method for the Estimation of Estrogens in Tissue Extracts

The method of McKerns and Nordstrand (1964, 1965) is presented in Flow-sheet 13. The method contains an interesting step; the TMSi derivatives of the steroids in ethyl acetate are purified by adding Silica gel G and centrifuging the mixture. The supernatant is removed, the Silica gel is washed with ethyl acetate and the extracts are pooled and evaporated to dryness. The TMSi derivatives are dissolved in hexane prior to gas chromatography.

Flow-sheet 13. *Method of* McKerns *and* Nordstrand *(1964, 1965) for the estimation of estrone, estradiol-17β and estriol and some neutral steroids in tissue extracts*

Tissue homogenate extracted with methylene chloride:methanol (2:1 v/v) with occasional stirring for 30 min. Extract filtered through a filter paper and the precipitate washed thoroughly with 30 ml of the methylene chloride: methanol mixture. Filtrate evaporated to dryness in a rotary evaporator at 60° C.

|

Dry residue dissolved in 60 ml of methylene chloride and transferred to a separatory funnel. Methylene chloride washed with 10 ml of water and the aqueous phase back-extracted with 30 ml of methylene chloride.

|

Water removed by addition of 10 g calcium chloride to the combined solvent fractions. Extract filtered and filtrate evaporated to dryness in a rotary evaporator.

|

Dry residue transferred to a 4 ml vial using methylene chloride:methanol (2:1) by a total vol. of 4 ml. Solvent evaporated at 60° C in stream of nitrogen.

|

TMSi ether formation by adding 1 ml of pyridine, 0.20 ml of hexamethyl-disilazane, and 0.05 ml trimethylchlorosilane. Reaction time 1 h at room temperature (26° C). Solvents evaporated in a stream of nitrogen and residue dissolved in 3 ml of ethyl acetate.

|

To the ethyl acetate extract 0.5 g of Silica gel G is added and the mixture centrifuged. Silica gel washed with 3 ml of ethyl acetate. Combined solvent fractions evaporated to dryness in nitrogen and dissolved in 50 µl of hexane. GLC: 4—6 ft×4 mm glass column with 3% XE-60 and 3% SE-30 in a 1:1 w/w ratio.

Comment: This very short procedure may prove useful for investigation of enzyme reactions involving estrogens in tissue homogenates. The recovery of the steroids is likely to be good. The gas chromatograms presented indicate some of the difficulties that may be encountered in the identification work. If both neutral and phenolic steroids are chromatographed simultaneously, so many compounds will have identical retention data that only very extensive studies, necessitating collection of the steroids emerging from the column or gas chromatographic-mass-spectrometric investigations, can solve the identification problem.

VI. Conclusion

At present the most pressing need in the GLC study of estrogens is not to find better derivatives for GLC or more sensitive instruments, but to develop more specific and convenient purification methods in order to permit higher specificity in estimates of the compounds. In this survey much attention has been paid to the purification procedures and to investigations on the specificity of the final estimation. During the course of the work in this laboratory it has frequently been impossible to predict which GLC column will give specific quantitation. In low-titer samples, especially those from patients, interfering compounds are often present which may give erroneous results if the samples are not chromatographed on at least two different columns (one selective and one nonselective). Urine samples from different individuals differ considerably and until the first GLC separation has been made it is impossible to anticipate what troubles may be encountered during quantification.

The use of stereoselective derivatives, such as the acetonides of the estrogens, during the purification procedure is a new approach to the problem of quantification of small amounts of estrogens in biological samples. The combination of several different derivatives and purification procedures, as used in many of the methods cited, has certain advantages, since in this way the estrogens are divided into fairly well-defined groups within which there is more likelihood of obtaining a specific estimate.

The proper use of all potentialities of GLC methods, in particular the recently developed method of investigating gas chromatographic effluents with a mass spectrometer, should in the future contribute significantly to our knowledge of the metabolism of steroid estrogens in all animal species including man.

References

AAKVAG, A., and K. B. EIK-NES: Metabolism *in vivo* of (7-^{3}H)pregnenolone by the ovary of dogs treated with follicle stimulating hormone. Biochim. biophys. Acta **86**, 380 (1964).

— — Metabolism *in vivo* of steroids in the canine ovary. Biochim. biophys. Acta **111**, 273 (1965 a).

— — Metabolism *in vitro* of steroids in the canine ovary. Biochim. biophys. Acta **111**, 286 (1965 b).

ADLERCREUTZ, H.: Studies on oestrogen excretion in human bile. Acta endocr. (Kbh.) **42**, Suppl. 72 (1962).

— A method for the separation and estimation of conjugated oestrogens in pregnancy blood. Acta med. scand. Suppl. **412**, 123 (1964 a).

— A comparison between conjugated oestrogens in late pregnancy blood and bile. Acta med. scand. Suppl. **412**, 133 (1964 b).

— Estimation of oestrogen sulphates in pregnancy urine. Scand. J. clin. lab. Invest. **17**, Suppl. 86, 121 (1965).

— Studies on the hydrolysis of gel-filtered urinary oestrogens. Acta endocr. (Kbh.) **57**, 49 (1968).

—, and T. LUUKKAINEN: Gas chromatography of oestrogens. Internationales Round-Table Gespräch über Analytik von Oestrogenen, Hormonen und Testosteron, Jena 1964, in press.

— — Isolation and identification of 17α-oestradiol in the bile of a pregnant cow. J. Reprod. Fertil. **9**, 137 (1965 a).

— — Determination of urinary estrogens by gas chromatography. In: Gas chromatography of steroids in biological fluids, ed. M. B. LIPSETT. New York: Plenum Press, 215 (1965 b).

— — Gas-chromatographic studies on oestrogens in the bile of pregnant women. Biochim. biophys. Acta **97**, 134 (1965 c).

— — Estimation and identification of metabolites of estrogens and progesterone in human bile. Excerpta Med. International Congress Series **111**, 129 (1966).

— — Biochemical and clinical aspects of the enterohepatic circulation of oestrogens. Acta endocr. (Kbh.) Suppl. **124**, 101 (1967).

—, and K.-O. SCHAUMAN: A note on the chemical estimation of oestrogens in the urine of patients with liver disease. Acta endocr. (Kbh.) **46**, 230 (1964).

The investigations presented for the first time in this chapter have been made with the aid of grants from The Population Council (No. M 65.110), the Sigrid Jusélius Foundation and The National Research Council for Medical Sciences, Finland. The permission of the Society for Endocrinology (London) to publish Figures Nos. 5, 7, 8, 9, 15, 17, 18, 19 and Table 2, which appeared in the Memoir of the Society No. 16, is acknowledged.

ADLERCREUTZ, H., S. LAIHO, and T. LUUKKAINEN: Preparation of steroid derivatives for gas chromatography, including studies of the gas chromatographic properties of steroidal acetonides. Proc. of meeting on gas chromatographic determination of hormonal steroids. Roma, 22—23 Sept., 1966, in press.

—, A. SALOKANGAS, and T. LUUKKAINEN: Measurement of oestrogens in biological material. In: Memoirs of the Society for Endocrinology, No. 16, 89 (1967 a).

—, A. SVANBORG and Å. ÅNBERG: Recurrent jaundice in pregnancy II. A study of the estrogens and their conjugation in late pregnancy. Amer. J. Med. **42,** 341 (1967 b).

ATTAL, J., S. M. HENDELES, and K. B. EIK-NES: Determination of free estrone in blood plasma by gas-phase chromatography with electron capture detection. Anal. Biochem. **20,** 394 (1967).

BEER, C. T., and T. F. GALLAGHER: Excretion of estrogen metabolites by humans. I. The fate of small doses of estrone and estradiol-17β. J. biol. Chem. **214,** 335 (1955).

BELING, C. G.: Gel filtration of conjugated urinary oestrogens and its application in clinical assays. Acta endocr. (Kbh.) Suppl. 79 (1963).

BEROZA, M., and M. C. BOWMAN: Identification of pesticides at nanogram level by extraction p-values. Anal. chem. **37,** 291 (1965).

BLOCH, E., and N. B. GIBREE: Hydrolysis of urinary 17-ketosteroid and estrogen conjugates by an intestinal extract from the snail *Helix pomatia*. Arch. Biochem. **79,** 307 (1959).

BREUER, H.: Vorkommen, Biogenese und Stoffwechsel der Östrogene. Z. Vitamin-, Hormon- u. Fermentforsch. **11,** 182 (1960).

— Occurrence and determination of the newer oestrogens in human urine. In Research on Steroids, vol. 1, 133. Roma: Tipografia Poliglotta Vaticana 1964.

—, und G. PANGELS: Isolierung von 17-epi-Östriol und 16,17-epi-Östriol aus dem Urin schwangerer Frauen. Hoppe Seylers Z. physiol. Chem. **322,** 177 (1961).

BRIGGS, L. H., L. D. COLEBROOK, H. M. FALES, and W. C. WILDMAN: Infrared absorption spectra of methylenedioxy and aryl ether groups. Anal. Chem. **29,** 904 (1957).

BROOKS, C. J. W., E. M. CHAMBAZ, W. L. GARDINER, and E. C. HORNING: Gas chromatographic determination of hormonal steroids in biological fluids in comparison to other methods of determinations. Proc. of Meeting on Gas-chromatgraphic determination of hormonal steroids. Roma, 22—23 Sept. 1966, in press.

BROWN, J. B.: A chemical method for the determination of oestriol, oestrone and oestradiol in human urine. Biochem. J. **60,** 185 (1955).

— The determination and significance of the natural estrogens. In: Advances in clinical chemistry, vol. 3, 158. New York-London: Academic Press 1960.

—, and H. A. F. BLAIR: The hydrolysis of conjugated oestrone, oestradiol-17β and oestriol in human urine. J. Endocrinol. **17,** 411 (1958).

Brown, J. B., R. D. Bulbrook, and F. C. Greenwood: An evaluation of a chemical method for the estimation of oestriol, oestrone and oestradiol-17β in human urine. J. Endocrinol. **16**, 41 (1957 a).

— — — An additional purification step for a method for estimating oestriol, oestrone and oestradiol-17β in human urine. J. Endocrinol. **16**, 49 (1957 b).

Brownie, A. C., H. J. van der Molen, E. E. Nishizawa, and K. B. Eik-Nes: Determination of testosterone in human peripheral blood using gas-liquid chromatography with electron capture detection. J. clin. Endocr. **24**, 1091 (1964).

Bugge, S., M. Nilsen, A. Metcalfe-Gibson, and R. Hobkirk: Hydrolysis of conjugated estrogen fractions in human pregnancy urine. Can. J. Biochem. Physiol. **39**, 1501 (1961).

Clark, S. J., and H. H. Wotiz: Separation and detection of nanogram amounts of steroids. Steroids **2**, 535 (1963).

Cox, R. I., and A. R. Bedford: The use of double derivatives in the gas chromatography of urinary estrogens. Steroids **6**, 663 (1964).

Diczfalusy, E., und C. Lauritzen: Oestrogene beim Menschen. Berlin-Göttingen-Heidelberg: Springer 1961.

Eik-Nes, K. B., A. Aakvaag, and L. J. Grota: Estimation of estradiol-17β by gas-liquid chromatography with electron capture detection. In: Gas chromatography of steroids in biological fluids, ed. M. B. Lipsett. New York: Plenum Press, 247 (1965).

Engel, L., W. R. Slaunwhite jr., P. Carter, and I. T. Nathanson: The separation of natural estrogens by counter-current distribution. J. biol. Chem. **185**, 255 (1950).

Exley, D., and J. Chamberlain: The ultramicro-determination of steroid Δ4—3 ketones in plasma by gas liquid chromatography with electron capture detection. Proc. of Meeting on Gas-chromatographic determination of hormonal steroids. Roma, 22—23 Sept. 1966, in press.

Fales, H. M., and T. Luukkainen: O-Methyloximes as carbonyl derivatives in gas chromatography, mass spectrometry and nuclear magnetic resonance. Anal. Chem. **37**, 955 (1965).

—, E. O. A. Haahti, T. Luukkainen, W. J. A. Vandenheuvel, and E. C. Horning: Milligram-scale preparative gas chromatography of steroids and alkaloids. Anal. Biochem. **4**, 296 (1962).

Fishman, J., and J. B. Brown: Quantitation of urinary estrogens by gas chromatography. J. Chromatog. **8**, 21 (1962).

Frandsen, V. A.: A clinical routine method for the simultaneous estimation of oestrone and 17β-oestradiol in human pregnancy urine. Acta endocr. (Kbh.) **50**, 418 (1965).

Givner, M. L., W. S. Bauld, and K. Vagi: A method for the quantitative fractionation of mixtures of 2-methoxyoestrone, oestrone, ring D α-ketolic oestrogens, oestradiol-17β, 16-epioestriol and oestriol by partition chromatography and the Girard reaction. Biochem. J. **77**, 400 (1960 a).

GIVNER, M. L., W. S. BAULD, and K. VAGI: A chemical method for the quantitative determination of 2-methoxyoestrone, oestrone, ring D α-ketolic oestrogens, oestradiol-17β, 16-*epi*oestriol and oestriol in human urine. Biochem. J. 77, 406 (1960 b).

GRUNDY, S. M., E. H. AHRENS, and T. A. MIETTINEN: Quantitative isolation and gas-liquid chromatographic analysis of total fecal bile acids. J. Lipid Res. 6, 397 (1965).

HOBKIRK, R., A. ALFHEIM, and S. BUGGE: Hydrolysis of estrogen conjugates in diabetic pregnancy urines. J. clin. Endocr. 19, 1352 (1959).

ITTRICH, G.: Eine Methode zur chemischen Bestimmung von Östrogenen Hormonen in Blut, Milch und Colostrum. Hoppe-Seylers Z. physiol. Chem. 320, 103 (1960).

KATZMAN, P. A., R. F. STRAW, H. J. BUEHLER, and E. A. DOISY: III. Estrogens. Hydrolysis of conjugated estrogens. Rec. Prog. Hormone Res. 9, 45 (1954).

KENNARD, O.: X-Ray analysis of steroids. Excerpta Medica. Internat. Congress Series 111, 112 (1966).

KOBER, S.: Eine kolorimetrische Bestimmung des Brunsthormons (Menformon). Biochem. Z. 239, 209 (1931).

KROMAN, H. S., S. R. BENDER, and R. L. CAPIZZI: The gas chromatographic separation and quantitation of estrogens from normal human plasma. Clin. chim. Acta 9, 73 (1964).

KUSHINSKY, S., and J. A. DEMETRIOU: Analysis of urinary metabolites of oestradiol-17β-4-14C. A rapid paper chromatographic method for obtaining a profile of urinary metabolites. Steroids 2, 253 (1963).

—, and I. OTTERNESS: Conjugated estrogens. IV: Separation of urinary estrogens by gel-filtration and the effect of endogenous inhibitor on the rate and extent of hydrolysis by β-glucuronidase. Steroids 3, 311 (1964).

—, J. A. DEMETRIOU, J. WU, and W. NASUTAVICUS: Analysis of urinary metabolites of oestradiol-4-14C. I. In human mammary carcinoma. J. clin. Endocr. 20, 719 (1960).

LISBOA, B. P.: Über die Dünnschichtchromatographie von neueren Oestrogenen an Kieselgel G. Clin. chim. Acta 13, 179 (1966 a).

— Formation and separation of Girard hydrazones on thin-layer chromatography by elatographic techniques. J. Chromatog. 24, 475 (1966 b).

—, and E. DICZFALUSY: Colour reactions for the *in situ* characterization of steroid oestrogens on thin-layer chromatograms. Acta endocr. (Kbh.) 43, 545 (1963).

LORAINE, J. A., and E. T. BELL: Hormone assays and their clinical application, 2nd ed. Edinburgh-London: Livingstone 1966.

LUUKKAINEN, T., and H. ADLERCREUTZ: Gas chromatography of methylated estrogens and application of the method to the analysis of human late pregnancy bile. Biochim. biophys. Acta 70, 700 (1963).

— — Isolation and identification of 11-dehydro-estradiol-17α, a new type of urinary steroid, in the urine of pregnant women. Biochim. biophys. Acta 107, 579 (1965).

LUUKKAINEN, T., and H. ADLERCREUTZ: Studies on estrogen metabolites in urine during the last half of pregnancy. Excerpta Med. International Congress Series 111, 129 (1966).
— — Mass spectrometric studies in the specificity of estriol determination in urine by gas-liquid chromatography. Ann. Med. exp. Fenn. 45, 264 (1967).
—, W. J. A. VANDENHEUVEL, E. O. A. HAAHTI, and E. C. HORNING: Gas-chromatographic behaviour of trimethylsilyl ethers of steroids. Biochim. biophys. Acta 52, 599 (1961).
MARSH, C. A.: Inhibition of β-glucuronidase by endogenous saccharate during hydrolysis of urinary conjugates. Nature 194, 974 (1962).
McKERNS, K. W., and E. NORDSTRAND: Simple method for tissue extraction and gas chromatographic separation of estrogens. Biochim. biophys. Acta 82, 198 (1964).
— — Gas chromatography of estrogens and other steroids from endocrine tissues. In: Gas chromatography of steroids in biological fluids (ed. M. B. LIPSETT). New York: Plenum Press 255, 1965.
MENINI, E.: Gas-liquid chromatography of urinary oestrogens. Biochem. J. 94, 15 P (1965 a).
— Analysis of estrogens in the urine of non-pregnant women by gas liquid chromatography. In: Gas chromatography of steroids in biological fluids, (ed. M. B. LIPSETT). New York: Plenum Press 233, 1965 b.
VAN DER MOLEN, H. J., and D. GROEN: Determination of progesterone in human peripheral blood using gas-liquid chromatography with electron capture detection. In: Gas chromatography of steroids in biological fluids (ed. M. B. LIPSETT). New York: Plenum Press 153, 1965.
NEHER, R.: Steroid chromatography. Amsterdam-London-New York: Elsevier 1964.
NOCKE, W.: A note on the chemical determination of 16-epioestriol. Clin. chim. Acta 6, 449 (1961).
O'DONNEL, V. J., and J. R. K. PREEDY: The oestrogens. In: Hormones in blood (ed. C. H. GRAY, and A. L. BACHARACH). London-New York: Academic Press, 303, 1961.
PAULSEN, C. A. (ed.): Estrogen assays in clinical medicine. Seattle: University of Washington Press 1965.
PREEDY, J.: Estrogens. In: Methods in hormone research, vol. 1 (ed. R. DORFMAN). New York-London: Academic Press p. 1, 1962.
ROY, E. J., and J. B. BROWN: A method for the estimation of oestriol, oestrone and oestradiol-17β in the blood of the pregnant woman and of the foetus. J. Endocrinol. 21, 9 (1960).
SCOMMEGNA, A., and S. C. CHATTORAJ: Gas chromatographic estimation of urinary estriol in pregnancy: A rapid and practical way to forecast fetal survival. Proc. of Meeting on Gas chromatographic determination of hormonal steroids. Roma, 22—23 Sept. 1966, in press.
SLAUNWHITE, W. R., JR., and A. A. SANDBERG: Studies on phenolic steroids in human subjects: evaluation of enzymatic hydrolysis of estrogen conjugates. Endocrinology 67, 815 (1960).

THOMAS, B. S., and D. R. M. WALTON: Halogenoalkylsilyl ether derivatives in steroid analysis by gas-liquid chromatography. Proc. of Meeting on Gas chromatographic determination of hormonal steroids. Roma, 22—23 Sept. 1966, in press.

—, C. EABORN, and D. R. M. WALTON: Preparation and gas chromatography of steroid chloromethyl dimethylsilyl ethers. Chem. Commun. 13, 408 (1966).

TOUCHSTONE, J. C., and T. MURAWEC: Gas chromatography of free and conjugated estrogens in blood plasma. In: Gas chromatography of steroids in biological fluids (ed. M. B. LIPSETT). New York: Plenum Press, 243, 1965.

—, J. W. GREENE, JR., R. C. MCELROY, and T. MURAWEC: Blood estriol conjugation during human pregnancy. Biochemistry 2, 653 (1963).

WAKABAYASHI, M., and W. H. FISHMAN: The comparative ability of β-glucuronidase preparations (Liver, Escherichia coli, Helix pomatia, and Patella vulgata) to hydrolyze certain steroid glucosiduronic acids. J. biol. Chem. 236, 996 (1961).

WOTIZ, H. H.: Studies in steroid metabolism. XIV. Modification of the analysis of urinary estrogens by gas chromatography. Biochim. biophys. Acta 74, 122 (1963).

—, and S. C. CHATTORAJ: Determination of estrogens in low and high titer urines using thin layer and gas liquid chromatography. Anal. Chem. 36, 1466 (1964).

— — Gas chromatography and its role in the versatile analysis of urinary estrogens. In: Gas chromatography of steroids in biological fluids (ed. M. B. LIPSETT). New York: Plenum Press, 195, 1965.

—, and S. J. CLARK: Gas chromatography in the analysis of steroid hormones. New York: Plenum Press 1966.

—, and H. F. MARTIN: Gas-chromatographic estimation of estrogens in pregnancy urines. Fed. Proc. 20, Suppl. 7, 99 (1961).

— — Studies in steroid metabolism. XI. Gas chromatographic determination of estrogens in human pregnancy urine. Anal. Biochem. 3, 97 (1962).

—, G. CHARRANSOL, and I. N. SMITH: Gas-chromatographic measurement of plasma estrogens using an electron capture detector. Proc. of Meeting on Gas chromatographic determination of hormonal steroids. Roma, 22—23 Sept. 1966, in press.

YOUSEM, H. L.: Simple gas chromatographic method for estimation of urinary estriol in pregnant women. Amer. J. Obst. Gyn. 88, 375 (1964).

Chapter 3

Gas Phase Chromatography of Progesterone and Related Steroids

H. J. VAN DER MOLEN

I. Introduction

The advantages of gas chromatography for steroid methodology are clearly reflected in some of the applications of this technique for the quantitative estimation of progesterone and related steroids.

General aspects of the application of gas chromatography to the separation of steroids as well as to steroid quantification are discussed in this monograph (see Chapter I) and in other publications (HORNING et al., 1963; VAN DER MOLEN and GROEN, 1967). In this chapter we will deal with qualitative and quantitative aspects pertinent to the specific steroids, or groups of steroids, under consideration.

1. "Metabolism" of Progesterone

In order to define "progesterone metabolism" for present purposes, we may consider the metabolism of progesterone as outlined in Fig. 1. Reduction of the C-4 double bond and of the ketone groups at carbon atoms 3 and 20 may theoretically result in 26 structurally different metabolites of progesterone, depending upon the sequence and completeness of these reactions. Not all of these metabolites have been isolated from human or other animal sources. The occurrence of specific metabolites in biological material appears to vary widely, both qualitatively and quantitatively. For example, the C_{21} Δ^4-3-keto structure of progesterone is hardly, if at all, present in the urine of normal human subjects; a relatively large proportion of the hormone is completely reduced, and 5β-pregnane-$3\alpha,20\alpha$-diol constitutes the major progesterone metabolite excreted by man.

In an evaluation of the potential usefulness of gas-phase chromatography for the study of the qualitative aspects of progesterone metabolism one must consider the possibilities and limitations of gas chromatography as a technical tool for the separation and identification of all metabolites that could theoretically occur. Our knowledge of progesterone metabolism rests largely on results not obtained with the aid of gas chromatography. Thus the possibility exists that

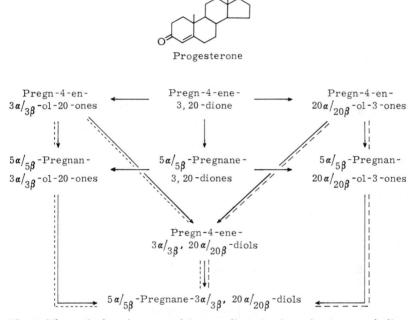

Fig. 1. Theoretical pathways and intermediates in the reductive metabolism of progesterone (pregn-4-ene-3,20-dione)

the high resolving power of gas chromatographic columns and the sensitive detection systems employed in this technique may reveal the presence of progesterone metabolites that can not be separated by other means (such as the separation of 3-hydroxypregnan-20-ones and 20-hydroxypregnan-3-ones), or that are present in amounts too small to be detected by other less sensitive detection methods. Hence, a complete qualitative analysis for products arising from reductive progesterone metabolism as outlined in Fig. 1 should include the 26 metabolites given in the first row of Table 1.

Table 1. *Metabolites originating from progesterone and several $C_{21}O_3$ pregnane* *that the relevant steroid has been isolated from a mammalian source. The addition*

Reduced steroid		Progesterone isolated H	6α-Hydroxy-progesterone
5-Pregnane-3,20-dione	5α-P-3,20-dione	isolated H	
	5β-P-3,20-dione	isolated H	
5-Pregnan-3-ol-20-ones	5α-P-3α-ol-20-one	isolated H	isolated H
	5α-P-3β-ol-20-one	isolated H	isolated H
	5β-P-3α-ol-20-one	isolated H	isolated H
	5β-P-3β-ol-20-one		
5-Pregnan-20-ol-3-ones	5α-P-20α-ol-3-one		
	5α-P-20β-ol-3-one		
	5β-P-20α-ol-3-one	isolated H	
	5β-P-20β-ol-3-one	isolated	
5-Pregnane-3,20-diols	5α-P-3α,20α-diol	isolated H	
	5α-P-3α,20β-diol	isolated H	
	5α-P-3β,20α-diol	isolated H	
	5α-P-3β,20β-diol	isolated	
	5β-P-3α,20α-diol	isolated H	
	5β-P-3α,20β-diol	isolated	
	5β-P-3β,20α-diol	isolated H	
	5β-P-3β,20β-diol	isolated	
Pregn-4-en-3-ol-20-ones	P-4-en-3α-ol-20-one		
	P-4-en-3β-ol-20-one		
Pregn-4-en-20-ol-3-ones	P-4-en-20α-ol-3-one	isolated H	
	P-4-en-20β-ol-3-one	isolated H	
Pregn-4-ene-3,20-diols	P-4-ene-3α,20α-diol		
	P-4-ene-3α,20β-diol		
	P-4-ene-3β,20α-diol		
	P-4-ene-3β,20β-diol		

Example: 3α,6α-dihydroxy-5α-pregnan-20-one was identified by SALOMON an 6α-hydroxyprogesterone on the line of 5α-P-3α-ol-20-one.

References to the original papers describing the identification of individua (1964); JAYLE and CRÉPY (1962); JAYLE et al. (1965); LEVY and SAITO (1966)

In addition to the reductive degradation of progesterone, the introduction of oxygen-containing functional groups (hydroxyl and ketone groups) at several carbon atoms of the progesterone molecule is also involved in progesterone metabolism. Inclusion of all theoretical introductions of one or more oxygen functions in progesterone

teroids through reduction of the Δ4-3,20-diketo structure. "Isolated" indicates
"H" indicates that the steroid has been isolated from human material

5β-Hydroxy-progesterone	11-Keto-progesterone	11β-Hydroxy-progesterone	16α-Hydroxy-progesterone	17α-Hydroxy-progesterone
isolated H	isolated	isolated	isolated H	isolated H
			isolated	isolated
				isolated
			isolated H	isolated H
			isolated	isolated
	isolated H	isolated H	isolated H	isolated H
			isolated H	isolated H
				isolated H
			isolated H	isolated
			isolated H	isolated
	isolated H	isolated H	isolated H	isolated H
				isolated
	isolated			isolated H
				isolated
			isolated	

ᴅᴏʀʙʀɪɴᴇʀ (1952) from human pregnancy urine and is indicated in the row under

teroids may be found in papers by: ᴅᴏʀꜰᴍᴀɴ and ᴜɴɢᴀʀ (1965); ꜰᴏᴛʜᴇʀʙʏ ᴜsᴇ and Sᴀʟᴏᴍᴏɴ (1966) and Zᴀɴᴅᴇʀ et al. (1962).

would make the number of its "metabolites" prohibitively large. This would also include metabolic routes leading to the corticosteroids and rare pregnane steroids with oxygen functions at carbon atoms 1, 7, 10, 14 and 15. The latter series of steroids has been demonstrated in microbiological systems. In a recent review ᴅᴏʀꜰᴍᴀɴ and ᴜɴɢᴀʀ

(1965), listed 36 structural modifications of progesterone through introduction of hydroxyl and ketone groups that have actually been isolated or inferred from animal systems. They have called such steroids "key steroids". During the present discussion we will limit progesterone metabolism to include C-21 key steroids (DORFMAN and UNGAR, 1966), that, in addition to the Δ^4-3,20-diketo structure, posses the oxygen functions found in pregnane steroids isolated from mammalian sources, namely 6α-hydroxyl, 6β-hydroxyl, 11-keto, 11β-hydroxyl, 16α-hydroxyl, 17α-hydroxyl, or a combination of these functions. All steroids carrying a C-21 hydroxyl group are considered members of the corticosteroids [*].

Table 2 shows the number of different key steroids that may be obtained by introduction of one or more of these oxygen functions in

Table 2. *Theoretical number of "key steroids" derived from progesterone ($C_{21}O_2$) through introduction of one or more of the following oxygen functions: 6α-hydroxyl, 6β-hydroxyl, 11-keto, 11β-hydroxyl, 16α-hydroxyl, and 17α-hydroxyl in the basic pregn-4-ene-3,20-dione structure. The theoretical number of progesterone is also included*

Number of oxygen functions introduced	Basic formula	Number of different key compounds
0	$C_{21}O_2$	1
1	$C_{21}O_3$	6
2	$C_{21}O_4$	13
3	$C_{21}O_5$	12
4	$C_{21}O_6$	4
total		36

the progesterone molecule. Since each of these 36 key steroids may give 26 different reduced metabolites, a complete discussion of possible products of progesterone metabolism should include the gas chromatographic behaviour of $36 + (36 \times 26) = 972$ steroids. Only a limited number of these steroids have been isolated from natural sources. The $C_{21}O_2$ and $C_{21}O_3$ pregnane steroids that have been isolated are listed in Table 1.

---

[*] This is an arbitrary selection based on steroid structure. It may well be argued that since compounds like 21-deoxycortisol and 5β-pregnane-3α, 17α, 20α-triol are predominantly of adrenal origin, these should be considered as corticosteroids, rather than as metabolites of progesterone.

2. Qualitative Considerations

Although many of the pregnane steroids occur as conjugates (glucosiduronates and sulfates) in biological material, the gas chromatographic behaviour of the conjugates has not been explored in detail (see Chapter 1).

Samples of biologic origin that have been subjected to gas chromatographic analysis for progesterone and related steroids have varied from very crude extracts containing numerous steroids to highly purified extracts containing a single steroid.

When estimating pregnanediol in a crude extract of urine from pregnant women the steroid under consideration is present in amounts so much larger than those of other steroids that satisfactory results may be obtained when the extract is subjected to gas chromatography without further purification. GARDINER and HORNING (1965) and HORNING and GARDINER (1966) worked with crude urinary extracts following treatment with O-methylhydroxylamine and hexamethyldisilazane. The steroids were converted to methoxime trimethylsilyl ethers and/or trimethylsilyl ethers. Under standardized conditions it is possible to obtain quantitative and qualitative data relating to the major components in such extracts following gas chromatography. Although this technique may have great value for the rapid screening of major steroids in a large series of biologic samples, no detailed information on minor compounds can be obtained when working with such complex mixtures.

Several approaches have been used for the systematic identification of unknown compounds through correlation of retention times with steroid structure. In addition to the simple, direct comparison of the behaviour of an unknown compound with that of reference compounds, these approaches have included the use of "group retention factors" (CLAYTON, 1962) or "separation factors" (BROOKS and HANAINEH, 1963), ΔR_{mg} and ΔR_{mr} values (KNIGHTS and THOMAS, 1962 a, b; 1963 a, b); "steroid numbers" (VANDENHEUVEL and HORNING, 1962; HAMILTON et al., 1963); and "T-values" (HAAHTI et al., 1961; VANDEKHEUVEL and HORNING, 1965). Although some of these parameters (most notably the steroid number, which is essentially independent of temperature) may have advantages over others, the observed correlations have in general been adequate for interlaboratory comparisons. It has been observed that supposedly similar column packings give differences in relative retention times for the same steroid. In some cases the retention sequence of closely related compounds as observed in different laboratories with similar column packings may be different, as will be illustrated in the present discussion by the behaviour of isomeric pregnanediols and pregnanolones. The preferred way to establish identity is by comparing the behaviour of unknown compounds to that of authentic reference compounds with different gas chromatographic columns. Extreme care should be exercised when compound identification is attempted by comparing retention time of an unknown "steroid" with published retention times of known structures (see Chapter 1). Derivatives and/or reaction products of unknown compounds should also be prepared. This is illustrated in publications dealing with the presence of progesterone (KUMAR et al., 1962; FUTTERWEIT et al., 1963; VAN DER MOLEN et al., 1965; RÜNNE-BAUM et al., 1965), 20α-hydroxypregn-4-en-3-one (VAN DER MOLEN and GROEN, 1965 a), pregnane-3α,6α,20α-triol (KNIGHTS et al., 1962), and 20α-hydroxy-5β-pregnan-3-one (VAN DER MOLEN et al., 1966) in biologic samples.

Other approaches to the qualitative analysis of progesterone metabolites have employed gas chromatography for the isolation of appropriate fractions. The identification of *isolated* compounds in such fractions has been carried out by means of mass spectrometry (ADLERCREUTZ and LUUKKAINEN, 1965), infrared spectrometry (BARNES et al., 1962; VAN DER MOLEN et al., 1965; 1966) and double isotope dilution assay (VAN DER MOLEN et al., 1965).

3. Quantitative Considerations

The gas chromatographic measurement of pregnanediol and pregnanetriol in urine and progesterone in blood has been widely explored. Much work in this field has been directed towards simplification of already existing techniques through substitution of sometimes time-consuming purification steps by a rapid gas chromatographic separation with the added advantage of a simultaneous quantitative determination. The estimation of pregnanediol in urine by gas chromatography is a good example of this approach.

On the other hand, the sensitivity of the detection systems that are employed in gas chromatographic work has several advantages. When the amount of biological material is too small to permit a quantitative determination by other techniques, as is the case for progesterone in normal blood, the methodology improvement provided by gas-liquid chromatography is often based on the sensitivity of the detection system. Effort spent on the purification of such samples prior to gas chromatography seems completely justified in light of the sensitivity and simplicity of the final detection. The sensitivity of detection, however, may not necessarily be decisive in the choice of a gas chromatographic technique, as long as sufficient material (as in the analysis of pregnanediol in urine) is available. In such circumstances it is often the combination of advantages, i. e. handling of a smaller sample size as a consequence of more sensitive detection, in addition to a faster and simpler system of purification, that may favour the use of a gas chromatographic technique.

II. Progesterone and Reduced Metabolites: Progesterone, 20α- and 20β-Hydroxypregn-4-en-3-one, 3α- and 3β-Hydroxypregn-4-en-3-one and Pregn-4-ene-3,20-Diols

Progesterone and both 20-hydroxypregn-4-en-3-ones have been isolated and identified in a variety of animals including man. 3-Hydroxypregn-4-en-20-ones and preg-4-ene-3,20-diols have not been isolated from animal sources. Tentative evidence for the formation of 3α- or 3β-hydroxypregn-4-en-20-one has been found in incubation experiments of progesterone with ovarian tissue (GRIFFITHS et al., 1964).

The important role of progesterone for cyclic ovarian function and maintenance of pregnancy in the human as well as in other animals is well established (ROTHSCHILD, 1965). Moreover, progesterone may be involved in numerous other physiological processes (FOTHERBY, 1964). 20α-Hydroxypregn-4-en-3-one and 20β-hydroxypregn-4-en-3-one are the only other naturally occurring compounds that possess a biological activity qualitatively similar to progesterone. 20α-Hydroxypregn-4-en-3-one may play an important role in the regulation of ovarian and gestagenic activity in certain animals such as the rat and rabbit. Progesterone in the human is present at approximately 10 times the level of 20α-hydroxypregn-4-en-3-one. The latter steroid has been shown to occur in equal or even larger quantity than progesterone in the rabbit. In the cow, both the normal corpus luteum and the corpus luteum of pregnancy are major sources of 20β-hydroxypregn-4-en-3-one. This steroid may be present in cow blood in concentrations 20—50% of that of progesterone (GORSKI et al., 1958).

Due to lack of adequate techniques for the direct measurement of these steroids in biological samples, their correlation with biological effects was for a long time largely based on pharmacological experiments or on indirect measurement through the estimation of metabolites such as pregnanediol in human urine. Interest has been expressed for measurement of plasma progesterone in the normal human, but the possible clinical value of this measurement is not too well defined. The lack of suitable methods has prevented the collection of sufficient data which might indicate that the measurement of progesterone in blood has definite advantages over that of pregnanediol estimation in urine. The data thus far obtained clearly indicate that the excretion of pregnanediol in urine reflects progesterone levels in blood. Whether, and to what extent, plasma progesterone estimations might offer better diagnostic aids in situations associated with disturbed ovarian or placental function remains to be investigated. Thus, gas phase chromatographic methods for the estimation of progesterone and 20α/20β-hydroxypregn-4-en-3-one in blood plasma and tissues of several animal species have largely been used for the study of basic control mechanisms for ovarian and placental function, rather than for well defined routine clinical problems.

1. Qualitative Observations

The identification and estimation of progesterone by GLC techniques was first applied by KUMAR et al. (1962) and BARNES et al. (1962) to the problem of progesterone in human myometrium. Following tissue digestion with 5 N sodium hydroxide solution, crude lipid material was extracted with ether and partially purified on silicic acid columns. An SE-30 column was employed for the GLC separation. Material with a retention corresponding to that of authentic progesterone showed ultraviolet absorption at 240 mμ and had biological activity similar to that of synthetic progesterone.

The presence of progesterone in the plasma of pregnant women was rigourously established by ZANDER and SIMMER (1954). FUTTERWEIT et al. (1963) extracted pregnancy plasma with a chloroform-ether mixture. The sample was purified by TLC on silica gel with benzene-ethylacetate (3 : 2) as a developing system. They demonstrated that when such purified extracts were subjected to gas chromatographic separation with an SE-30 column, a peak corresponding to that of authentic progesterone was observed. VAN DER MOLEN et al. (1965) employed a gas chromatographic separation to isolate progesterone from plasma from normal women for further identification by infrared spectrometry and double isotope dilution derivative analysis. RÜNNEBAUM et al. (1965) used gas chromatographic methods for the identification of the following purified compounds isolated from peripheral blood of normal women: progesterone, 20α-hydroxypregn-4-en-3-one and 20β-hydroxypregn-4-en-3-one. A mean concentration during the 16—25th day of the menstrual cycle of 0.69, 0.13 and 0.04 μg/100 ml plasma for progesterone, 20α-dihydroprogesterone and 20β-dihydroprogesterone respectively, was reported by these authors. McKERNS and NORDSTRAND (1964; 1965 a; 1965 b) developed a simple method for the extraction, separation and tentative identification by gas-phase chromatography on XE-60, SE-30 or mixed SE-30/XE-60 columns of several steroids, including progesterone and the 20-dihydroprogesterones. They successfully applied this technique in studies on the regulation of steroid synthesis in vitro in the rat ovary and in the human placenta. Since in the gas chromatographic tracings of McKERNS and NORDSTRAND several peaks may overlap each other, quantitative estimations by this method may be of limited precision.

2. Excretion in Urine

Biologically active steroids like testosterone, corticosteroids and estrogens are present in the urine of normal human subjects, but progesterone and other biologically active progestins have not been identified in this source in comparable amounts. DROSDOWSKY et al. (1965) using a GLC method with flame ionization detection were not able to detect progesterone in the urine of pregnant women. They concluded that the amount of progesterone excreted must be on the order of from < 0.6 to < 11 μg/day. ISMAIL and HARKNESS (1961) used gas chromatography for the first identification of small amounts of progesterone in urine from pregnant women. In a similar study, using pooled urine obtained from normal women during the menstrual cycle, VAN DER MOLEN et al. (1966) have on several occasions been able to detect progesterone in amounts of approximately 1 µg/24 hrs. The urine was extracted with ether at pH 7.4; the extract was purified by thin-layer and paper chromatography, and progesterone was determined by gas chromatography with either flame ionization or electron capture detection (VAN DER MOLEN et al., 1965).

3. Quantitative Estimation in Blood and Tissue

Techniques for the measurement of unconjugated progestins in blood have usually included the following steps:
1. Extraction.
2. Removal of lipids.
3. Chromatographic purification of steroids, including derivative formation.
4. Quantitative measurement of the isolated progestins.

The first reliable chemical method for the determination of progesterone in human blood was introduced by ZANDER (1964). SHORT (1961), ZANDER (1962), HENDELES (1965) and VAN DER MOLEN and AAKVAAG (1967) have extensively reviewed the methods for progesterone measurement. Newer methods employing gas chromatography have mainly relied on specific compound purification by gas chromatographic separation and sensitive quantitative estimation. The use of gas chromatography for the determination of progestins in blood and tissue has not influenced to any significant extent the nature of the extraction and preliminary purification of the biological samples.

4. Sensitivity of Detection

Prior to the introduction of gas-liquid chromatography, spectrophotometric techniques were widely used for the measurement of progesterone. UV absorption at 240 mµ (ZANDER and SIMMER, 1954; SHORT, 1958), and the absorption of the dinitrophenylhydrazone derivative (HINSBERG et al., 1956), the thiosemicarbazone derivative (SIMMER and SIMMER, 1959; SOMMERVILLE et al., 1963), and isonicotinic acid hydrazone derivative (SOMMERVILLE and DESHPANDE, 1958) have been used for this purpose. Using microcells (capacity 0.2—0.3 ml), the smallest amounts of progesterone that can be measured in this way fall in the range 0.1—0.5 µg.

Sulphuric acid fluorescence techniques were employed by SHORT and LEVITT (1962) and HEAP (1964). Although as little as 0.005 to 0.05 µg of pure compounds can be estimated, the general drawback of fluorescence reactions is lack of specificity at low concentrations of steroids.

Recently, double isotope derivative techniques have been developed for the measurement of plasma progesterone (WOOLEVER and GOLDFIEN, 1963; RIONDEL et al., 1965; WIEST et al., 1966). The most sensitive of these techniques, employing the ^{35}S-labeled thiosemicarbazide derivative of progesterone, permits the measurement of approximately 0.002 µg of the hormone (RIONDEL et al., 1965).

In a number of publications on progesterone estimation following GLC, existing methods for isolation have been retained and a less sensitive detection technique has been replaced by detection following gas chromatography. SHORT et al. (1964) and DEANE et al. (1966) used SHORT's (1958) method for the estimation of progesterone in ovarian vein blood. Instead of the final ultraviolet spectrophotometric quantification step, gas-liquid chromatography on an SE-30 column (flame ionization detection) was employed. This approach may of course be applied to any extract that is sufficiently pure for GLC work.

The sensitivity of GLC detection systems is given in Table 3. Electron capture methods permit the detection of as little as 0.001 µg or less of suitable derivatives.

Progesterone is relatively easy to separate from other steroids present in extracts from biological material. It has been reported that difficulties may be encountered in the separation of progesterone from sterols like cholesterol and cholestadiene (DROSDOWSKY et al., 1965). It is possible, however, to obtain relatively clean samples of progesterone from human blood following thin-layer or paper chromatography. Selection of a satisfactory stationary phase for the gas chromatography of progesterone has not been discussed extensively. Some workers have expressed a preference for one phase over another with regard to the ability to separate progesterone from nonsteroidal contaminants.

The isolation of individual 20-dihydroprogesterones from plasma or tissue extracts can be performed without too great difficulties using paper chromatography (ZANDER, 1962). Separation of the 20α- and 20β isomers by thin-layer chromatography is, however, less efficient.

Table 3. *Sensitivity of detection of some physico-chemical techniques that have been used for the quantitative estimation of progesterone isolated from biological sources*

Principle of detection	Sensitivity (μg)	References
U.V absorption of progesterone ($\varepsilon_{240} = \pm 17.000$)	0.3—0.5	ZANDER and SIMMER (1954); SHORT (1958)
Absorption of dinitrophenylhydrazone derivative ($\varepsilon_{380} = \pm 40.000$)	0.1—0.2	HINSBERG et al. (1956)
Absorption of isonicotinic acid hydrazide derivative ($\varepsilon_{380} = \pm 12.000$)	0.5—1.0	SOMMERVILLE and DESHPANDE (1958)
Absorption of sulphuric acid-ethanol chromogen ($\varepsilon_{290} = \pm 20.000$)	0.3—0.5	OERTEL et al. (1959)
Absorption of thiosemicarbazide derivative ($\varepsilon_{300} = \pm 40.000$)	0.1—0.2	PEARLMAN and CERCEO (1953); SIMMER and SIMMER (1959)
KOH-sulphuric acid fluorescence	0.05—0.10	TOUCHSTONE and MURAWEC (1960); SHORT and LEVETT (1962)
Sulphuric acid fluorescence after conversion to 20β-dihydroprogesterone	0.003—0.005	HEAP (1964)
Double isotope derivative (^{3}H and ^{14}C) measuring 20-[3]H-20β-dihydroprogesterone	0.10	WOOLEVER and GOLDFIEN (1963)
Double isotope derivative (^{3}H and ^{35}S) measuring progesterone-^{35}S-thiosemicarbazide-2',4'-diacetate	0.002	RIONDEL et al. (1965)
Double isotope derivative (^{3}H and ^{14}C) measuring 20β-dihydroprogesterone-20-^{3}H-acetate	0.01—0.02	WIEST et al. (1966)
Argon ionization detection after gas liquid chromatography	0.01—0.10	COLLINS and SOMMERVILLE (1962); CARLSON et al. (1964)

Table 3 (continued)

Principle of detection	Sensitivity (µg)	References
Flame ionization detection after gas liquid chromatography	0.005—0.10	YANNONE et al. (1964); LUISI et al. (1965); LURIE et al. (1966)
Electron capture detection of the chloroacetate derivative of 20β-dihydroprogesterone	$\leq$0.001	VAN DER MOLEN and GROEN (1965)

Several stationary phases that have been used in gas chromatography will often adequately separate these isomers, and in cases where both isomers are present in a mixture, gas-liquid chromatography may be used to separate both compounds. Attempts to separate and measure progesterone, 20α-hydroxypregn-4-en-3-one and 20β-hydroxypregn-4-en-3-one by GLC techniques when present in a mixture have not been published. When working with samples containing these three steroids, it should be kept in mind that progesterone and 20α-hydroxy-pregn-4-en-3-one are better separated on QF-1 columns than on either XE-60 or SE-30 columns (Table 4). It may also be seen from the data of Table 4 that a good separation of 3-dihydroprogesterone from both progesterone and the 20-dihydroprogesterones can be obtained on SE-30, XE-60 or QF-1 columns.

5. Methods for Estimation in Human Peripheral Blood

Early methods that demonstrated the possibility of using gas chromatography for the serial measurement of progesterone in biological samples include those that have already been mentioned (BARNES et al., 1962; KUMAR et al., 1962; KUMAR et al., 1964; KUMAR and BARNES, 1965; and FUTTERWEIT et al., 1963). A similar technique was employed by NIENSTEDT (1963, 1966).

Method of YANNONE et al. (1963)

The chief stages of the method for the estimation of plasma progesterone as described by YANNONE et al. (1964) and GOLDFIEN et al. (1965) are:

Table 4. *Range of relative retention times of progesterone and reduced metabolites. All values are expressed relative to the retention time of cholestane = 1.00*

| | Liquid phase | | | | | |
| | SE-30 | | QF-1 | | XE-60 | |
	Free steroids	Acetates	Free steroids	Acetates	Free steroids	Acetates
Progesterone	0.80		9.9		9.7	
Pregnane-3,20-diones (5β-5α)	0.60—0.66		5.4—6.0		5.2—5.7	
Pregnan-3-ol-20-ones	0.60—0.66	0.80—0.93	2.5—3.3	4.1— 4.9	3.5—4.3	4.2— 5.0
Pregnan-20-ol-3-ones	0.65—0.70	0.90—1.00	3.6—4.6	6.2— 6.8	4.8—5.9	5.7— 7.0
Pregnane-3,20-diols	0.60—0.72	1.14—1.45	1.7—2.3	3.9— 5.1	3.1—4.3	4.3— 5.8
Pregn-4-en-3-ol-20-ones (3α-3β)	0.62—0.67		3.6—3.9	6.4— 6.7	4.5—5.0	5.7— 6.0
Pregn-4-en-20-ol-3-ones (20β-20α)	0.98—1.05	1.28—1.34	6.0—6.9	10.5—11.7	7.8—9.2	9.8—11.2
Pregn-4-ene-3,20-diols	0.60—0.85					

See: BROOKS and HANAINEH (1963); CHAMBERLAIN and THOMAS (1964); CHAMBERLAIN et al. (1964); HAMMOND and LEACH (1965); VAN DER MOLEN et al. (unpublished observations).

1. Addition of ³H-progesterone to plasma.

2. Extraction of plasma with diethylether (YANNONE et al., 1964) or methylene dichloride (GOLDFIEN et al., 1965).

3. Removal of lipid material ("freezing" at −15° C from 70⁰/₀ methanol, followed by a heptane-70⁰/₀ methanol partition).

4. Isolation of progesterone by paper chromatography in the system heptane-70⁰/₀ methanol.

5. Sampling for counting of radioactivity.

6. Gas chromatography with a 1⁰/₀ XE-60 column in combination with flame ionization detection.

The authors used a special solid injector (McCOMAS and GOLDFIEN, 1963) for introduction of the purified sample on the gas chromatograph. Thus they prevented the occurrence of a broad solvent peak that might otherwise have interfered with the analysis. The sensitivity of this method was reported to be 0.02 μg of progesterone.

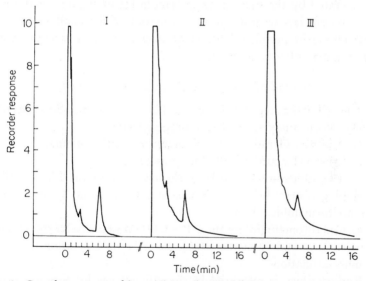

Fig. 2. Gas chromatographic tracings obtained by YANNONE et al. (1964) in the analysis of: I. 5 ml of plasma from a woman 34 weeks pregnant. Attenuation 300. Peak area is equal to 0.25 μg of progesterone. II. 10 ml of plasma from a woman 10 weeks pregnant. Attenuation 100. Peak area is equal to 0.12 μg of progesterone. III. 5 ml of plasma from the luteal phase of the menstrual cycle. Attenuation 30. Peak area is equal to 0.02 μg of progesterone. The retention time of progesterone is 6 minutes. (Reprinted with permission of the authors and the editors of the Journal of Gas Chromatography)

By the addition of known amounts of progesterone to male plasma, the precision of the determination was found to be about 10% when working with 0.02—0.115 µg of pure steroid. The technique was applied mainly to the study of progesterone levels in the blood of pregnant women. The average deviation from the mean of duplicate samples in the range of 3.0—20.0 µg/100 ml plasma was 6%. The few levels that the authors have published on plasma progesterone in normal ovulating women fall in the range of values reported by others using non-GLC techniques. The method has also been applied to the study of progesterone in rat ovarian vein blood and dog adrenal vein blood (GOLDFIEN et al., 1965). An example of the gas chromatographic tracings that the authors obtained after the injection of their plasma extracts is shown in Fig. 2. This tracing indicates the absence of impurities that might interfere with quantitative evaluation of the progesterone peak. The sensitivity of detection as illustrated by the small peak in sample III of Figure 2 may make this technique less accurate for the estimation of the small amounts of progesterone in peripheral blood of normal men or women unless large plasma volumes are used.

Method of COLLINS *and* SOMMERVILLE *(1964)*

The following steps have been used by COLLINS and SOMMERVILLE (1962) for the analysis of plasma progesterone:

1. Addition of radioactive progesterone to the plasma.
2. Ether extraction of alkaline plasma.
3. Two dimensional thin-layer chromatography on silica gel (first developing system: benzene-ethylacetate, 3 : 2; second system: ether-dimethylformamide, 99 : 1.
4. Gas chromatography on a 1% CHDMS or 2% XE-60 column (SOMMERVILLE and COLLINS, 1965), using argon ionization detection for mass estimation.

Radioactivity is measured in the effluent gas by a proportional counter after combusting the gas leaving the argon ionization detector. Introduction of the sample into the column was carried out by depositing the samples on a metal gauze (MENINI and NORYMBERSKI, 1965) or by use of a HAMILTON solid injection syringe. The sensitivity of detection with the argon ionization detector as described in the original procedure was in the order of 0.01 µg. The main drawback of this method (use of the argon detector) has limited the application mainly to studies involving plasma progesterone during human pregnancy. A later publication (SOMMERVILLE, 1966) described the use of flame ionization detection; the sensitivity of the estimation was increased to 0.01—0.005 µg. This method would be expected to offer one of the best ways to correct for sample losses, in that the added internal standard (labeled progesterone) is taken through every step, including gas phase chromatography. It has been recognized that losses or differences in behaviour of an effluent gas stream in the different detectors (for mass and radioactivity respectively) may influence the accuracy and precision of the final result. Since such difficulties arise mainly from problems of instrumentation and not from false theoretical assumptions, it may be expected that with increasing use of such instruments these problems will eventually be solved. The method as originally published (Collins and SOMMERVILLE, 1964) used approximately 0.25 µg of 4-^{14}C-progesterone as an internal standard. This tends to overestimate progesterone in peripheral blood obtained from male subjects and from female subjects during the follicular phase of the menstrual cycle (SOMMERVILLE, 1965). Moreover, as discussed by TAIT (1965), the use of such large amounts of internal standard might lead to serious errors (50—60%) for the values estimated in samples containing small amounts of progesterone. Accordingly, the 4-^{14}C-progesterone was replaced as an internal standard by ^{3}H-progesterone of higher specific activity. This would reduce the error of estimation for small amounts to approximately 3% for 0.1 µg of pure progesterone (SOMMERVILLE, 1965; SOMMERVILLE and COLLINS, 1965). Detailed data for biological samples giving the accuracy and precision of the technique incorporating these modifications have not yet been published.

Problems of instrumentation associated with the continuous monitoring of radioactivity in the effluent gas prevented the precise estimation of progesterone in plasma of non-pregnant human subjects. These difficulties led this group to develop another method using gas chromatography for the serial analysis of plasma progesterone. The estimation of recovered radioactivity was performed with liquid scintillation counting of a sample removed prior to gas chromatography (WYMAN and SOMMERVILLE, 1966). Moreover, to correct for losses due to sampling for radioactivity and other losses prior to gas chromatographic detection, they followed the outline initially applied by BROWNIE et al. (1964) and VAN DER MOLEN and GROEN (1965) to include a non-radioactive second internal standard for detection following gas chromatography of the samples.

Method of WYMAN and SOMMERVILLE (1966)

1. Addition of 0.025 µg 4-^{14}C-progesterone to the plasma.

2. Ether extraction of alkaline plasma.

3. Thin-layer chromatography on silica gel using the solvent system benzene-ethyl acetate, 3 : 2.

4. Acetylation (for conversion to acetyl derivatives of contaminating impurities).

5. Thin-layer chromatography on silica gel using the solvent system chloroform-acetone, 9 : 1.

6. Addition of estrone acetate as an internal standard for gas chromatography.

7. Counting of radioactivity in an aliquot of the sample.

8. Gas chromatographic estimation with flame ionization detection.

An automatic electronic digital integrator with base-line drift corrector was used to estimate the detector response. Quantitative determination involves comparison of area units of standard and unknowns with recoveries calculated from both liquid scintillation counting and the area units of the second reference standard (estrone acetate).

Recoveries of the labeled progesterone just prior to gas chromatography were found to be 60—80%.

This relatively simple method derives its importance from the increased sensitivity (0.005—0.010 µg) of the flame ionization detection system employed under rigidly standardized conditions. Although results of serial analysis for plasma samples throughout several menstrual cycles have been estimated using this technique, detailed data relating to the accuracy and precision of the method have not yet been published. The specificity of this technique is based on the similar behaviour of the compound in unknown samples with standard progesterone throughout all steps. Indirect evidence for the specificity of the procedure may be derived from the agreement between the values obtained for samples during a study of the menstrual cycle by another gas chromatographic technique (VAN DER MOLEN and GROEN, 1965) and an isotope derivative formation technique (RIONDEL et al., 1965).

Method of van der Molen *and* Groen *(1965)*

The chief stages in the method developed by van der Molen and Groen for the measurement of plasma progesterone are:

1. Addition of 7-^{3}H-progesterone to the plasma.
2. Extraction of alkaline plasma with ether.
3. Isolation of progesterone by thin-layer chromatography.
4. Reduction of progesterone with 20β-hydroxysteroid dehydrogenase.
5. Formation of the chloroacetate of 20β-hydroxypregn-4-en-3-one.
6. Thin-layer chromatography of 20β-hydroxypregn-4-en-3-one chloroacetate.
7. Addition of testosterone chloroacetate as an internal standard.
8. Counting of radioactivity in an aliquot of the sample.
9. Gas chromatography on a 3 ft 1% XE-60 column with electron capture detection.

The recovery of progesterone up to the gas chromatographic step is calculated from the recovery of the radioactive compound. Other losses prior to detection, including sampling for measurement of radioactivity, losses during transference into the gas chromatographic column and during gas chromatographic separation, are corrected for by recovery values for the second internal standard added prior to sampling for radioactivity measurements. In Chapter 4 Eik-Nes has discussed details of a similar technique (Brownie et al., 1964) for the measurement of testosterone in human peripheral blood. The tracings in Fig. 3 illustrate the sensitivity of electron capture detection as compared with that of flame ionization detection for progesterone, 20α- and 20β-hydroxypregn-4-en-3-ones and the chloroacetate derivatives of the latter steroids chromatographed under identical conditions.

Amounts of 0.001—0.005 µg of the chloroacetate derivatives may easily be detected with good precision. The precision for routine application to human peripheral blood analyses ranges from 10 to 25% for samples containing less than 0.01 µg progesterone to from 10—15% for samples containing more than 0.01 µg, and is 5—6% for samples containing 0.1 µg or more (van der Molen and Groen, 1965; 1967).

For most samples the final precision of assay is mainly dependent on the accuracy and precision of preparation of standards and

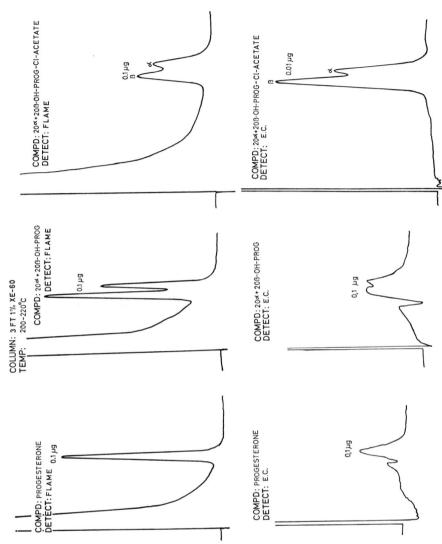

Fig. 3. Electron capture and flame ionization detection of free steroids and the chloroacetate derivatives of 20α- and 20β-hydroxypregn-4-en-3-one *(20α- +20β-OH-prog).* Chromatography was done on a 3 ft 1% XE-60 column. *E. C.:* electron capture detection. A mixture of 0.1 μg each of 20α- and 20β-hydroxypregn-4-en-3-one was chromatographed in experiment *B.* In experiment *C* a mixture of 0.1 *μg* each of 20α- and 20β-hydroxypregn-4-en-3-one chloroacetate was chromatographed for detection by flame ionization. For the electron capture detection of the chloroacetate derivatives of these steroids a mixture containing 0.01 *μg* of each was chromatographed. (Reprinted with permission of the editors of the Journal of Clinical Endocrinology and Metabolism). VAN DER MOLEN and GROEN (1965 b)

measurement of peak areas. Triangulation or planimetry of peak areas introduces an error of approximately 3—5%. This might be reduced by using automatic means (electronic integration including proper correction for baseline drift) for measurement of the detector response. Pure progesterone added to plasma and water in amounts of from 0.005 to 0.100 µg was accurately recovered. Difficulties inherent in the application of this method have mainly involved the use of appropriate instrumentation for electron capture detection (BROWNIE et al., 1964) and the problems related to the handling of small amounts of steroids (VAN DER MOLEN and GROEN, 1967). In this respect, the use of a non-radioactive internal standard for gas-liquid chromatography has been stressed (see Chapter 1). Minor differences in operation of the detector or small amounts of impurities may occasionally influence the sensitivity of detection. Thus, even chromatographing a standard immediately prior to injection of an unknown sample may render quantification (based upon measurement of absolute peak areas and recovery of radioactivity in the effluent gas) less precise than quantification based on the ratio of peak areas that are obtained using a non-radioactive internal standard. Accordingly, the non-radioactive internal standard should be as similar to the unknown as possible with respect to sensitivity of detection and gas chromatographic behaviour (VAN DER MOLEN and GROEN, 1967. See Chapter 1).

Since steroid chloroacetates are relatively polar, their gas chromatographic separation may require a relatively high temperature if polar phases are used. When short columns (3 feet) are used with a low concentration of stationary phase (about 1%), satisfactory separation can be obtained. XE-60 and QF-1 have given better results than SE-30.

Recently (VAN DER MOLEN et al., 1967), the use of heptafluorobutyrates instead of chloroacetates has been explored. Although steroid heptafluorobutyrates may require special methods with regard to preparation and handling, they offer definite advantages in gas chromatography. The retention times are much shorter (Table 5), and the sensitivity of electron capture detection of these derivatives of testosterone and 20β-hydroxypregn-4-en-3-one is approximately five times higher than that for the chloroacetates. The increased sensitivity of detection should permit the more precise determination of samples containing small amounts of progesterone.

Table 5. *Relative retention times and sensitivity of electron capture detection of some steroid chloroacetates and heptafluorobutyrates. The retention times are given relative to the retention time of cholestane = 1. E.A. = electron absorbing activity, expressed as observed peak area relative to the peak area of an aequimolecular amount of testosterone chloroacetate = 100*

	Relative Retention Times on:			E.A.
	SE-30	XE-60	QF-1	
Testosterone chloroacetate	1.70	21.4	17.9	100
Testosterone heptafluorobutyrate	0.52	2.8	5.5	500
20β-dihydroprogesterone chloroacetate	2,41	29,7	22.0	100
20β-dihydroprogesterone heptafluorobutyrate	0.84	4.2	7.7	375
20α-dihydroprogesterone chloroacetate	2,65	33.2	24.5	60
20α-dihydroprogesterone heptafluorobutyrate	1.07	5.0	10.8	475

The technique as originally published has been applied successfully to the measurement of progesterone in peripheral blood obtained from male and female subjects (VAN DER MOLEN and GROEN, 1965), as well as in canine peripheral and testicular vein blood (VAN DER MOLEN and EIK-NES, 1966). Representative examples of analytical records are presented in Fig. 4. Values found for plasma progesterone in human subjects (VAN DER MOLEN and GROEN, 1965) are in good agreement with those obtained with sensitivity techniques not employing gas chromatography (RIONDEL et al., 1965).

The principle used for the estimation of progesterone has also been used for the measurement of testosterone and 20α- and 20β-hydroxy-pregn-4-en-3-ones in the same blood sample (VAN DER MOLEN et al., 1965 a). The 20α- and 20β-isomers may be isolated from the silica gel after the first thin-layer chromatographic separation employed in the testosterone method of BROWNIE et al. (1964), and they can subsequently be separated using paper chromatography (BUSH A or hexane-65% methanol). After derivative formation (chloroacetates or heptafluorobutyrates) and addition of appropriate internal standards, quantification is accomplished using gas phase chromatography with electron capture detection. Examples of the gas chromatographic records that have been obtained in analyses for 20α-hydroxypregn-4-en-3-one are shown in Fig. 5.

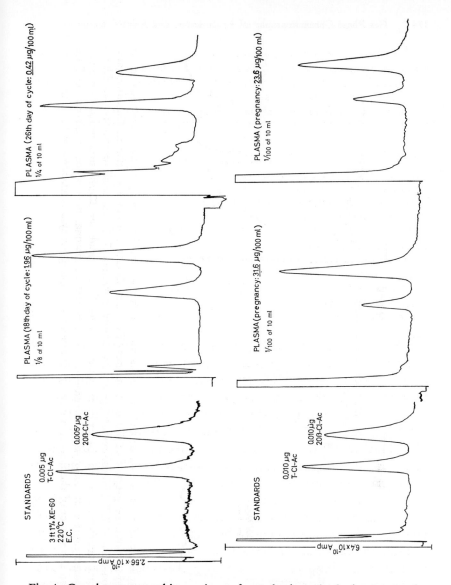

Fig. 4. Gas chromatographic tracings of standards and of plasma samples from normal women taken through the method for the estimation of plasma progesterone (VAN DER MOLEN and GROEN, 1965 a, b). Gas chromatography was performed on a 3 ft 1% XE-60 column using electron capture detection. *T-Cl-Ac:* peak of testosterone chloroacetate (added as internal standard prior to gas chromatography). *20β-Cl-Ac:* peak of 20β-hydroxypregn-4-en-3-one chloroacetate. The estimated progesterone content in 100 ml plasma, the volume of plasma used for estimation and the aliquot of the final residue subjected to gas chromatography are indicated in the figure

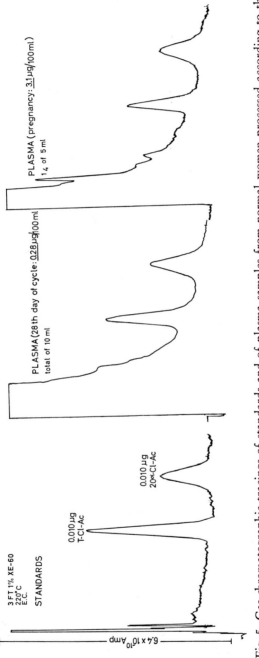

Fig. 5. Gas chromatographic tracings of standards and of plasma samples from normal women processed according to the method for estimation of 20α-hydroxypregn-4-en-3-one in plasma (VAN DER MOLEN and GROEN, 1965 a). Gas chromatography was performed on a 3 ft 1% XE-60 column using electron capture detection. *T-Cl-Ac*: Peak of testosterone chloroacetate (added as internal standard prior to gas chromatography). *20α-Cl-Ac*: peak of 20α-hydroxypregn-4-en-3-one chloroacetate. The estimated content of 20α-hydroxypregn-4-en-3-one in 100 ml plasma, the volume of plasma used for the estimation and the aliquot of the final residue subjected to gas chromatography are indicated in the figure

The sensitivity, precision and accuracy of the estimation of plasma 20α- and 20β-hydroxypregn-4-en-3-ones are the same as for the progesterone method (VAN DER MOLEN and GROEN, 1966). Application of this technique to the study of peripheral blood samples from normal women during the corpus luteum phase of the menstrual cycle has revealed the presence of 20α-hydroxypregn-4-en-3-one in quantities approximately one-fifth to one-tenth those of progesterone. In plasma of pregnant women the amount of 20α-hydroxypregn-4-en-3-one was estimated to be approximately one-tenth that of progesterone, whereas 20β-hydroxypregn-4-en-3-one was present in amounts one-fiftieth to one-hundredth those of progesterone. Cyclic variations of 20α-hydroxypregn-4-en-3-one levels in the plasma of non-pregnant women and the increase in plasma levels of both 20α- and 20β-hydroxypregn-4-en-3-ones in pregnant women appear to parallel those of progesterone.

Method of LURIE et al. (1966)

LURIE et al. (1966) measured progesterone by the following method:

1. Addition of acetone to alkaline plasma and subsequent removal of the precipitated proteins following centrifugation.

2. Ether extraction of the water residues obtained after evaporation of the acetone.

3. Celite column chromatography (trimethylpentane-90% methanol).

4. Thin-layer chromatography on silica gel (chloroform-acetone, 9 : 1).

5. Gas-liquid chromatography on a 3% XE-60 column in combination with flame ionization detection.

A dry injector device (LURIE and VILLEE, 1966 a) eliminates the solvent front during gas phase chromatography and allows the whole sample to be transferred quantitatively to the column. In an addendum to their paper the authors state that the accuracy and reproducibility of the analysis may be increased by the addition of radioactive progesterone to the plasma prior to any handling. Correction for losses can then be made on the basis of the recovery estimated following elution from the silica gel after thin-layer chromatography. The authors stress the importance of preventing contamination of the final samples for gas chromatography with sebum from human skin.

In a separate publication (LURIE and VILLEE, 1966 b) they investigated the problem in greater detail. The prevention of contamination

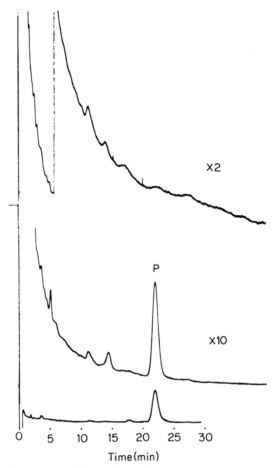

Fig. 6. Gas chromatographic tracings obtained by LURIE et al. (1966). The
lowermost curve is a sample of 0.3 μg progesterone standard. Corresponding to the elution time of the standard is a progesterone peak (marked P)
in the middle curve which represents a sample of an extract of plasma taken
from a patient in the 40th week of a normal pregnancy. The upper curve
is derived from a water sample which was taken through the identical
procedure as the plasma sample. Conditions for GLC: 6 ft 3% XE-60
column; column temp. 230° C; helium carrier gas approximately 60 ml/min;
injector temp. 280° C; detector temp. 250° C; hydrogen flame detector.
(Reprinted with permission of the authors and the editors of the Journal of
Clinical Endocrinology and Metabolism)

appeared, however, to be very difficult. Typical gas chromatographic tracings obtained with this procedure are shown in Fig. 6.

The authors applied their method to the assay of plasma from pregnant women during all stages of pregnancy. Multiple measurement of 0.1 µg of progesterone added to male plasma gave an average recovery of 78.6%; the precision of the method at this hormone concentration was found to be 14.8%. When amounts of from 0.02—0.08 µg of progesterone were added to male plasma, the recovery ranged from 109—145% and hormone overestimation occurred. The application of the method to samples containing very small amounts of progesterone, (10—20 ml of plasma samples of peripheral blood from normal men and women) might therefore result in too high progesterone values.

Recently RAISINGHANI et al. (1966) reported the use of electron capture detection for the estimation of nanogram quantities of progesterone. Gas phase chromatography of the 20β-chlorodifluoroacetyl-pregn-4-en-3-one was employed. Following chemical reduction of progesterone to pregn-4-ene-3,20-diol, this compound was reoxidized with dichlorodicyanobenzoquinone to 20β-hydroxypregn-4-en-3-one. This steroid was subsequently esterified with chlorodifluoroacetic anhydride.

Other techniques that have been described for the measurement of progesterone in human blood (LUISI et al., 1965; KUMAR et al., 1962; BARNES et al., 1963) have not used new principles. The reliability of these techniques may be debated since no determination of the precision of assay has been given (BARNES et al., 1963). The sensitivity of measurement of progesterone in plasma from non-pregnant subjects by these methods is such that at least 100 ml of blood would be required (LUISI et al., 1965).

6. Measurement of Progestins in Laboratory Animals

Representative examples of the application of gas-liquid chromatography to the study of progesterone and 20α- and 20β-hydroxypregn-4-en-3-one in laboratory animals have been reported by NEILL et al. (1964), by CARLSON et al. (1964, 1965), by NISHIZAWA and EIK-NES (1964) and by HEAP et al. (1966). In these investigations relatively high levels of steroids were present and the objective was to measure relatively large differences in steroid concentrations. Thus the requirements of sensitivity, precision and accuracy were in general less extreme than those for measurement of the same steroids in human blood. The speed of analysis was increased through the use of simple steps for purification, since the large amounts of steroids present in the biological samples gave acceptable results under conditions where measurement of small amounts would have been impossible. Nothing, however, precludes the use of the techniques that have been described for progesterone measurement in human blood in animal studies.

Method of NEILL *et al. (1964)*

These workers employed:

1. Ether extraction of alkaline plasma or tissue homogenates.

2. Thin-layer chromatography (cyclohexane-ethylacetate, 1 : 1) to separate progesterone and 20α-hydroxypregn-4-en-3-one.

3. Addition of cholestane as an internal standard.

4. Gas chromatography on a 1% SE-30 column with a flame ionization detection system.

These investigators estimated progesterone and 20α-hydroxypregn-4-en-3-one for kinetic studies of the action of luteotrophin in such diverse samples as porcine ovarian tissue, guinea pig ovarian vein blood, rabbit ovarian vein blood and rabbit ovarian tissue. The sensitivity of detection was approximately 0.1 µg for biological samples. This permitted the use of minimal (1—2 ml) plasma samples containing high concentrations of the progestins.

Method of CARLSON *et al. (1964)*

CARLSON et al. (1964, 1965) developed a method for the analysis of the progestin content of ovarian blood and systemic blood of the laboratory rat. The procedure included:

1. Acetone extraction of blood.

2. Methylene dichloride extraction of the aqueous residues of the acetone extract.

3. Gradient column chromatography on silica gel to remove extraneous lipid material.

4. Thin-layer chromatography (chloroform-ethylacetate, 13 : 1) for the separation of progesterone from 20-dihydroprogesterone, followed by thin-layer chromatography of the isolated fractions using the same solvent system.

5. Addition of testosterone as an internal standard.
6. Gas liquid chromatography on either XE-60, QF-1 or SE-30 columns with an argon ionization detection system.

Method of Nishizawa *and* Eik-Nes *(1964)*

Nishizawa and Eik-Nes (1964) measured progesterone in extracts from canine ovarian vein blood. Their approach (see chapter 4) involved:
1. Extraction of plasma with methylene dichloride.
2. Removal of estrogens (toluene/sodium hydroxide partition).
3. Removal of lipid material (ligroin/70% methanol partition).
4. Paper chromatography (methylcyclohexane-propyleneglycol).
5. Gas chromatography of the purified progesterone sample on a 6 ft 0.75% SE-30 column using argon ionization detection.

The quantitative data were found to agree well with results obtained by a method employing ultraviolet absorption at 240 mμ. The average recovery of progesterone applied to the column for gas chromatography, as estimated in the collected effluent gas, was 70%. Losses during the purification procedure, however, limited the sensitivity of estimation to 0.2 μg of progesterone in the original plasma samples. Even this rather low sensitivity permitted the estimation of progesterone in several ovarian vein plasma samples of normal dogs treated with large doses of human gonadotrophin.

7. Conclusion

Several of the methods employing gas chromatography for the quantitative measurement of progesterone in biological samples are competitive in all respects with procedures based on methods not employing gas chromatography (Table 6). Moreover, the combination of gas chromatographic and thin-layer chromatographic techniques may have distinct advantages leading to faster, and frequently more specific and more sensitive, measurement. For the assay of progesterone in human blood plasma, it is also desirable to have a method that will permit reliable measurement in a reasonable volume (20 ml or less) of blood, especially if repeated determinations in the same subject are required.

The *sensitivity* of detection by GLC methods, in all procedures reviewed, may permit the analysis of progesterone in "physiological"

Table 6. *Some characteristics of methods using GLC for the estimation of progesterone in human peripheral blood*

Reference	Principle of detection	Phase for GLC	Useful sensitivity of detection (µg) *	Precision (coefficient of variation) **
COLLINS and SOMMERVILLE (1964) SOMMERVILLE and COLLINS (1965)	Argon ionization of progesterone	1% CHDMS or 2% XE-60	0.01	?
YANNONE et al. (1964)	Flame ionization of progesterone	1% XE-60	0.02	10%: 0.02—0.115 µg
VAN DER MOLEN and GROEN (1965 a, b)	Electron capture of 20β-hydroxypregn-4-en-3-one chloro-acetate	1% XE-60	0.002—0.005	10—25%: <0.01 µg 10—15%: 0.01—0.10 µg 5%: $\geqq$0.10 µg
LUISI et al. (1965)	Flame ionization of progesterone	3% SE-30 or 1% QF-1	0.02	10%: 0.5 µg
LURI et al. (1966)	Flame ionization of progesterone	3% XE-60	0.02	15%: 0.1 µg

* Expressed as the smallest amount, that may be measured after isolation from biological samples.
** The coefficient of variation is given in per cent of estimated values within the indicated range.

volumes of blood from pregnant women and women during the second half of the menstrual cycle, where the hormone concentration may be on the order of 1 μg/100 ml of plasma or higher. Some of the techniques may lack sensitivity, however, for the accurate measurement of progesterone in male plasma or in plasma of female subjects before ovulation (or else may require large volumes of blood for accurate estimation). In this respect, a technique employing sensitive electron capture detection of appropriate derivatives may offer distinct advantages. A sensitivity as good as that of the most sensitive and reliable technique not using gas chromatography (the double isotope derivative technique using ^{35}S-thiosemicarbazide, RIONDEL et al., 1964) can be achieved. RIONDEL et al. reported progesterone concentrations in human plasma of 0.028 ± 0.013 μg/100 ml for normal adult males, and 0.113 ± 0.049 μg/100 ml and 1.04 ± 0.32 μg/100 ml for women during the follicular and luteal phase of the cycle. These values are in good agreement with those found by the gas chromatographic technique of VAN DER MOLEN and GROEN (1965), who found: < 0.015—0.048 μg/100 ml for normal male subjects, < 0.015—0.42 (mean: 0.09) and 0.10—2.06 (mean: 1.15) μg/100 ml blood plasma for women during the follicular and luteal phases of the menstrual cycle.

The *specificity* of gas chromatographic techniques may to some extent be judged by the nature of the chromatographic elution patterns. Although identity of retention time behaviour and theoretical peak shape for a compound in a biological sample do not offer absolute proof of identity, the chromatographic record may lead to conclusions about specificity of the method which are as adequate as those based on spectrophotometric absorption curves. GLC methods, in fact, provide definitely better evidence for specificity than data based on detection techniques using a single physicochemical parameter. The absorption of ultraviolet radiation at 240 mμ is a common property shared by most Δ4-3-keto steroids, including progesterone, and the final estimation in methods based on double isotope labeling techniques rests only upon the amounts of radioactivity in the final sample. No indication of specificity can be obtained from the observed absorption of UV radiation or from the number of counts. Additional evidence, such as the constancy of isotope ratio following further (and sometimes tedious) purification must be presented as proof of specificity in methods of the latter type.

Definite proof of specificity may be obtained in techniques employing gas chromatography by collecting the effluent product and by identification of the compounds under consideration by a variety of methods including mass spectrometry, and infrared spectrometry (see Chapter 2).

The *precision* for several of the gas chromatographic techniques for the measurement of even relatively large amounts of progesterone has been estimated at about 10%. This is lower than the precision (3—5%) that has been claimed for other techniques at the same level of estimation. Although electron capture detection of large amounts (> 0.1 µg) of progesterone may be as precise as double isotope techniques, the precision at low levels (≦0.01 µg/sample) is probably less. The precision of estimation in methods employing gas chromatography is partly dependent upon the precision of measurement of the detector response. The peak area is frequently determined by measurement of peak height and width at half height, or by peak area measurement by planimetry. It may be expected that more widespread use of digital integrating systems will be applied to progesterone methodology and thus increase the precision of estimation, as indicated by SOMMERVILLE (1965). Finally, acceptance of the use of an internal standard will probably improve the accuracy and precision of many GLC methods.

III. Pregnanolones

The study of pregnanolones in biological media has mainly added to our knowledge of the pathways by which progesterone is metabolized. Prior to the introduction of gas chromatography the separation of individual pregnanolone isomers was difficult, and methods which were sensitive and/or specific were lacking. The 3-hydroxy-pregnan-20-one isomers isolated from human urine are listed in Table 1. From these data it may be concluded that reductive progesterone metabolism takes place mainly via the route: progesterone → pregnane-3,20-diones → pregnan-3-ol-20-ones → pregnane-3,20-diols. The few quantitative studies of the occurrence of 5β-pregnan-3α-ol-20-one, as the major pregnanolone in human urine, show that the excretion of this steroid parallels the excretion of pregnanediol but at a lower level (VAN DER MOLEN, 1962 b; LACHESE et al., 1963).

CHAMBERLAIN and THOMAS (1964) were the first to use a gas chromatographic approach for the systematic identification of preg-

Table 7. Relative retention times of the isomeric pregnanolones as the free compounds (free) and as the acetates (acetate) on different phases. Retention times are expressed relative to the retention time of cholestane = 1.00. (VAN DER MOLEN et al., unpublished observations 1966)

	SE-30 6 ft 3%		XE-60 6 ft 1%		QF-1 6 ft 3%	
	220 C Free*	220 C Acetate**	215 C Free	215 C Acetate	225 C Free	225 C Acetate
1 5α-Pregnan-3α-ol-20-one	0.65	0.81	3.78	4.37	2.74	4.36
2 5α-Pregnan-3β-ol-20-one	0.66	0.93	4.26	4.91	3.06	4.96
3 5β-Pregnan-3α-ol-20-one	0.60	0.81	3.83	4.33	2.80	4.08
4 5β-Pregnan-3β-ol-20-one	0.60	0.78	3.48	4.17	2.49	4.40
5 5α-Pregnan-20α-ol-3-one	0.76	1.13	5.92	7.02	4.29	7.28
6 5α-Pregnan-20β-ol-3-one	0.70	1.00	5.13	6.29	4.04	6.80
7 5β-Pregnan-20α-ol-3-one	0.72	0.96	5.48	6.21	4.06	6.80
8 5β-Pregnan-20β-ol-3-one	0.67	0.89	4.78	5.70	3.60	6.24

* Free steroid
** Steroid acetate

nanolone (either 3-hydroxy-20-keto or 20-hydroxy-3-keto) isomers. Their analyses were based on the following observations:

1. The 3-hydroxypregnan-20-ones as a group may be separated from the 20-hydroxypregnan-3-ones by employing gas chromatography with QF-1 as the stationary phase.

2. The 17β side chain of 3-hydroxypregnan-20-ones is in part epimerized to the 17α-configuration following treatment of these steroids with hot methanolic potassium hydroxide or with boiling acid (see page 224). The resulting 3-hydroxy-17α-pregnan-20-ones invariably show shorter retention times than the original corresponding 17β-isomeres during chromatography on QF-1.

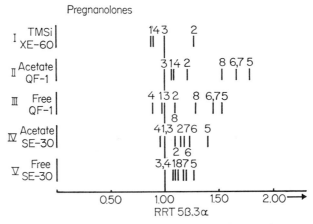

Fig. 7. Graphic representation of retention data of isomeric pregnanolones as the free steroids *(Free)*, as the acetates *(Acetate)* and as the trimethyl silyl ether *(TMSi)* on different stationary phases. All data are presented relative to the retention time of 3α-hydroxy-5β-pregnan-20-one (compound number 3) or the relevant derivative of this compound = 1.00. The numbers (1—8) in the graphs correspond with the different isomers given in Table 7

Retention times for the isomeric pregnanolones and their acetates (VAN DER MOLEN et al., unpublished data, 1966) are recorded in Table 7. From these data and the retention times reported by other investigators (CHAMBERLAIN and THOMAS, 1964; ADLERCREUTZ and LUUKKAINEN, 1964; BROOKS and HANAINEH, 1963; ADLERCREUTZ et al., 1966) (see Figs. 7, 8, 9) it is clear that a reasonable separation of both the free and acetylated pregnanolone isomers can be obtained by using QF-1 and XE-60 phases.

ADLERCREUTZ et al. (1966) used gas chromatography to demonstrate the presence of 3α-hydroxy-5β-pregnan-20-one in "sodium
pregnanediol glucuronidate" isolated according to VENNING (1937).

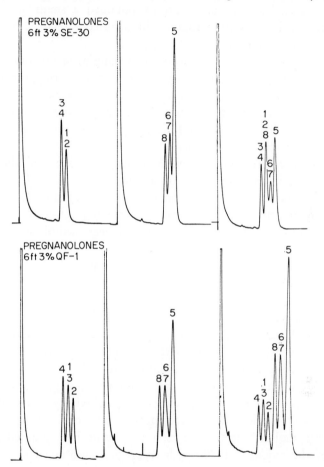

Fig. 8. Chromatographic tracings of mixtures of the isomeric free
pregnanolones following gas chromatography on 6 ft 3⁰/₀ SE-30 and 6 ft
3⁰/₀ QF-1 columns. The numbers (1—8) in the tracings correspond with
the different isomers given in Table 7

In studies (CHAMBERLAIN et al., 1963) on steroid metabolites in
human pregnancy urine, tentative evidence was found for the presence
of a small amount of 20α-hydroxy-5β-pregnan-3-one. The only other
indication for the occurrence of a 20-hydroxypregnan-3-one in humans

is in the work of THYSSEN and ZANDER (1966), which involved the injection of 4-^{14}C-progesterone intravenously in non-pregnant women. Following the extraction of blood samples and hydrolysis with β-glucuronidase, THYSSEN and ZANDER obtained a small amount of radioactivity in a fraction that might have contained 20-hydroxy-pregnan-3-one isomers.

VAN DER MOLEN et al. (1966) routinely employed a method for the determination of 3α-hydroxy-5β-pregnan-20-one in urine; the method was largely based on a modification of previous work (VAN DER MOLEN, 1962 a). A gas chromatographic technique was used for quantitative estimation. This method includes the following steps:

1. Acid hydrolysis of urine,
2. Toluene extraction and washing of the extract with alkali,
3. Column chromatography on alumina,
4. Acetylation of the fraction containing pregnanolone,
5. Column chromatography of the acetylated steroids on alumina,
6. Addition of an internal standard (pregnanediol diacetate) to the eluate containing pregnanolone acetate:
7. Gas chromatographic determination using a 6 ft 3% SE-30 or a 6 ft 3% QF-1 column in combination with a flame ionization detector.

The final samples were expected to contain isomeric pregnanolones (VAN DER MOLEN, 1962 a). Other metabolites of progesterone or 20α-hydroxypregn-4-en-3-one, such as pregnane-3,20-diones or pregnandiols, were excluded by the isolation process.

During metabolic clearance rate studies involving 20α-hydroxy-pregn-4-en-3-one, a larger amount of radioactivity from injected radioactively labeled 20α-hydroxypregn-4-en-3-one was isolated in the "pregnanolone" acetate fraction than could be explained on the basis of the amount of 20α-hydroxypregn-4-en-3-one converted to progesterone. It was moreover observed that the gas chromatographic tracings (SE-30 column) of occasional samples from this experiment showed invariably a shoulder just preceding the main peak (3α-hydroxy-5β-pregnan-20-one acetate peak, Fig. 9, left panel) and occasionally an extra peak just behind the main peak. The shoulder preceding the 3α-hydroxy-5β-pregnan-20-one acetate peak was shown to result from 3α-hydroxy-5β, 17α-pregnan-20-one acetate formed during acid hydrolysis of the urine samples. Gas chromatography of the same samples on QF-1 columns (Fig. 9, right panel) shifted the

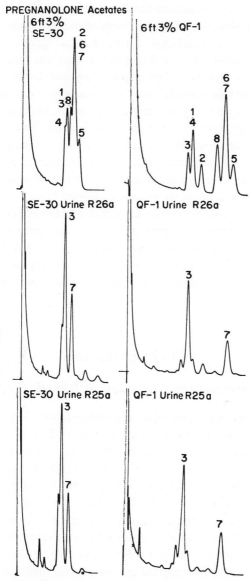

Fig. 9. Chromatographic tracings of mixtures of the eight isomeric pregnanolone (acetates) and samples isolated from term pregnancy urines following gas chromatography on a 6 ft 3% SE-30 column and a 6 ft 3% QF-1 column. The numbers (1—8) in the tracings correspond with the acetates of the different isomers given in Table 7. For further explanations see text

peak with the longer retention time than pregnanolone acetate into the area of the 20-hydroxypregnan-3-one acetates. Further analysis of effluent gas fractions collected during chromatography of such urine samples on a QF-1 column has proved that the material in these fractions is 20α-hydroxy-5β-pregnan-3-one acetate (VAN DER MOLEN et al., 1966). In this work infrared spectrometry and specific chemical transformations resulting in changes of retention time during gas phase chromatography were used for the identification. This peak has only been observed in some urine samples of pregnant women. In five out of six subjects this compound was not found in urine collected during a 6 day period. In the sixth subject the compound was found invariably in all urine samples, in amounts varying from 0.5—3.0 mg/day. Whether the occurrence of this pregnanolone isomer reflects a specific pattern of progesterone metabolism remains an unanswered question.

HAMMOND and LEACH (1967) recently reported the combined estimation of pregnanediol and pregnanolone using gas chromatography of the trimethylsilyl ether derivatives for extracts from pregnancy urine.

IV. Pregnanediols

1. Gas Chromatographic Separation of Isomeric Pregnanediols

Data about the qualitative gas chromatographic behaviour of isomeric pregnanediols have been reported by KNIGHTS and THOMAS (1962 a; 1963 a; 1963 b), BROOKS and HANAINEH (1963), NELSON (1963), CHAMBERLAIN et al. (1964), ADLERCREUTZ and LUUKKAINEN (1964), HAMMOND and LEACH (1965 a; 1965 b), and ADLERCREUTZ et al. (1966). Tables 8, 9 and 10 contain retention data for these steroids. There is not complete agreement between the results obtained under presumably comparable conditions in different laboratories; the values of the retention times expressed relative to the retention time of cholestane vary. Although slight variations might be expected as a result of either temperature dependence of (relative) retention times or differences in column preparation, some of the published values from chromatography on QF-1 or on XE-60 phases (ADLERCREUTZ and LUUKKAINEN, 1964) differ considerably from those obtained by others (see Chapter 1).

Table 8. *Relative retention times of isomeric pregnanediols on* **SE-30** *columns. Retention times are expressed relative to the retention time of cholestane* = *1.00*

		Free steroids			Acetates	
		1 *	2 *	3 *	4 *	5 *
		6 ft, 3%	6 ft, 1%	4.5 ft, 1 %	6 ft, 3%	6 ft, 1%
		210 C	224 C	200 C	220 C	224 C
1	5α-Pregnane-3α,20α-diol	0.71	0.75	—	1.26	1.23
2	5α-Pregnane-3α,20β-diol	0.66	—	—	1.20	—
3	5α-Pregnane-3β,20α-diol	0.72	0.76	0.65	1.45	1.43
4	5α-Pregnane-3β,20β-diol	0.66	0.71	0.60	1.36	1.30
5	5β-Pregnane-3α,20α-diol	0.65	0.70	0.59	1.29	1.21
6	5β-Pregnane-3α,20β-diol	0.62	0.63	0.54	1.20	1.15
7	5β-Pregnane-3β,20α-diol	0.63	—	—	1.24	—
8	5β-Pregnane-3β,20β-diol	0.60	—	—	1.14	—

1*: VAN DER MOLEN et al. (1966); *2**: ADLERCREUTZ and LUUKKAINEN (1964); *3**: BROOKS and HANAINEH (1963); *4**: VAN DER MOLEN et al. (1966); *5**: ADLERCREUTZ and LUUKKAINEN (1964).

Moreover, the sequence of elution for the various isomers chromatographed under apparently similar conditions differ. Fig. 10 presents some of these data in a graphic form. This illustrates more clearly that the elution sequence of the same four pregnanediols as the free steroids on QF-1 columns has been reported as: 1-4-5-3, 4-5-1-3 as well as 4-1-5-3. It may thus be hazardous to identify a pregnanediol isomer, or mixture of isomers, by comparison with retention data from the literature. Comparisons should be made with authentic reference steroids under identical conditions of gas chromatography.

There appears to be little difference between the resolution of the isomeric pregnanediols whether chromatographed as the free compounds or as any one of several derivatives on different stationary

Table 9. *Relative retention times of isomeric pregnanediols on* **XE-60** *columns. Retention times are expressed relative to the retention time of cholestane = 1.00*

	Free steroids			Acetates		TMSi-ethers	
	1* 6 ft, 1% 213 C	2* 5 ft, 3% 245 C	3* 6 ft, 1% 215 C	4* 6 ft, 1% 218 C	5* 6 ft, 1% 215 C	6* 5 ft, 3% 225 C	7* 6 ft, 1% 205 C
1 5α-Pregnane-3α,20α-diol	2.22	3.40	3.87	3.04	5.00	0.78	0.80
2 5α-Pregnane-3α,20β-diol	—	—	3.32	—	4.78	—	—
3 5α-Pregnane-3β,20α-diol	2.47	3.91	4.27	3.36	5.62	1.08	1.13
4 5α-Pregnane-3β,20β-diol	2.17	3.44	3.79	3.21	5.24	1.00	1.05
5 5β-Pregnane-3α,20α-diol	2.11	3.58	3.87	2.93	4.89	0.90	0.90
6 5β-Pregnane-3α,20β-diol	1.98	3.12	3.39	2.70	4.54	0.81	0.78
7 5β-Pregnane-3β,20α-diol	—	—	3.56	—	4.62	—	—
8 5β-Pregnane-3β,20β-diol	—	—	3.08	—	4.31	—	—

1: ADLERCREUTZ and LUUKKAINEN (1964); *2*: HAMMOND and LEACH (1965 a); *3*: VAN DER MOLEN et al. (1966);
4: ADLERCREUTZ and LUUKKAINEN (1964); *5*: VAN DER MOLEN et al. (1966); *6*: HAMMOND and LEACH (1965 b);
7: ADLERCREUTZ and LUUKKAINEN (1964).

Table 10. *Relative retention times of isomeric pregnanediols on* QF-1 *columns. Retention times are expressed relative to the retention time of cholestane* $= 1.00$

	Free steroids				Acetates			TMSi-ethers	Pro-pionates
	1* 6 ft 3% 210 C	2* 6 ft 1% 175 C	3* 4.5 ft 1% 200 C	4* 3 ft 6% 250 C	5* 6 ft 3% 210 C	6* 6 ft 1% 175 C	7* 3 ft 6% 250 C	8* 3 ft 6% 250 C	9* 3 ft 6% 250 C
1 5α-Pregnane-3α,20α-diol	2.04	0.83	—	2.09	5.36	2.20	4.62	0.79	6.17
2 5α-Pregnane-3α,20β-diol	1.88	—	—	1.91	5.05	—	4.47	0.78	5.37
3 5α-Pregnane-3β,20α-diol	2.30	0.90	2.27	2.29	6.16	2.53	4.13	1.05	7.24
4 5α-Pregnane-3β,20β-diol	2.04	0.80	2.01	2.04	5.73	2.28	5.01	1.00	6.46
5 5β-Pregnane-3α,20α-diol	2.07	0.81	2.06	2.19	5.15	2.15	4.31	0.82	5.82
6 5β-Pregnane-3α,20β-diol	1.90	0.75	1.81	1.87	4.77	2.00	3.89	0.76	5.13
7 5β-Pregnane-3β,20α-diol	1.93	—	—	1.93	5.40	—	4.47		6.03
8 5β-Pregnane-3β,20β-diol	1.67	—	—	1.76	5.01	—	4.17		5.43

1: VAN DER MOLEN et al. (1966); *2*: ADLERCREUTZ et al. (1966); *3*: BROOKS and HANAINEH (1963); *4*: CHAMBERLAIN et al. (1964); *5*: VAN DER MOLEN et al. (1966); *6*: ADLERCREUTZ and LUUKKAINEN (1964); *7, 8,* and *9*: CHAMBERLAIN et al. (1966).

phases, as illustrated in Fig. 11. Whenever maximal resolution for pregnanediols is required, the use of the propionate derivatives on QF-1 columns might lead to the best separations. Although the numerical retention data, or their representation as in Figs. 10 and 11, may give the impression that individual isomers can always be

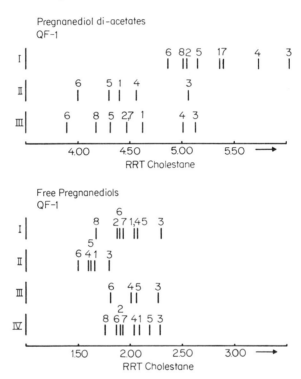

Fig. 10. Graphic representation of retention data of the free and acetylated pregnanediol isomers on **QF-1** columns (see also Table 10). All data are presented relative to the retention time of cholestane = 1. The numbers (1—8) in the graphs correspond to the different isomers given in Table 10. The data on the separation of the *free pregnanediols* in row I are from: VAN DER MOLEN et al. (1966), in row II from: ADLERCREUTZ and LUUKKAINEN (1964). To permit comparison on the same graph, published values of relative retention times (column 2, Table 10) have been multiplied by a factor of 2 and in row III from: BROOKS and HANAINEH (1963); and in row IV from: CHAMBERLAIN et al. (1964). The data on separation of the *acetylated pregnanediols* in row I are from: VAN DER MOLEN et al. (1966); in row II from: ADLERCREUTZ and LUUKKAINEN (1964), (published values, column 6, Table 10, have been multiplied by a factor of 2). Data in row III from: CHAMBERLAIN et al. (1964)

resolved, it should be noted that resolution for any group of derivatives depends upon column efficiency and nature of the liquid phase. This is illustrated by the record of separation (Fig. 12) for free and acetylated pregnanediol isomers chromatographed on 6 ft 3% QF-1 and 6 ft 3% SE-30 columns. It should be recalled, however, that these

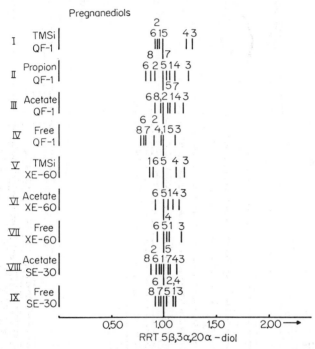

Fig. 11. Graphic representation of retention data of the free isomeric pregnanediols and several derivatives on different phases. All data are presented relative to the retention time of 5β-pregnane-3α,20α-diol (compound number 5) or the relevant derivative of this compound. The numbers (1—8) in the graphs correspond with the different isomers given in Table 10. The data in row I are from: CHAMBERLAIN et al. (1964); II: CHAMBERLAIN et al. (1964); III: VAN DER MOLEN et al. (1966); IV: VAN DER MOLEN et al. (1966); V: HAMMOND and LEACH (1965 a); VI: ADLERCREUTZ and LUUKKAINEN (1964); VII: ADLERCREUTZ and LUUKKAINEN (1964); VIII: VAN DER MOLEN et al. (1966); IX: VAN DER MOLEN et al. (1966)

isomers are even more difficult to separate using paper chromatography (EBERLEIN and BONGIOVANNI, 1958) or column chromatography (KLOPPER et al., 1955). Unambiguous characterization of any pregnanediol isomer can be obtained if the gas chromatographic

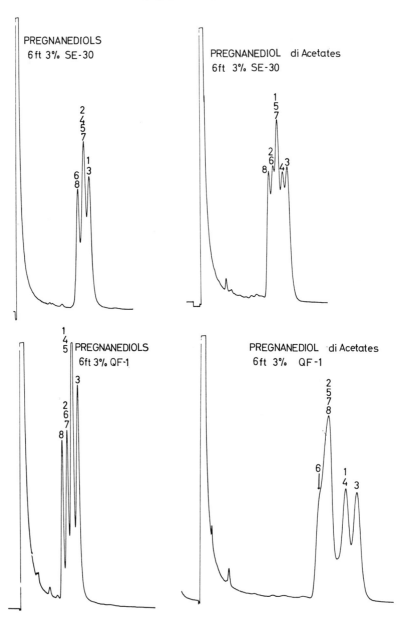

Fig. 12. Chromatographic tracings of a mixture of the eight isomeric pregnanediols and their diacetates following gas chromatography on 6 ft 3% SE-30 and 6 ft QF-1 columns. The numbers (1—8) in the tracings correspond with the different isomers given in Table 10

behaviour of free compounds, derivatives (acetate, trimethylsilyl ethers) and/or oxidation products are studied. CHAMBERLAIN et al. (1964) identified several pregnanediols in the urine of man, monkey, rabbit and guinea-pig with the aid of this technique, and ADLER-CREUTZ et al. (1966) used gas chromatography with different stationary phases in the analysis of sodium pregnanediol glucosiduronate isolated according to VENNING (1937).

In a preliminary communication SHEERIN and SOMMERVILLE (1966) described a quantitative estimation procedure involving gas chromatography of the diacetate of pregnanediol isolated from human blood samples.

2. Quantitative Estimation of Pregnanediol in Human Urine

5β-Pregnan-3α, 20α-diol (pregnanediol) is quantitatively the most important pregnanediol in human urine. It is excreted as a glucosiduronate. In addition, much smaller amounts of 5α-pregnan-3α, 20α-diol (allopregnanediol) and 5α-pregnan-3β, 20α-diol have been isolated from the urine of pregnant women.

The level of excretion of pregnanediol in urine has been generally accepted as a reflection of circulating progesterone, and it should therefore be a useful parameter in the study of ovarian function (i. e. the existence of corpus luteum producing increased amounts of progesterone). Numerous studies have been made of the excretion of pregnanediol in urine during pregnancy, since such measurements are believed to reflect placental progesterone production.

Even prior to the introduction of gas chromatography numerous techniques for the assay of urinary pregnanediol were available, and the methodological pattern for the estimation of pregnanediol in urine is well established. Although in some of the early methods the estimation of conjugated pregnanediol was attempted, most methods have routinely employed:

1. Hydrolysis of the conjugate (boiling with acid or incubation with β-glucuronidase),

2. Extraction of the free steorid,

3. Purification of the extracts to separate pregnanediol from other compounds, by means of solvent partition, column, paper or thin-layer chromatography, including or not including, the chromatographic separation of derivatives,

4. Quantitative measurement of the isolated pregnanediol.

Variations in these steps have resulted in a large number of methods that frequently differ only in detail. The methods developed by KLOP-PER et al. (1955) using a column chromatographic purification procedure, and by EBERLEIN and BONGIOVANNI (1958) involving paper chromatographic purification, have been widely applied and may be considered adequate for clinical purposes in so far as sensitivity, specificity, precision and accuracy are concerned.

In addition, simpler and less time consuming techniques have been applied successfully to the estimation of the larger amounts of pregnanediol in urine during pregnancy (WALDI, 1962). Extensive reviews dealing with the estimation of pregnanediol have recently been published by KLOPPER (1962 a), LORAINE and BELL (1966) and BORTH (1965).

The first applications (COOPER et al., 1962; COOPER and CREECH, 1962) of gas chromatography to the measurement of urinary pregnanediol mainly tried to exploit the specificity of gas chromatographic separations in combination with the sensitivity of detection, in order to increase the speed of analysis. Relatively crude urine extracts were applied to the column. Many of these attempts did not improve or even equal the reliability of already existing techniques. This approach to methodology, however, should be viewed in light of the rapid development of gas chromatography during the time that the application of this technique to steroids was being explored. Many of the stationary phases were not yet fully studied in 1961—1962, and detailed investigations of the quantitative aspects of gas chromatographic detection were still to come. The possibilities and limitations of gas chromatography have been more clearly defined since that time. Thus, it has been recognized that not every problem involving pregnanediol estimation may be solved by a determination based on tracings obtained following gas chromatography of a crude urinary extract.

3. Sensitivity of Detection

The quantitative estimation of isolated pregnanediol, in techniques not employing GLC, during the last 20 years has almost universally been performed with the sulphuric acid reaction according to TALBOT et al. (1941). The corrected molecular absorbancy of the absorption peak at 425 mμ (using ALLEN's correction at 460 and 390 mμ) is in

Table 11. *Relative retention times of several free and acetylated steroids on different stationary phases, employed for the analysis of pregnanediol or pregnanediol diacetate in urinary extracts. Unless otherwise indicated, retention times are expressed relative to the retention time of cholestane = 1.00*

	Free Steroids						Steroid Acetates		
	1* XE-60 6 ft 2% 205 C	2 SE-30 6 ft 1% 200 C	3 QF-1 4.5 ft 1% 200 C	4** SE-52 6 ft 1% 210 C	5 Embaph. 4 ft 3% 240 C	6 NGA 4 ft 220 C	7 XE-60 6 ft 1% 205 C	8 SE-30 6 ft 1% 200 C	9 QF-1 4.5 ft 1% 220 C
1 Androsterone	0.71	0.34	1.96	1.11	0.39	2.39	3.2	0.53	3.3
2 Etiocholanolone	0.71	0.32	2.05	1.00	0.38	2.39	3.3	0.53	3.0
3 Dehydroepiandrosterone	0.76	0.34	1.99	1.13	0.38	2.64	3.6	0.55	3.3
4 11-Ketoetiocholanolone	1.52	0.40	3.98	1.43	0.44	5.36	6.6	0.84	6.4
5 11β-Hydroxyandrosterone	2.29	0.61	4.04	2.22	0.73	10.1	—	0.95	6.6
6 5β-Pregnane-3α,20α-diol	1.00	0.62	2.06	1.92	0.68	4.31	4.4	1.32	4.3
7 5β-Pregnan-3α-ol-20-one	1.01	0.56	2.82	1.74	0.66	3.32	4.4	0.83	3.6
8 5β-Pregnane-3α,17α,20α-triol	—	0.96	—	—	—	—	—	1.92	—

* All values expressed relative to the retention time of pregnanediol = 1.00
** All values expressed relative to the retention time of etiocholanolone = 1.00

The data in column *1*. are from: TURNER et al. (1963); *2*: KIRSCHNER and LIPSETT (1964); *3*: BROOKS and HANAINEH (1963); *4*: PATTI et al. (1963); *5*: COX (1963); *6*: COX (1963); *7*: VAN DER MOLEN et al. (1966); *8*: KIRSCHNER and LIPSETT (1964); *9*: BROOKS and HANAINEH (1963).

Table 12. *Retention times of* **trimethyl silyl ether** *derivatives of several derivative of pregnanediol in extracts from human urine. Unless otherwise* cholestane = 1.00

		1 XE-60 6 ft 3% 262 C	2 XE-60 5 ft 3% 225 C	3 XE-60 6 ft 3% 225 C	4 XE-60 6 ft 2% 215 C	5 XE-60 6 ft 2.8% —
1	Androsterone	1.02	0.96	0.96	1.56	0.94
2	Etiocholanolone	1.18	1.13	1.16	1.81	1.14
3	Dehydroepiandrosterone	1.36	1.33	1.44	2.20	1.30
4	11-Ketoetiocholanolone	2.40	2.51	—	4.10	2.66
5	11β-Hydroxyandrosterone	2.57	3.34	—	4.53	—
6	5β-Pregnane-$3\alpha,20\alpha$-diol	0.78	0.90	0.88	1.53	0.97
7	5β-Pregnan-3α-ol-20-one	1.44	1.55	1.57	2.52	1.50
8	5β-Pregnane-$3\alpha,17\alpha,20\alpha$-triol	—	—	1.88	3.75	1.98

* Values expressed relative to the retention time of androstan-17-one
** Values expressed relative to the retention time of the trimethyl silyl
*** Values expressed relative to the retention time of the trimethyl silyl
from: HARTMAN and WOTIZ (1963); 2: HAMMOND and LEACH (1965 a); (1965); 6: CREECH (1964); 7: VAN DEN HEUVEL et al. (1962); 8: KIRSCHNER LUUKKAINEN (1964); 10: RAMAN et al. (1965); 11: HARTMAN and WOTIZ et al. (1965).

the order of 6.000. This permits the measurement of minimal amounts of ± 5 µg/3 ml of reagent (1—2 µg/ml). Since the lowest excretion of pregnanediol in urine of normal adult human subjects is frequently about 1 mg/day, the sensitivity of detection using the sulphuric acid reaction has not led to difficulties. The sensitivity of detection using gas chromatography (in the order of 0.001—0.1 µg) is much higher and this may lead to the use of smaller urine samples.

4. Specificity

It is clear from the foregoing discussion on separation of isomeric pregnanediols and from the discussion by HORNING (Chapter 1), that the gas chromatographic separation of a single steroid from an un-fractionated urinary extract is still rather involved and may not be successful in all instances.

steroids on different phases employed for analysis of the trimethyl silyl ether
indicated, retention times are expressed relative to the retention time of

6 **	7	8 *	9	10	11	12	13	14 ***
NGS	NGS	NGS	SE-30	QF-1	NGSeb	DC-200	Hi-Eff	STAP
6 ft	6 ft	6 ft	6 ft	4 ft	6 ft	4 ft	6 ft	6.8 ft
2%	1%	1%	1%	1.4%	1%	1.5%	1%	3%
210 C	212 C	200 C	205 C	—	231 C	222 C	242 C	233 C
1.27	1.09	1.44	0.37	1.25	0.60	0.56	0.78	0.67
1.70	1.34	1.87	0.39	1.25	0.73	0.60	0.98	0.80
2.00	1.57	2.20	0.46	1.30	0.84	0.52	1.14	1.00
4.30	—	4.15	—	2.14	1.36	0.63	2.03	1.63
5.40	—	5.25	—	—	1.87	—	2.59	0.78
1.00	0.93	1.85	0.98	1.00	0.70	1.00	0.68	0.54
—	—	—	0.54	1.51	1.08	0.79	1.38	—
2.78	—	—	1.32	1.94	—	1.52	—	1.16

= 1.
ether derivative of pregnanediol = 1.
ether derivative of dehydroepiandrosterone = 1. The data in colum *1.* are
3: Curtius (1966); *4:* Kirschner and Lipsett (1964); *5:* Raman et al.
and Lipsett (1964); *9:* van den Heuvel et al. (1962), and Adlercreutz and
(1963); *12:* Raman et al. (1965); *13:* Hartman and Wotiz (1963); *14:* Oaks

If, as is the case for pregnanediol in pregnancy urine, the steroid
is present in large excess over other steroids, it may be possible to
obtain an isolated peak in the gas chromatographic tracing. The
compound of interest may under these conditions be measured without
much interference from other compounds that are present in much
smaller amounts.

The retention data of the free compounds, acetates and trimethylsilyl ethers of pregnanediol and some other steroids that might be
present in comparable amounts in crude extracts of urine are listed in
Tables 11 and 12. Figs. 13, 14 present a graphic representation of
these retention data relative to the retention time of pregnanediol
or that of the relevant pregnanediol derivative.

It is evident from these data that the separation reported by
different authors on similar stationary phases are not always in
agreement. Although Hartman and Wotiz (1963) observed an

excellent separation of pregnanediol ditrimethylsilyl ether from several other steroid trimethylsilyl ethers using a 6 ft 3% XE-60 column at 262°, the separations obtained by KIRSCHNER and LIPSETT (1964) on a 6 ft 2% XE-60 column at 215°, by HAMMOND and LEACH (1965 a) on a 5 ft 3% XE-60 column at 225°, and CURTIUS (1966) on

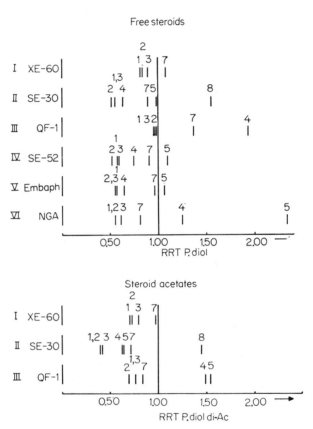

Fig. 13. Graphic representation of retention data of pregnanediol and other steroids, that may be present in extracts of human urine. All data are presented relative to the retention time of pregnanediol or pregnanediol diacetate = 1.00. The numbers (1—8) in the graphs correspond with the different steroids given in Table 12. The data on the separation of the *free steroids* in row I are from: VAN DER MOLEN et al. (1966); II: KIRSCHNER and LIPSETT (1964); III: BROOKS and HANAINEH (1964); IV: PATTI et al. (1963); V: COX (1963); VI: COX (1963). The data on the separation of the *acetylated steroids* in row I are from: VAN DER MOLEN et al. (1966); II: KIRSCHNER and LIPSETT (1964); III: BROOKS and HANAINEH (1964)

a 6 ft 3% XE-60 column at 225° were less specific. In the latter studies the peak for androsterone trimethylsilyl ether might interfere with the peak of pregnanediol ditrimethylsilyl ether.

The same remark applies to the separation of steroid trimethylsilyl ethers on NGS columns. KIRSCHNER and LIPSETT (1964) using a 6 ft 1% NGS column at 200° observed a retention sequence definitely

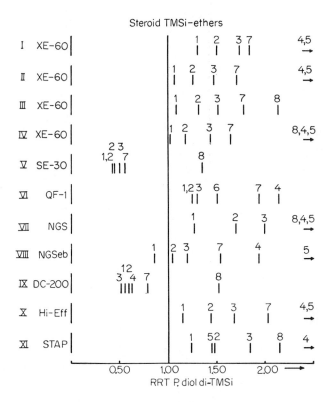

Fig. 14. Graphic representation of retention data of the *trimethyl silyl ethers* of pregnanediol and other steroids that may be present in extracts of human urine. All data are presented relative to the retention time of pregnanediol di-(trimethylsilyl ether) = 1.00. The numbers (1—8) in the graphs correspond with the different steroids given in Table 12. The data in row I are from: HARTMAN and WOTIZ (1963); II: HAMMOND and LEACH (1965 a); III: CURTIUS (1966); IV: KIRSCHNER and LIPSETT (1964); V: VANDENHEUVEL et al. (1962); VI: RAMAN et al. (1965); VII: CREECH (1964); VIII: HARTMAN and WOTIZ (1963); IX: RAMAN et al. (1965); X: HARTMAN and WOTIZ (1963); XI: OAKS et al. (1965)

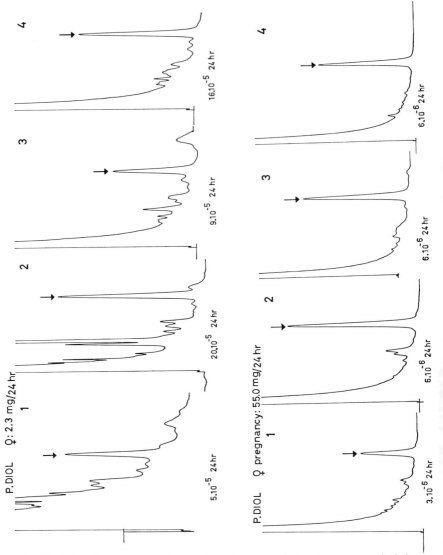

Fig. 15. Gas chromatographic tracings from analysis of pregnanediol in urine. Urine was hydrolyzed with hydrochloric acid and extracted with toluene according to KLOPPER et al. (1955). The toluene extract was washed with 1 N NaOH solution and water and subsequently evaporated to dryness. *Experiment 1:* the residue was acetylated and subjected to gas chromatography (see: WOTIZ 1963); *Experiment 2:* the residue was acetylated, subjected to thin-layer chromatography on silica gel using the solvent system benzene-ethylacetate 8—2; the pregnanediol diacetate area was eluted, evaporated and subjected to gas chromatography (see: KIRSCH-NER and LIPSETT 1964, 1965); *Experiment 3:* the residue was chromatographed on an alumina column according to KLOPPER et al. (1955); the

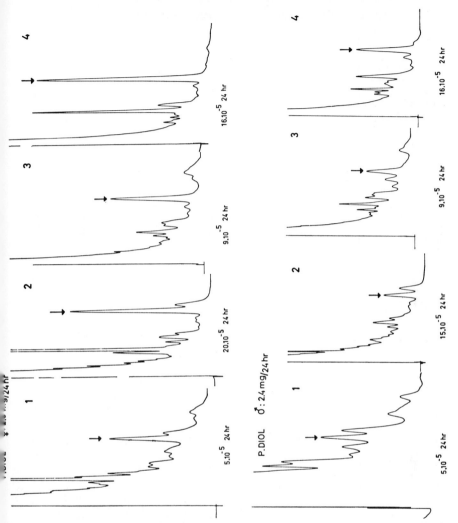

Fig. 16. Gas chromatographic tracings obtained for the analysis of pregnanediol in urine. For explanation see Fig. 15

pregnanediol containing fraction was collected, evaporated to dryness, acetylated and subjected to gas chromatography; *Experiment 4:* the residue was purified using the complete procedure according to KLOPPER et al. (1955); the final pregnanediol diacetate containing residue was subjected to gas chromatography.

Gas chromatography was performed using a 6 ft 3% SE-30 column (on 80/100 mesh Gas Chrom Q); column temperature: 225° C; carrier gas: nitrogen (70 ml/min). Detection: flame ionization. The arrows in the figure indicate the peaks corresponding in retention time to those of authentic pregnanediol diacetate

Table 13. *Methods for quantitative estimation of pregnanediol in human urine*

References	Extraction and purification following hydrolysis	Free steroid or derivative used for GLC	Stationary phase used for GLC	Other steroids estimated from chromatographic tracing
JONES et al. (1962) and TURNER et al. (1963) LAU and JONES (1964)	Toluene extraction; no further purification, thin-layer chromatography	Free steroid	Poly siloxane	
PATTI et al. (1963 a, b, c)	Compared several techniques for hydrolysis and extraction; no purification	Free steroid	SE-52	
JANSEN (1963)	Benzene extraction of precipitate obtained after boiling urine with HCl	Free steroid	SE-30	
COX (1963)	*Low titre:* toluene extraction, NaOH wash, column chromatography *High titre:* toluene extraction, NaOH wash	Free steroid	NGA	
BARRY et al. (1966)	Extraction, silica gel column chromatography	Free steroid	SE-30/XE-60	
WOTIZ (1963)	Toluene extraction, NaOH wash, acetylation	Acetate	SE-30	
KIRSCHNER and LIPSETT (1964, 1965); KIRSCHNER et al. (1964)	Toluene extraction, acetylation, thin-layer chromatography	Acetate	SE-30	
VANDENHEUVEL et al. (1962)	Extraction, TMSi-ether preparation	Trimethyl silyl ether	XE-60	17-Ketosteroids

References	Extraction and purification following hydrolysis	Free steroid or derivative used for GLC	Stationary phase used for GLC	Other steroids estimated from chromatographic tracing
CREECH (1964)	Extraction, TMSi-ether preparation	Trimethyl silyl ether	NGS	Pregnanetriol and 17-ketosteroids
KINOSHITA and ISURUGI (1964) KINOSHITA et al. (1966)	Extraction, alumina column chromatography. TMSi-ether preparation	Trimethyl silyl ether	XE-60	
RAMAN et al. (1965)	Extraction, 1st thin-layer chromatography, 2nd thin-layer chromatography, TMSi-ether preparation	Trimethyl silyl ether	DC-200	
CURTIUS (1966)	Extraction, TMSi-ether preparation	Trimethyl silyl ether	XE-60	Pregnanetriol, pregnanetriolone and 17-ketosteroids
RIVERA et al. (1967)	Extraction, NaOH wash, silicagel column chromatography, TMSi-ether preparation	Trimethyl silyl ether	XE-60	
HAMMOND and LEACH (1967)	Extraction, TMSi-ether preparation	Trimethyl silyl ether	XE-60	Pregnanolone
GARDINER and HORNING (1965)	Extraction, preparation of methoxim-TMSi derivatives	Trimethyl silyl ether	SE-30	Complete spectrum of all steroids using temperature programmed GLC
MENINI and NORYMBERSKI (1965)	Extraction, KBH_4 reduction, HIO_4 oxidation, Girard separation, t. butylchromate oxidation	Pregnanedione	SE-30	Other reduction and/or oxidation products

different from the sequence for the same steroid trimethylsilyl ethers reported by CREECH (1965) on a 6 ft 2% NGS column at 210°, and by VAN DEN HEUVEL et al. (1962) on a 6 ft 1% NGS column at 212°. This might be due to differences in column temperature and to differences in the silanization treatment of the support.

Direct measurement of free pregnanediol in crude urine extracts may be feasible as shown by COX (1963) for urine containing large amounts of pregnanediol as compared to other steroids. A neopentyl-glycol adipate (NGA) column was used. The acetylation of crude extracts and subsequent gas chromatography on an SE-30 phase may be preferred in some instances. For samples obtained during pregnancy, no other purification may be necessary, and peaks for pregnanediol diacetate may easily be used for quantitative measurements. For samples from nonpregnant subjects a simple thin-layer chromatographic purification of the acetylated samples will routinely permit isolation of pregnanediol diacetate; this purification may not be necessary, however, for all samples. For those samples containing very small amounts (less than 1 mg/24 hr) this chromatographic step may significantly improve specificity and accordingly the accuracy of the estimation.

The gas chromatographic tracings recorded in Fig. 15 and 16 illustrate work from our own laboratory (VAN DER MOLEN et al., 1966) which is in complete agreement with the data of WOTIZ (1963), of KIRSCHNER and LIPSETT (1964; 1965) and of BRUSH et al. (1966).

For the estimation of pregnanediol alone, the gas chromatographic separation of the trimethylsilyl ether derivative of the steroid does not have significant advantages over the separation of the acetate. Both derivatives may be adequately separated from other steroids on an SE-30 column. The steroid acetates are stable derivatives, while the trimethylsilyl ethers are easily hydrolyzed. If, however, the simultaneous estimation of individual 17-ketosteroids and pregnanediol is attempted in the same sample, more efficient separations may be obtained between the trimethylsilyl ethers of the individual compounds using a number of stationary phases (Tables 11 and 12). This is in agreement with the results obtained by HORNING and GARDINER (1965), by CREECH (1965) and by CURTIUS (1966).

Table 13 summarizes some of the approaches that have included gas chromatography for measurement of urinary pregnanediol.

5. Routine Estimations of Free Pregnanediol

JONES et al. (1962) and TURNER et al. (1963) attempted to estimate pregnanediol in urine following hydrolysis and toluene extraction, using a gas chromatographic separation of an aliquot of the extract on a polysiloxane column. They reported quantitative recoveries when as little as 0.25 mg of pregnanediol was added to a 24 hr urine specimen. The percentage recovery of free pregnanediol and sodium pregnanediol glucosiduronate added to urine samples ranged from 69—95%. The method was not completely specific for pregnanediol in that allopregnanediol and pregnanolone could not be separated on this column. In a subsequent publication, LAU and JONES (1964) reported the use of preparative thin-layer chromatography for the isolation of pregnanediol prior to gas chromatography. Their chart for a gas chromatographic separation of an extract of acid-hydrolyzed pregnancy urine, after thin-layer chromatographic purification, still shows a shoulder of allopregnanediol on the pregnanediol peak.

PATTI et al. (1963 a, b), using gas chromatography on an SE-30 column, measured pregnanediol as the free compound in samples of urine following various hydrolytic and extraction procedures. Although the separation of pregnanediol from etiocholanolone and androsterone might have been acceptable, other steroids (pregnanolone, 11β-hydroxyandrosterone) could interfere with the quantification of the pregnanediol peak. Prior to gas chromatography hydrolysis and extraction according to KLENDSHOJ et al. (1953), (boiling with 30% hydrochloric acid and extraction with ethylene dichloride) were adequate for qualitative screening. The authors indicated, however, that precise analysis under their condition of gas chromatography was only possible after further purification of the extracts.

JANSEN (1963) reported the gas chromatographic analysis of a benzene solution containing material that precipitated after boiling urine with hydrochloric acid. This precipitate is believed to contain pregnanediol. The limitations of this procedure are those related to gas chromatographic separation of such extracts on a SE-30 column show a main peak corresponding in retention time to that of authentic pregnanediol. The limitations of this procedure are more over related to the specificity of gas chromatography of the free steroids on a SE-30 column, and the limited accuracy that may be obtained as a result of the initial precipitation of the pregnanediol. For four urine samples containing from 3.7—10.6 mg pregnanediol/100 ml benzene, the authors showed that the direct sulphuric acid reaction of such precipitates results in up to 50% higher estimates than detection following gas chromatography. Repeated estimation of a urine extract containing 3.67 mg pregnanediol/100 ml benzene had a precision of 0.26 mg per 100 ml. Recoveries of authentic pregnanediol added to the benzene extract prior to gas phase chromatography were 80—110%. Cox (1963) measured pregnanediol in extracts of urine following gas chromatography on NGA and Embaphase as stationary phases. The NGA phase was preferred because of better separations from contaminating steroids. The author carried out a gas chromatographic evaluation of extracts from different stages in the method of KLOPPER et al. (1955). When the toluene extract obtained from pregnancy urines was subjected to gas chromatography, a distinctly isolated peak corresponding in retention time to pregnanediol was obtained, without interference from other steroids. Crude extracts from different pregnancy urines gave 37.0—28.0—8.9—7.5 and 4.2 mg pregnanediol per 24 hr versus 38.0—30.0—9.0—8.3 and 3.8 mg/24 hr when the same urinary samples were subjected to the complete KLOPPER procedure. The recovery of pregnanediol added to pregnancy urine was 92—103%. In urine from nonpregnant subjects, acceptable results were obtained following purification of the urine extracts using the first alumina column chromatography of the method of KLOPPER et al. (1955). Gas chromatography on NGA of such samples gave tracings with a major peak corresponding to that of pregnanediol. Similar observations were made by BRUSH et al. (1966) employing QF-1 columns.

BARRY et al. (1966) undertook an evaluation of several methods for determining urinary pregnanediol using gas chromatography. For purification of their samples prior to gas chromatography they compared: 1) toluene-acid hydrolysis and extraction; 2) extraction of conjugates with ether-ethanol followed by perchloric acid-tetrahydrofuran solvolysis; 3) enzymic hydrolysis, chloroform extraction and silica gel column chromatography. Gas chromatography of the final extracts was carried out on mixed 1% XE-60 — 1% SE-30 columns. Such columns will not separate pregnanediol efficiently from other free steroids (Table 11). Purification of extracts prior to gas chromatography was found essential. They concluded that a method using enzymic hydrolysis, with preliminary purification using silica gel column chromatography and quantification of the free pregnanediol by gas chromatography, is to be preferred. Recovery of free pregnanediol at a level of 0.3 mg/l was reported to be 83%. The recovery decreased at high concentration of pregnanediol in urine because of insufficient elution from the silica gel column. The precision of estimation using measurement of peak heights of unknown samples as compared to those of standards was 5—10% (1.1—13.9 mg/l).

6. Routine Estimations of Pregnanediol Diacetate

WOTIZ (1963) and WOTIZ and CHATTORAJ (1966) acetylated the steroids extracted with toluene from acid-hydrolyzed urine. Gas chromatography on a 6 ft 3% SE-30 column was employed to isolate the pregnanediol diacetate. The material corresponding in retention time to that of an authentic reference standard was shown to be pregnanediol diacetate by infrared spectrophotometric analysis of the collected gas fraction. The reproducibility of this technique was estimated to be in the order of 6%, whereas the lower limit of sensitivity was given as 50 μg/24 hr.

CHATTORAJ et al. (1966) have recently reported simultaneous estimation of pregnanediol and pregnanetriol following gas chromatography of acetylated crude extracts. The method used for urine from men and non-pregnant women involved precipitation of free and conjugated steroids by ammonium sulphate, enzymic hydrolysis, ether extraction, sodium hydroxide and water washes, acetylation and gas chromatographic estimation.

KIRSCHNER and LIPSETT (1964; 1965; KIRSCHNER et al., 1964) acetylated the ether extractable steroids obtained from acid-hydrolyzed urine. They isolated the pregnanediol diacetate-containing area of a thin-layer plate after chromatography in the solvent system benzene-ethyl acetate, 8 : 2. It was reported that pregnanediol (diacetate) could be measured without significant interference from other steroids after chromatography on an SE-30 column. Appreciable amounts of allopregnanediol (diacetate) might interfere slightly with the estimation of pregnanediol diacetate. The sensitivity of the technique was given as 50 μg/24 hr using 10—20% of a 24 hr urine sample. For randomly selected urine samples, the precision was estimated as 3% at a 24 hr excretion level of 0.55 mg and 5% at a level of 1.9 mg/24 hr. The accuracy was tested following the addition of pregnanediol to urine; a recovery of 80—108% of 0.5 mg of preg-nanediol was reported.

7. Routine Estimations of Pregnanediol Trimethylsilyl Ether

Steroid trimethylsilyl ether derivatives are easily hydrolyzed by traces of moisture. To avoid possible decomposition, steroids con-verted to trimethylsilyl ethers are frequently subjected to gas chro-matographic analysis without further purification. Although excess reagent does not generally interfere with the gas chromatographic analysis, such techniques may be criticized from a fundamental point of view since it is assumed that derivative formation is quantitative. Free steroid present in the reaction mixture, either because the steroid is not converted to a derivative or as a result of decomposition of the derivative, is separated only during gas chromatography. Whenever an internal standard behaving similarly to the steroids under investi-gation is added to the sample prior to derivative formation, incom-pleteness of reaction or decomposition of the product(s) can be cor-rected. As long as radioactively labeled pregnanediol is not generally available, non-radioactive substances may be used as internal stan-dards in such experiments. For this purpose VANDEN HEUVEL et al. (1962) and HORNING et al. (1963) used β-sitosterol, CREECH (1965) used coprostan-3α-ol, and CURTIUS (1966) used pregnanolone. It should be stressed once more that standard amounts of authentic free steroids used for calibration in any method should be treated in exactly the same ways as the unknown sample. Whenever this is done, the same internal standards should be used to evaluate conversion and/or decomposition. Ample proof has been presented that complete, quantitative conversions to the trimethylsilyl ethers of steroids can be obtained under appropriate circumstances (LUUKKAINEN et al., 1961; CREECH, 1964; RAMAN et al., 1965; CURTIUS, 1966). (See also Chapter 1.)

RAMAN et al. (1965) prepared pregnanediol ditrimethylsilyl ether from samples obtained after fractionation of extracts from enzy-matically hydrolyzed urine. Using thin-layer chromatography on alumina with an ethanol-benzene (1 : 66) mixture as developing sol-vent, the 17-ketosteroids were separated from a fraction containing pregnanediol, pregnanetriol and pregnanetriolone. A second thin-layer chromatographic separation on alumina (solvent system: ethanol-benzene, 1 : 8) separated pregnanediol from the other two steroids. Following preparation of the trimethylsilyl ether, aliquots were injected on a DC-200 column. Although ³H-labeled pregnanediol was used to correct for losses up to the stage of gas chromatography, no internal standard was used to validate the trimethylsilyl ether preparation and analysis. The sensitivity of this determination was reported to be on the order of 20 µg/24 hrs, whereas the precision was estimated to be in the order of 5%. For routine analysis, pregnanetriol and pregnanetriolone in the same urine samples were analyzed along the same lines.

CURTIUS (1966) used trimethylsilyl ether derivatives of the residue from an alkali-washed ether extract of hydrolyzed urine. The gas chromatographic tracings were used for the simultaneous measurement of 17-ketosteroids, pregnanediol, pregnanetriol and pregnanetriolone. To correct for losses throughout the complete procedure, pregnanolone was added as an internal standard to the urine prior to hydrolysis. The gas chromatographic tracings of urine samples did not indicate complete separation of different peaks; some overlap of neighbouring peaks was observed. Although such overlap may have affected the quantification, the precision of measurement at a level of 1.9 mg pregnanediol/l was estimated as 10%.

RIVERA et al. (1967) described a method for the estimation of 17-ketosteroids, pregnanediol and pregnanetriol in urine, involving preliminary separation of the steroids on a silica gel column. This separation resulted in a first fraction containing the 17-ketosteroids, a second containing pregnanediol and a third containing pregnanetriol. After formation of the trimethylsilyl ethers, the individual fractions were analyzed separately by gas chromatography on a 6 ft XE-60 column. Tritium-labeled steroids were added prior to extraction of the urines to check for recoveries up to the gas chromatography stage. Cholesterol was added as an internal standard to check the efficiency of trimethylsilyl ether formation and to aid in quantification of the gas chromatographic separation. The authors emphasize the necessity of a proper separation of etiocholanolone and pregnanediol prior to gas chromatography, because the trimethylsilyl ethers of these steroids are not well separated by GLC on XE-60 columns. Using a 1/25 aliquot of a 24 hr urine, levels of 100 µg/24 hr could be determined, whereas with larger urine fractions the sensitivity might be increased. The coefficient of variation at a level of 4.32 mg pregnanediol/24 hrs was reported to be 0.14 mg (13.2%). The method has been applied to steroid measurement in urine from normal and abnormal human subjects. HAMMOND and LEACH (1967) reported the combined estimation of pregnanediol and pregnanolone in extracts from pregnancy urine. Following acid hydrolysis and toluene extraction, trimethylsilyl ethers of the extracted steroids were prepared. Gas chromatography of these derivatives was done on a 6 ft 3% XE-60 column. According to the authors this permitted adequate separation of the derivatives of pregnanediol and pregnanolone; for these samples (during pregnancy) the resolution from ketosteroid trimethylsilyl ethers was reported to be satisfactory.

In their systematic analysis of urinary steroids using sequential oxidations and reductions, MENINI and NORYMBERSKI (1965) estimated 5β-pregnane-3,20-dione following gas chromatography of the final extract. This 5β-pregnanedione originated from urinary 3,20-disubstituted pregnanes and may therefore be expected to reflect the combined excretion of 5β-pregnane-3,20-diols and 5β-pregnanolone as well as 5β-pregnane-3,20-dione in urine.

8. Accuracy and Precision

The *accuracy* and *precision* of several gas chromatographic methods for the estimation of pregnanediol in urine are comparable with those of techniques not employing gas-liquid chromatography. Recoveries of appropriate steroids (either free pregnanediol or the pregnanediol glucosiduronate) added to water or urine have been reported from 80 to 100% (JONES et al., 1962; KIRSCHNER and LIPSETT, 1964).

The precision of a complete method involving detection and quantification following gas-liquid chromatography depends on variable losses that may occur prior to gas chromatography and also on the specificity of the final gas chromatographic analysis. The precision attained with the most commonly employed detection system, the flame ionization detector, may be on the order of 3—5% (RAMAN et al., 1965; KIRSCHNER and LIPSETT, 1964).

For a large series of urines, no difference was observed (VAN DER MOLEN, 1965) between the precision using flame ionization detection following gas chromatography and spectrophotometric detection of

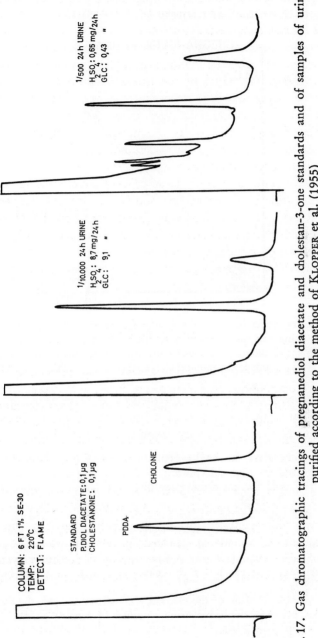

COLUMN: 6 FT 1% SE-30
TEMP: 220°C
DETECT: FLAME

STANDARD
P.DIOL DIACETATE: 0,1 μg
CHOLESTANONE: 0,1 μg

PDDA·

CHOLONE

1/10.000 24 h URINE
H_2SO_4: 8,7 mg/24 h
GLC: 9,1 "

1/500 24 h URINE
H_2SO_4: 0,65 mg/24 h
GLC: 0,43 "

Fig. 17. Gas chromatographic tracings of pregnanediol diacetate and cholestan-3-one standards and of samples of urine purified according to the method of KLOPPER et al. (1955)

the sulphuric acid chromogen of pregnanediol diacetate isolated according to the method of KLOPPER et al. (1955) *.

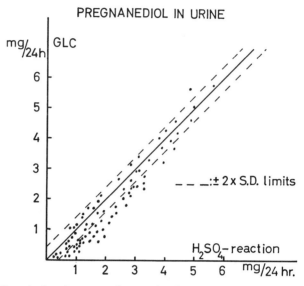

Fig. 18. Correlation between the results for measurement of pregnanediol diacetate using the sulphuric acid reaction and flame ionization detection following gas chromatography using the same urine samples purified according to the method of KLOPPER et al. (1955)

In addition, the increase in *specificity* that might be obtained using gas chromatographic isolation of pregnanediol diacetate isolated according to KLOPPER et al. may favourably influence the accuracy of

---

* Residues after the final chromatography of pregnanediol diacetate were dissolved in 1 ml chloroform; 1/10th of the sample was taken to dryness and used for gas chromatography. The remainder was evaporated and used for the sulphuric acid reaction (measuring the peak absorption at 420 mμ and applying the ALLEN correction at 380 and 460 mμ). To the samples for gas chromatography were added appropriate amounts of 5α-cholestan-3-one as internal standard and aliquots were injected on a 6 ft 3% SE-30 column (Fig. 17). A flame ionization detector was employed. The precision using gas liquid chromatography was shown to be on the order of 5%.

The overall precision of the method was calculated from the differences in results between duplicate urine samples (Table 14) as the standard

$$\text{deviation} = \sqrt{\frac{(\text{differences})^2}{2\,N}}$$

Table 14. *Precision of estimation of pregnanediol in urine containing 0.10—5.53 mg/24 hr. 1/20th of the 24 hr urine sample was analyzed according to* KLOPPER *et al. (1955). The pregnanediol diacetate in the final residue was measured using the sulphuric acid reaction or by flame ionization detection following gas chromatography*

Method of quantification	Number of duplicate analysis	Standard deviation (mg/24 hr)
Sulphuric acid reaction	64	0.19
Flame ionization detection	68	0.20

the result. It appears (Fig. 18) that at low levels in the urine a large number of samples show significantly lower concentrations when determined by flame ionization detection and gas chromatography than after quantification with the sulphuric acid reaction. This may indicate the presence of impurities in the final residue that may cause inflated results when the sulphuric acid reaction is used.

9. Conclusion

From these data it is evident that several methods are available for gas chromatographic measurement of pregnanediol in urine. Although crude urinary extracts may be used in a gas chromatographic separation for the detection of pregnanediol, this does not necessarily imply adequate reliability of the quantitative result. However, it may safely be predicted that it will be possible to select or modify a technique for the measurement of urinary pregnanediol that will more frequently than not result in either a faster, a more sensitive, or a more specific assay than could have been obtained without the use of gas chromatography. Gas chromatography on SE-30 or QF-1 columns of pregnanediol-containing samples, isolated from urine following acetylation or trimethylsilyl ether preparation, will lead to adequate information about the specificity of the estimation and will indicate the extent of interference by major 17-ketosteroids whenever these are present. Both the SE-30 and QF-1 columns, however, may tend to give a single peak of the acetates of pregnanediol and allopregnanediol (Figs. 11 and 12). Since 5β-pregnane-$3\alpha,20\alpha$-diol is normally present in so much larger amounts than 5α-pregnane-$3\alpha,20\alpha$-diol this may influence the final quantitative result only slightly. If the determination is carried out to obtain an estimate of progesterone production, the combined estimate including both pregnanediol isomers may be as good a parameter as the estimate of either isomer alone. A technique for pregnanediol estimation in urine as outlined in Table 15 may suffice for most clinical purposes. It may be expected that simple estimations may be completely automated using devices for automatic solid sample application (PODMORE, 1966) and automatic digital print-out of the gas chromatographic elution pattern.

Table 15. *Technique for serial and routine analysis of pregnanediol in urine*
Pregnant subjects:
1. Acid or enzymic hydrolysis of urine
2. Toluene extraction of urine
3. Washing of toluene extract with 1 N NaOH solution and water; evaporation to dryness
4. Acetylation of residue
5. Addition of a known amount of internal standard, f. i. cholestanone
6. Gas chromatography on a 6 ft 3% SE-30 column, using flame ionization detection
Non-pregnant subjects:
Same procedure, with addition of:
4a. Thin-layer chromatography on silica gel, using the solvent system benzene-ethylacetate 8—2 for isolation of pregnanediol diacetate

V. 17α-Hydroxyprogesterone and Reduced Metabolites

17α-Hydroxyprogesterone is produced mainly in the adrenal cortex, and it is an intermediate in the biosynthetic sequence leading to the formation of corticosteroids. In certain clinical disorders associated with increased 17α-hydroxyprogesterone secretion the excretion of metabolites of 17α-hydroxyprogesterone, such as 5β-pregnane-3α,17α,20α-triol and 3α,17α-dihydroxy-5β-pregnan-20-one (17α-hydroxypregnanolone) may be increased and the estimation of these compounds in urine may be of diagnostic value.

Several authors (ROSENFELD et al., 1962; CHAMBERLAIN and THOMAS, 1964; BROOKS, 1965) have observed that 17α-hydroxyprogesterone and other 17α-hydroxypregnan-20-one steroids are structurally altered at the temperatures employed during gas chromatography. Homoannulation of the D-ring occurs (Fig. 19). This was expected on the basis of the earlier observations of VON EUW and REICHSTEIN (1941) with respect to heating such steroids above their melting points.

ROSENFELD et al. (1962) report quantitative conversion of 3β,17α-dihydroxy-5β-pregnan-20-one to 17α-hydroxy-17β-methyl-D-homo-5β-androstan-17α-one (structure II, Fig. 19) during gas chromatography. In addition CHAMBERLAIN and THOMAS (1964) have found evidence for the formation of the 17aα-hydroxy-17aβ-methyl-D-

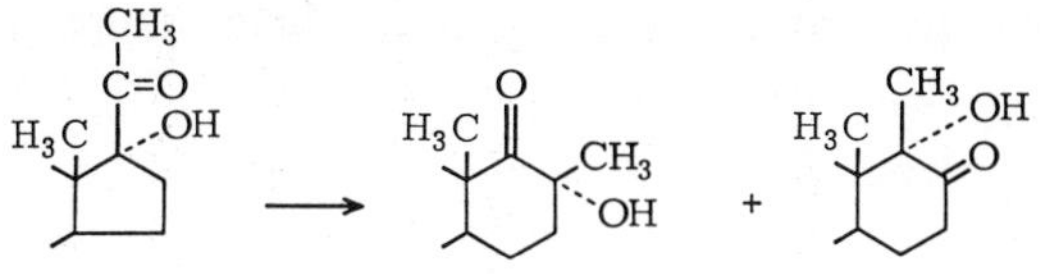

Fig. 19. Rearrangement of 17α-hydroxypregnane-20-ketosteroids during gas chromatography. I: 17α-hydroxypregnane-20-keto steroid; II: 17α-hydroxy, 17β-methyl-D-homoandrostan-17α-keto steroid; III: 17α-hydroxy, 17aβ-methyl-D-homoandrostan-17-keto steroid

homoandrostane-17-one isomer (structure III, Fig. 19). Treatment of such 17α-hydroxypregnan-20-one steroids with hot alkali or acid followed by gas chromatography results in both 17β → 17α epimerization and D-homoannulation, giving 17aβ-hydroxy-17aα-methyl-D-homoandrostan-17-one as the major product seen in the gas chromatographic tracing (CHAMBERLAIN and THOMAS, 1964). BROOKS (1965) reported that 17α-acetoxy-20-keto steroids (unsubstituted at C-21) are stable during gas chromatography and give well-defined single peaks. Acetylation of the 17α-hydroxyl groups may be achieved in good yield by using acetic anhydride containing p-toluenesulfonic acid rather than the usual acetic anhydride-pyridine mixture.

VAN DER MOLEN and EIK-NES (see chapter 4) estimated 17α-hydroxyprogesterone isolated from dog spermatic vein blood and testicular tissue. 17α-Hydroxyprogesterone-containing extracts were purified by paper and thin-layer chromatographic techniques. After the oxidation of 17α-hydroxyprogesterone-containing fractions using chromium trioxide, the resulting 4-androsten-3,17-dione was purified by thin-layer chromatography and, following the addition of suitable internal standards, subjected to gas chromatography on a 6 ft 1% XE-60 column. As a result of the relatively low recoveries of the steroid through several stages of this procedure, the overall sensitivity of this approach was limited to the detection of 0.1—0.2 µg 17α-hydroxyprogesterone. The precision of the estimation was 3—5%.

VI. Pregnanetriol in Human Urine

Since pregnanetriol and related steroids (such as $3\alpha,17\alpha,20\alpha$-trihydroxy-$5\beta$-pregnan-11-one and $3\alpha,17\alpha$-dihydroxy-5β-pregnan-20-one) are destroyed during acid hydrolysis at elevated temperatures, the conjugates of these steroids in urine must be hydrolyzed by enzymic means. Techniques for the estimation of these compounds in urine (Table 16) have generally included:

1. Enzymic hydrolysis.

2. Extraction.

3. Purification of extracts (i. e., isolation of individual compounds).

4. Quantitative estimation.

The behaviour during gas chromatography of *free* pregnanetriol may be less ideal than that of its derivatives, such as the acetate or the trimethylsilyl ether. KIRSCHNER and LIPSETT (1964) observed that free pregnanetriol may occasionally be adsorbed into certain stationary phases and supports, thus resulting in loss of sensitivity for estimation of the compound isolated from urine. ROSENFELD (1965) reported that 1—2 µg of the trimethylsilyl ether derivative of pregnanetriol may give a response equivalent to 5—8 µg of the free steroid using flame ionization detection. Therefore, derivative formation prior to gas chromatography of such polar steroids must be considered the method of choice.

Acetates were employed by ROSENFELD et al. (1962; ROSENFELD, 1965; CHATTORAJ et al., 1966) as were the trimethylsilyl ethers. The trimethylsilyl ethers were also used by KIRSCHNER and LIPSETT (1964; 1965), RAMAN et al. (1965), CREECH (1965), CURTIUS (1966), KINOSHITA et al. (1966) and RIVERA et al. (1967) for the analysis of pregnanetriol. CREECH (1965) and CURTIUS (1966) in attempting serial analyses for pregnanetriol in urine, discussed the possibility of isolating the trimethylsilyl ether derivative of pregnanetriol from crude urinary extracts using suitable columns for the gas chromatographic step. In the foregoing discussion of pregnanediol (see Figs. 11 and 12) we reviewed the gas chromatographic separation of pregnanetriol (derivatives) from several other steroids that are normally present in crude extracts of urine. Retention times of isomeric pregnanetriol trimethylsilyl ethers (5β-$3\alpha,17\alpha,20\alpha$; 5β-$3\alpha,17\alpha,20\beta$; 5α-$3\beta,17\alpha,20\alpha$, and

Table 16. *Quantitative estimation of pregnanetriol in human urine*

References	Extraction and purification following hydrolysis	Free steroid or derivative used for GLC	Stationary phase used for GLC	Other steroids estimated from chromatographic tracing
ROSENFELD et al. (1962) ROSENFELD (1965)	Extraction; paper chromatography	Acetate or trimethyl silyl ether	SE-30	
KIRSCHNER and LIPSETT (1964; 1965)	Extraction; thin-layer chromatography	Free steroid or trimethyl silyl ether	SE-30 XE-60	
RAMAN et al. (1965)	Extraction; thin-layer chromatography	Trimethyl silyl ether	DC-200	Pregnanetriolone
CREECH (1965)	Extraction; TMSi-ether preparation	Trimethyl silyl ether	NGS	Pregnanediol and 17-ketosteroids
CURTIUS (1966)	Extraction; TMSi-ether preparation	Trimethyl silyl ether	XE-60	Pregnanediol, pregnanetriolone and 17-ketosteroids
CHATTORAJ et al. (1966)	Extraction following hydrolysis of precipitated steroids; acetylation	Acetate		Pregnanediol
KINOSHITA and ISURUGI (1964); KINOSHITA et al. (1966)	Extraction; column chromatography on alumina; TMSi-ether preparation	Trimethyl silyl ether	SE-30	
RIVERA et al. (1967)	Extraction; NaOH wash, silica gel column chromatography, TMSi-ether preparation	Trimethyl silyl ether	XE-60	
MENINI and NORYMBERSKI (1965)	Extraction, KBH_4 reduction, HIO_4 oxidation, Girard separation, t.butyldichromate oxidation	5β-Androstane-3.17-dione	SE-30	Other reduction and oxidation products

5α-3β,17α,20β) on 3% XE-60 were reported by HAMMOND and LEACH (1966).

CURTIS (1966) used gas chromatography of the *trimethylsilyl ethers* of the steroids in urine extracts on a 6 ft 3% XE-60 column. He reported a precision of ±5% for the repeated estimation of a sample containing 27.1 mg (s. d. 1.18 mg) of pregnanetriol/l urine from a patient showing signs of the adrenogenital syndrome.

ROSENFELD et al. (1962; ROSENFELD, 1965) described a method for the determination of pregnanetriol, 17α-hydroxypregnanolone and pregn-5-ene-3β,17α,20α-triol in partially purified urinary extracts. Following paper chromatographic isolation, pregnanetriol was acetylated or trimethylsilylated and chromatographed on a 6 ft 3% SE-30 column. The infrared spectra of material collected following gas chromatography showed that the acetylated pregnanetriol fractions gave peaks corresponding to those of authentic pregnanetriol-3,20-diacetate. It was observed that 17α-hydroxypregnanolone was quantitatively rearranged to 3α,17α-dihydroxy, 17β-methyl-D-homo-5β-androstan-17-one during the gas chromatographic separation. Since this conversion appeared to be quantitative, the authors employed the peak of the D-homo steroid for quantitative estimation of the 17α-hydroxypregnanolone in the sample subjected to gas chromatography. The excretion values for 17α-hydroxypregnanolone in the urine of normal adults varied between 0 and 0.26 mg/24 hr. The pregnanetriol values found for urine samples containing from 0.75—25.2 mg of the steroid/day were approximately 10% lower than the values estimated in the same purified extracts as acetaldehydogenic steroids according to the method of Cox (1959). Pregn-5-ene-3β,17α,20α-triol was estimated by an essentially similar technique. Values in the range of from 0.25—35.5 mg/day were on the average 5% lower than when estimated as the acetaldehydogenic steroids. In occasional samples the gas chromatographic results were considerably lower and an additional peak could be observed in the gas chromatographic tracings. The authors could not decide whether this discrepancy was caused by the presence of an additional compound that would lead to erroneous results when estimated by the method of Cox, or that the pregnanetriol decomposed during gas chromatography, resulting in an extra peak and giving too low values.

KIRSCHNER and LIPSETT (1964; 1965) isolated pregnanetriol from urine after glucuronidase hydrolysis, extraction and thin-layer chromatography. Excretion levels were calculated from the tracings obtained after gas chromatography of either the free pregnanetriol on an SE-30 column, or of the pregnanetriol trimethylsilyl ether on SE-30 or XE-60 columns. Pregnanetriol fractions for gas chromatography were more contaminated with impurities when the urine was treated with β-glucuronidase followed by solvolysis. Thus the accuracy of the pregnanetriol measurement was increased by using the glucosiduronate fraction alone. At an excretion level of 0.55 mg/24 hr, they determined a coefficient of variation of 3% for the estimation of pregnanetriol in urine. The recovery of pregnanetriol added to several urine samples in amounts of 0.5 mg/24 hr was close to 100%. No differences were observed when either free pregnanetriol or trimethylsilyl ether derivative were used for the final gas chromatographic separation. Urinary excretion values for pregnanetriol for normal adult subjects (0.20 to 2.00 mg/24 hr) are in agreement with those obtained by conventional techniques.

RAMAN et al. (1965) devised a method for the simultaneous isolation of pregnanediol, pregnanetriol and pregnanetriolone from a single urine sample. The procedure for pregnanetriol isolation involved: addition of ^{3}H-labeled pregnanetriol to the urine; β-glucuronidase hydrolysis; extraction with dichloromethane and thin-layer chromatographic isolation of a fraction containing both pregnanetriol and pregnanetriolone. Following trimethylsilylation, the pregnanetriol and pregnanetriolone trimethylsilyl ethers were separated by gas chromatography on a 4 ft 1.5% DC-200 column. For quantification a flame ionization detector was used. The sensitivity of this method was reported to be on the order of 20 μg/24 hr of urine, whereas the precision was such that individual values from triplicate analysis of urine samples did not vary more than 5%. The excretion values estimated with this method for five normal human subjects are comparable with those obtained by methods not involving gas chromatography. Some of the clinical results that the authors obtained with this technique are difficult to explain, and some of their conclusions are not in agreement with the data presented; this does not, of course, effect the potential usefulness of their methodology. It would be of interest to compare this method with that of KINOSHITA and ISURUGI (1964) (KINOSHITA et al., 1966) also employing gas chromatography for the estimation of urinary pregnanediol, pregnanetriol, pregnanetriolone and pregnanetetrol. Following enzymic hydrolysis and ether extraction of the urine, the dried extract was chromatographed on alumina and separated into a pregnanediol-containing fraction and a fraction containing pregnanetriol, pregnanetriolone and pregnanetetrol (KINOSHITA and ISURUGI, 1964). After formation of the trimethylsilyl ethers of the steroids, a 5 ft 1.5% SE-30 column was used for the separation of the trimethylsilyl ethers of pregnanetriol, pregnanetriolone and pregnanetetrol. This gave acceptable separation. Trimethylsilyl ethers of steroids in the pregnanediol fraction were best separated on an XE-60 column. Using a hydrogen flame ionization detector, the sensitivity of detection was 10 µg/24 hr for each steroid using 1/10th aliquots of 24 hr urine samples. No internal standards for correction of losses throughout the method were employed. In four duplicate determinations following the addition of 100 µg of each steroid to 100 ml of urine, mean recoveries of 89%, 89% and 87% were obtained for pregnanetriol, pregnanetriolone and pregnanetetrol respectively. Detailed data establishing the precision of this method have not been published. The estimated values for excretion of pregnanetriol in urine are in the same range as those reported by other investigators, whereas the excretion of both pregnanetriolone and pregnanetetrol was consistently found to be lower than 0.01 mg/day for normal human subjects.

In their attempts to approach the systematic analysis of steroids in urine using gas chromatography, MENINI and NORYMBERSKI (1965) converted 5β-pregnan-$3\alpha,17\alpha,20\alpha$-triol by reduction and oxidation to 5β-androstan-3,17-dione. The 5β-androstan-3,17-dione was separated from other steroidal diones and triones on a 1% SE-30 column. A disadvantage of this approach is the loss of information about the original side chain at C-17. Strictly speaking the 5β-androstanedione might be derived from urinary metabolites of 17α-hydroxyprogesterone (including pregnanetriol and 17α-hydroxypregnanolone) as well as from 11-deoxycortisol.

Data on the excretion of pregnanetriol estimated by techniques employing gas chromatography are generally comparable with the values obtained by non-GLC methods (BONGIOVANNI and EBERLEIN, 1958; COX, 1959; FOTHERBY and LOVE, 1960; HARKNESS and LOVE, 1966). Although the sensitivity of the sulfuric acid colour reaction for pregnanetriol measurement will permit the estimation of small amounts (1 µg of pregnanetriol), this reaction is less specific than the combination of gas chromatographic separation and sensitive detection. Moreover, gas chromatographic detection is certainly simpler and faster than techniques employing fluorescence, acetaldehydogenic conversions (Cox, 1963) or conversion to 17-ketosteroids (HARKNESS and LOVE, 1966). Pregnanetriol isolated from crude urinary extracts by column chromatography on alumina is pure enough to be subjected to the sulfuric acid reaction. Most methods using gas chromatography have included a chromatographic step for the isolation of pregnanetriol prior to gas chromatography, and thus the time saving of such techniques as compared to the more conventional methods of analysis is small (if it exists at all). This the more so, if it is realized that only one sample at a time can be subjected to gas chromatography on a single instrument, and that each analysis may take at least 10—15 minutes. On the other hand, 10—20 samples can easily be treated with the sulfuric acid reagent at the same time, and the time necessary for spectrophotometric measurement of such samples is certainly less than 10 minutes/sample. If, however, the techniques used by CREECH (1965), CURTIUS (1966), HORNING and GARDINER (1965) and CHATTORAJ et al. (1966) employing gas chromatography of crude urinary extracts will permit adequate measurement of pregnanetriol simultaneously with a number of other steroids, such methods may eventually be the preferred ones.

VII. 6-Oxygenated Progesterone and Reduced Metabolites

Working with a QF-1 column CHAMBERLAIN et al. (1963) obtained tentative evidence that 3α,6α-dihydroxy-5α-pregnan-20-one and 3α,6α-dihydroxy-5β-pregnan-20-one occurred as minor metabolites in an extract of pregnancy urine. In addition, small amounts of the corresponding 17α-pregnane steroids might have been present as artifacts from acid hydrolysis.

KNIGHTS et al. (1962) investigated the gas chromatographic behaviour of the free 5α,20α-5α,20β-5β,20α- and 5β,20β-isomers of pregnan-3α,6α,20-triol as well as the acetates and propionates on a QF-1 column. They demonstrated the occurrence of 5α-pregnane-3α,6α,20α-triol in the urine of both male and female rabbits injected with progesterone.

VIII. 11-Oxygenated Progesterone and Reduced Metabolites

Retention data for 11-keto and 11β-hydroxypregnanes have been reported on QF-1 and SE-30 columns by CHAMBERLAIN et al. (1963), KNIGHTS and THOMAS (1962 b, 1963 a, b), BROOKS and HANAINEH (1963) and BROOKS (1965).

The gas chromatographic behaviour of some 11α-hydroxypregnanes on an SE-30 column was studied by TSUDA et al. (1962), and HEAP et al. (1966) measured 11β-hydroxyprogesterone in adrenal venous blood of pigs and dogs using a gas chromatographic separation of samples from purified plasma extracts.

IX. 16-Oxygenated Progesterone and Reduced Metabolites

VAN DER MOLEN et al. (1966) on several occasions observed the decomposition of free and acetylated 16α-hydroxyprogesterone on both QF-1 and SE-30 columns.

ROSENFELD (1962; 1965) reported the possibility of measuring quantitatively pregn-5-ene-3α,16α,20α-triol, as well as pregn-5-ene-3α,16α,20β-triol and pregn-5-ene-3β,16α,20β-triol isolated from purified urinary extracts. Gas chromatographic separation (SE-30 column) of the trimethylsilyl ether derivatives was used.

X. 17α-Pregnanes

It has been shown that treatment of 17,21-deoxypregnan-20-ones with hot alkali or hot acid will result in partial rearrangement to the corresponding 21-deoxy-17α-pregnan-20-ones. LIEBERMAN et al. (1948) isolated 17α-pregnanolone from human pregnancy urine. This substance may, however, have been an artifact of isolation, since it might have originated from pregnanolone (the normally occurring 17β compound) by acid-catalyzed epimerization (MOFFET and HOEHN, 1944). Following the administration of randomly labeled ^{3}H-16α-hydroxyprogesterone to a normal male subject, CALVIN and LIEBERMAN (1962) isolated tritium in urinary 17α-pregnanolone; urinary 17β-pregnanolone was devoid of radioactivity in this experiment. Rearrangement of the 17β-to the 17α isomer was unlikely in this work.

Thus it was concluded that the isolated 17α-pregnanolone is derived from 16α-hydroxyprogesterone, possibly via 16-dehydroprogesterone as an intermediate. Similar results were obtained by RUSE and SOLOMON (1966). A detailed review of 17α,20-keto pregnanes has been published by RUBIN (1963).

CHAMBERLAIN, THOMAS and coworkers described in several papers the gas chromatographic behaviour of 17α-pregnanes. They studied the retention behaviour of 5α and 5β, 17α-pregnan-3,20-dione (CHAMBERLAIN et al., 1963), 5α and 5β, 17α-pregnan-3-ol-20-ones (CHAMBERLAIN and THOMAS, 1964), 5α and 5β, 17α-pregnanediols (CHAMBERLAIN et al., 1964), as well as that of several 6-oxygenated, 11-oxygenated and 16-oxygenated, 5α and 5β, 17α-pregnanes (CHAMBERLAIN et al., 1963; KNIGHTS et al., 1963).

It was observed that the free or acetylated 17α-isomers are invariably separated from the corresponding 17β-steroids on QF-1 columns, since the 17α-compounds have a slightly shorter retention time. Retention sequences appear to be similar for the 17α-pregnanes when compared to the normal steroids. In extracts from acid-hydrolyzed human urine the occurrence of 17α-pregnanedione, 17α-pregnanolones and other 21-deoxy-17α-pregnane-20-ones has in fact been indicated by gas chromatographic records (CHAMBERLAIN et al., 1963).

XI. Other Pregnanes

The retention times of several 7-, 14- and 15-substituted pregnanes on SE-30 columns were studied by TSUDA et al. (1962). The 7α- and 7β-hydroxy-Δ^4-3-keto steroids as well as the 7α- and 7β-acetoxy-Δ^4-3-keto steroids were shown to be transformed into the $\Delta^{4.6}$-dione-3-ketosteroids at the high temperatures employed during gas chromatography. The corresponding 7-hydroxylated and 7-oxygenated saturated pregnanes were stable during gas chromatography.

The author is most grateful to Drs. O. CREPY (Paris), E. FORCHIELLI (Syntex Research, Palo Alto), F. O. KADRNKA (Upjohn International, Kalamazoo). W. KLYNE (M. R. C. Steroid Reference Collection, London), W. TAYLOR (New Castle Upon Tyne) and W. G. WIEST (St. Louis) for generous gifts of some of the steroids that were used for his personal work reported in this review.

He is also indebted to Drs. A. GOLDFIEN (San Francisco) and A. O. LURIE (Boston) for permission to use figures from their original publications.

References

ADLERCREUTZ, H., and T. LUUKKAINEN: Gas chromatographic identification of pregnanediol and some of its isomers in bile of pregnant women. Ann. med. exp. Fenn. 42, 161 (1964).
— —, and W. TAYLOR: Gas chromatographic and mass spectrometric investigations of "sodium pregnanediol glucuronidate". Europ. J. Steroids 1, 117—134 (1966).
BARNES, A. C., D. KUMAR, and J. A. GOODNO: Studies in human myometrium during pregnancy. Amer. J. Obstr. Gyn. 84, 1207—1212 (1962).
BARRY, R. D., M. GUARNIERI, P. K. BESCH, W. RING, and N. F. BESCH: Comparison of four methods of determining urinary pregnanediol. Anal. Chem. 38, 983—986 (1966).
BONGIOVANNI, A. M., and W. R. EBERLEIN: Critical analysis of methods for measurement of pregnane-3α,17α,20α-triol in human urine. Anal. Chem. 30, 388—393 (1958).
BORTH, R.: Die Methodik der Pregnandiolbestimmung im Urin. In: H. KRAATZ (ed.): Internationales Symposium der Gynäkologischen Endokrinologie. Abhandlungen der Deutschen Akademie der Wissenschaften zu Berlin, Klasse für Medizin 1965, Nr. 1. Berlin: Akademie-Verlag 1965, p. 57—63.
BROOKS, C. J. W.: Studies of acetylated corticosteroids and related 20-oxopregnane derivatives by gas liquid chromatography. Anal. Chem. 37, 636—641 (1965).
—, and L. HANAINEH: The correlation of gas-liquid chromatographic behaviour and structure of steroids. Biochem. J. 87, 151—161 (1963).
BROWNIE, A. C., H. J. VAN DER MOLEN, E. E. NISHIZAWA, and K. B. EIK-NES: Determination of testosterone in human peripheral blood using gas-liquid chromatography with electron capture detection. J. clin. Endocr. 24, 1091—1102 (1964).
BRUSH, M. G., R. W. TAYLOR, and R. MAXWELL: Gas chromatographic determination of urinary pregnanediol in toxaemia of pregnancy and suspected dysmaturity. J. Obstet. Gynaec. Brit. Cwlth 73, 954—960 (1966).
CALVIN, H. I., and S. LIEBERMAN: Studies on the metabolism of 16α-hydroxyprogesterone in humans; conversion to urinary 17-isopregnanolone. Biochem. 1, 639—645 (1962).
CARLSON, I. H., R. K. MEYER, and A. J. BLAIR: The analysis of progestational compounds by gas chromatography. J. clin. Res. 12, 351 (1964).
—, J. BLAIR, and R. K. MEYER: The analysis of plasma progesterone by gas chromatography. In: M. B. LIPSETT (ed.): Gas chromatography of steroids in biological fluids. New York: Plenum Press 1965, p. 169—176.
CHAMBERLAIN, J., and G. H. THOMAS: Characterization of 20-oxosteroids by gas chromatography. Anal. Biochem. 8, 104—115 (1964).
—, B. A. KNIGHTS, and G. H. THOMAS: Analysis of steroid metabolites by gas chromatography. J. Endocrin. 26, 367—387 (1963).

CHAMBERLAIN, J., B. A. KNIGHTS, and G. H. THOMAS: A system of analysis by gas chromatography of 17α- and 17β-pregnane-3,20-diols and their identification as metabolites of progesterone in man, the monkey, rabbit and guinea-pig. J. Endocrin. 28, 235—246 (1964).

CHATTORAJ, S. C., A. SCOMMEGNA, and H. H. WOTIZ: Simultaneous urinary determination of pregnanediol and pregnanetriol by gas chromatography. Abstract, Meeting on Gas chromatographic Determination of Hormonal Steroids. Rome, September (1966).

CLAYTON, R. B.: Gas liquid chromatography of sterol methyl ethers and some correlations between molecular structure and retention data. Biochemistry 1, 357—366 (1962).

COLLINS, W. P., and I. F. SOMMERVILLE: Quantitative determination of progesterone in human plasma by thin-layer and gas-liquid radiochromatography. Nature 203, 836—839 (1964).

COOPER, J. A., and B. G. CREECH: The application of gas-liquid chromatography to the analysis of urinary 17-ketosteroids. Anal. Biochem. 2, 502 (1962).

—, J. P. ABBOTT, B. K. ROSENGREEN, and W. R. CLAGGET: Gas chromatography of urinary steroids. I. A preliminary report on the demonstration and identification of pregnanediol in pregnancy urine by means of gas chromatography. Amer. J. clin. Path. 38, 388 (1962).

COX, R. I.: The separation and quantitative estimation of pregnane-3,17,20-triol, pregnane-3,17,20-triol-11-one and other urinary acetaldehydrogenic steroids. J. biol. Chem. 234, 1693—1697 (1959).

— Gas chromatography in the analysis of urinary pregnanediol. J. Chromatog. 12, 242—245 (1963).

CREECH, B. G.: Separation and determination of ketosteroids, pregnanediol and pregnanetriol on one column. J. Gas Chromatog. 21, 194—195 (1964).

CURTIUS, H. CH.: Gaschromatographische Bestimmung von Pregnandiol, Pregnantriol und Pregnantriolon im Urin. Z. klin. Chem. 4, 114—119 (1966).

DEANE, H. W., M. F. HAY, R. M. MOOR, I. E. A. ROWSON, and R. V. SHORT: The corpus luteum of the sheep. Relationship between morphology and function during the oestrus cycle. Acta endocr. (Kbh.) 51, 245—263 (1966).

DORFMAN, R. I., and F. UNGAR: Metabolism of steroid hormones. New York-London: Academic Press 1965.

DROSDOWSKY, M., A. DESSYPRIS, N. L. MCNIVEN, R. I. DORFMAN, and C. GUAL: A search for progesterone in human urine. Acta endocr. 49, 553—557 (1965).

EBERLEIN, W. R., and A. M. BONGIOVANNI: A paper chromatographic method for the measurement of pregnanediol in urine. J. clin. Endocr. 18, 300—309 (1958).

EUW, J. VON, und T. REICHSTEIN: Über Bestandteile der Nebennierenrinde und verwandte Stoffe. Helv. Chim. Acta 24, 879—889 (1941).

FOTHERBY, K.: The biochemistry of progesterone. Vitam. and Horm. **22,** 153—204 (1964).

—, and D. N. LOVE: A modified method for the determination of pregnanetriol in urine. J. Endocr. **20,** 157—162 (1960).

FUTTERWEIT, W., N. L. McNIVEN, and R. I. DORFMAN: Gas chromatographic determination of progesterone in human pregnancy plasma. Biochim. biophys. Acta **71,** 474—476 (1963).

GARDINER, W. L., and E. C. HORNING: Gas-liquid chromatographic separation of C_{19} and C_{21} human urinary steroids by a new procedure. Biochim. biophys. Acta **115,** 524—526 (1966).

GOLDFIEN, A., M. E. YANNONE, D. B. McCOMAS, and C. BRAGO: The application of gas-liquid chromatography to the measurement of plasma progesterone. In: M. B. LIPSETT (ed.): Gas chromatography of steroids in biological fluids. New York: Plenum Press 1965, p. 143—151.

GORSKI, J., R. E. ERB, W. M. DICKSON, and H. G. BUTLER: Sources of progestin in the pregnant cow. J. Dairy Sci. **41,** 1380 (1958).

GRIFFITHS, K., J. K. GRANT, and T. SYMINGTON: Steroid biosynthesis "in vitro" by granulose-theca cell tumor tissue. J. Endocr. **30,** 247—254 (1964).

HAAHTI, E. O., W. J. A. VANDENHEUVEL, and E. C. HORNING: Separation of urinary 17-ketosteroids by gas chromatography. Anal. Biochem. **2,** 182 (1961).

HAMILTON, R. J., W. J. A. VANDENHEUVEL, and E. C. HORNING: An extension of the "Steroid number" concept to relationships between the structure of steroids and their gas chromatographic retention times observed with selective phases. Biochim. biophys. Acta **70,** 679—687 (1963).

HAMMOND, K. B., and H. LEACH: The gas chromatography of human steroids as the trimethylsilyl ethers. Clin. chim. Acta **11,** 363—364 (1965 a).

— — The gas chromatography of pregnane series steroids. Clin. chim. Acta **11,** 584—585 (1965 b).

— — The gas chromatography of pregnanetriol and some pregnanetriol isomers. Clin. chim. Acta **14,** 569—570 (1966).

— — A routine method for the determination of urine pregnanediol and pregnanolone by gas chromatography. Clin. chim. Acta **15,** 145—148 (1967).

HARKNESS, R. A., and D. N. LOVE: From: LORAINE, J. A., and E. T. BELL: Hormone assays and their clinical application. Edinburgh and London: E. S. Livingstone Ltd. 1966, p. 398.

HARTMAN, I. S., and H. H. WOTIZ: A method for simultaneous separation of $C_{19}O_2$ and $C_{19}O_3$ 17-ketosteroids and progesterone metabolites by gas chromatography. Steroids **1,** 33—38 (1963).

HEAP, R. B.: A fluorescent assay of progesterone. J. Endocr. **30,** 293—305 (1964).

HEAP, R. B., M. HOLZBAUER, and H. M. NEWPORT: Adrenal secretion rates of C-19 and C-21 steroids before and after hypophysectomy in the pig and the dog. J. Endocr. 33, 159—176 (1966).

HEITZMAN, R. J., and G. H. THOMAS: Evaluation by gas chromatography of the urinary steroids of the pregnant dairy cow. J. Endocr. 33, 455—467 (1965).

HENDELES, S. M.: Evaluation des méthodes de dosage de la progestérone. Bull. Soc. roy. belge Gynéc. Obstét. 5, 395—381 (1965).

HINSBERG, K., H. PELZER und A. SEUKEN: Bestimmung sehr kleiner Mengen Progesterone im menschlichen Plasma. Biochem. Z. 328, 117 (1956).

HORNING, E. C., and W. J. A. VANDENHEUVEL: Gas chromatography. Ann. Rev. Biochem. 32, 709—753 (1963).

—, and W. L. GARDINER: Estimation of human steroids by gas-liquid chromatographic methods. In: C. GASSANO (ed.): Research on steroids. Vol. II. Rome: Il Pensiero Scientifico 1966, 121.

—, W. J. A. VAN DEN HEUVEL, and B. G. CREECH: Separation and determination of steroids using gas chromatography. In: D. GLICK (ed.): Methods of biochemical analysis. New York-London: Interscience Publishers, Vol. II, 69 (1963 a).

—, T. LUUKKAINEN, E. O. A. HAAHTI, B. G. CREECH, and W. J. A. VAN DEN HEUVEL: Studies of human steroidal hormones by gas chromatographic techniques. Rec. Prog. Horm. Res. 19, 57—92 (1963 b)

—, K. C. MADDOCK, K. V. ANTHONY, and W. J. A. VAN DEN HEUVEL: Quantitative aspects of gas chromatographic separations in biological studies. Anal. Chem. 35, 526—532 (1963 c).

ISMAIL, A. A. A., and R. A. HARKNESS: The isolation of progesterone from human pregnancy urine. Biochem. J. 98, 15 p (1966).

JANSEN, A. P.: Determination of pregnanediol in urinary extracts by gas-liquid chromatography. Clin. chim. Acta 8, 785—787 (1963).

JAYLE, M. F., et O. CRÉPY: Analyse du Prégnandiol, du Prégnantriol et des stéroïdes apparantés. In: M. F. JAYLE (ed.): Analyse des stéroïdes hormonaux. Paris: Masson et Cie Editeurs 1962, Tome II, 270—329.

—, R. SCHOLLER, J. BEQUE et L. HANNS: Oestrogènes, progestérone et leurs métabolites dans le sang et les urines de grossesses normales. In: M. F. JAYLE (ed.): Hormonologie de la grossesse humaine. Paris: Gauthier 1965, 49—104.

JONES, G. E., D. TURNER, I. J. SARLOS, A. C. BARNES, and R. COHEN: The determination of urinary pregnanediol by gas liquid chromatography. Fertil. and Steril. 13, 544—549 (1962).

KINOSHITA, K., and K. ISURUGI: Gas chromatographic determination of pregnanediol, pregnanetriol, pregnanetriolone and pregnanetetrol. Folia endocrin. (Jap.) 40, 978—981 (1964).

— — Y. KUMAMATO, and H. TAKAYASU: Gas chromatographic estimation of urinary pregnanetriol, pregnanetriolone and pregnanetetrol in congenital adrenal hyperplasia. J. clin. Endocr. 26, 1219—1226 (1966).

KIRSCHNER, M. A., and M. B. LIPSETT: The analysis of urinary steroids using gas-liquid chromatography. Steroids 3, 277—294 (1964).

— — Analysis of urinary pregnanediol and pregnanetriol by gas-liquid chromatography. In: M. B. LIPSETT (ed.): Gas chromatography of steroids in biological fluids. New York: Pergamon Press 1965, 135—142.

— —, and D. R. COLLINS: Analysis of steroids in urine and blood using gas liquid chromatography. J. Gas Chromatog. 2, 360—364 (1964).

KLENDSJOH, M. D., M. FELDSTEIN, and A. SPKAQUE: Determination of 17-ketosteroids in urine. J. clin. Endocr. 13, 922—927 (1953).

KLOPPER, A. I.: Pregnanediol and pregnanetriol. In: R. I. DORFMAN (ed.): Methods in hormone research. New York-London: Academic Press 1962, 139, 168, Vol. I.

—, E. A. MITCHIE, and J. B. BROWN: A method for the determination of urinary pregnanediol. J. Endocr. 21, 209—219 (1955).

KNIGHTS, B. A., and G. H. THOMAS: ΔR_{Mg} values in the gas-liquid chromatography of steroids. Nature 4831, 833—835 (1962 a).

— — Effect of substituents on relative retention times in gas chromatography of steroids. Anal. Chem. 34, 1046—1048 (1962 b).

— — ΔR_{mg} values in the gas chromatography of steroids. Chem. and Ind. (Lond.) 43—44 (1963 a).

— — Gas chromatography of steroids. ΔR_{mg} values for hydroxy and acyloxy groups. J. Chem. Soc. 652, 3477—3480 (1963 b).

—, A. W. ROGERS, and G. H. THOMAS: 5α-Pregnane-3α,6α,20α-triol, a metabolite of progesterone in the rabbit. Biochem. biophys. Res. Comm. 8, 253—258 (1962).

KUMAR, D., and A. C. BARNES: Studies in human myometrium during pregnancy. VI. Tissue progesterone profile of the various compartments in the same individual. Amer. J. Obstet. Gynec. 92, 717—719 (1965).

—, J. A. GOODNO, and A. C. BARNES: Isolation of progesterone from human pregnant myometrium. Nature 195, 1204 (1962).

—, E. F. WARD, and A. C. BARNES: Serial plasma progesterone levels and onset of labor. Amer. J. Obstet. Gynec. 90, 1360—1361 (1964).

LACHÈSE, H., O. CRÉPY, and M. F. JAYLE: Séparation chromatographique et dosage de la pregnanolone. Clin. chim. Acta 8, 538—546 (1963).

LAU, H. L., and G. E. S. JONES: The value of preparative thin-layer chromatography for the routine determination of pregnanediol. Amer. J. Obstet. Gynec. 90, 132—135 (1964).

LEVY, H., and T. SAITO: Conversion of 17-hydroxyprogesterone into 3α, 17-dihydroxypregn-4-en-20-one, 17,20β-dihydroxypregn-4-en-3-one and other substances by bovine adrenal perfusions. Steroids 7, 250—259 (1966).

LIEBERMAN, S., K. DOBRINER, B. R. HILL, L. F. FIESER, and C. P. RHOADS: Studies in steroid metabolism. Identification and characterization of ketosteroids isolated from urine of healthy and diseased persons. J. biol. Chem. 172, 263—295 (1948).

LORAINE, J. A., and E. T. BELL: Hormone assays and their clinical application. Edinburgh and London: E. and S. Livingstone Ltd. 1966, 303 to 348.

LUISI, M., G. GAMBASSI, V. MARESCOTTI, C. SAVI, and F. POLVANI: A gas-chromatographic method for the quantitative determination of progesterone in human plasma. J. Chromatog. 18, 278—284 (1965).

LURIE, A. O., and C. A. VILLEE: A device for the injection of dry samples prepared for gas liquid chromatography. J. Gas Chromatog. 4, 160 to 161 (1966 a).

— — Sebum: A common contaminant of samples for gas-liquid chromatography. J. Chromatog. 21, 113—115 (1966 b).

— —, and D. E. REID: Progesterone in the blood: A quantitative method employing gas liquid chromatography. J. clin. Endocr. 26, 742—749 (1966).

MARESCOTTI, V., M. LUISI, and G. GAMBASSI: Plasma progesterone and 17α-hydroxyprogesterone: gas chromatographic determination. Abstract, meeting on Gas-chromatographic determination of hormonal steroids. Rome, September 1966.

McCOMAS, D. B., and A. GOLDFIEN: A device for the introduction of sub-microgram quantities of solids into a gas chromatograph. Anal. Chem. 35, 263—264 (1963).

McKERNS, K. W., and E. NORDSTRAND: Simple method for tissue extraction and gas chromatographic separation of estrogens. Biochim. biophys. Acta 82, 198—200 (1964).

— — Stimulation of the rat ovary by gonadotrophin and separation of steroids by gas chromatography. Biochim. biophys. Acta 104, 237—249 (1965 a).

— — Gas chromatography of estrogens and other steroids from endocrine tissues. In: M. B. LIPSETT (ed.): Gas chromatography of steroids in biological fluids. New York: Plenum Press 1965 b, 255—261.

MENINI, E.: In: M. B. LIPSETT (ed.): Gas chromatography of steroids in biological fluids. New York: Plenum Press 1965, 117—118.

—, and J. NORYMBERSKI: An approach to the systematic analysis of urinary steroids. Biochem. J. 95, 1—16 (1965).

MOFFETT, R. B., and W. M. HOEHN: 17-Isopregnan-3α-ol-20-one. J. Amer. Chem. Soc. 66, 2098—2100 (1944).

MOLEN, H. J. VAN DER: Determination of micro amounts of 5β-Pregnan-3α-ol-20-one in urine using infrared spectrometry. Acta endocr. (Kbh.) 41, 234—246 (1962 a).

— 5β-Pregnan-3α-ol-20-one in urine. Acta endocr. (Kbh.) 41, 247—258 (1962 b).

—, and K. B. EIK-NES: Estimation of total mass and specific radioactivity of several steroids in canine testicular vein blood and testicular tissue following "in vivo" infusion of 4-¹⁴C-3β-hydroxypregn-5-en-20-one via the spermatic artery. Abstracts Second International Congress on Hormonal Steroids, Milan, Excerpta Med. Int. Congress Series 111, 264 (1966).

MOLEN, H. J. VAN DER, and D. GROEN: Determination of progesterone in human peripheral blood using gas liquid chromatography with electron capture detection. In: M. B. LIPSETT (ed.): Gas chromatography of steroids in biological fluids. New York: Plenum Press 1965 a, 153—168.

— — Determination of progesterone in human peripheral blood using gas-liquid chromatography with electron capture detection. J. clin. Endocr. 25, 1625—1639 (1965 b).

— — Quantitative determination of submicrogram amounts of steroids in blood using electron capture and flame ionization detection following gas-liquid chromatography. In: J. K. GRANT (ed.): Steroid gas chromatography. Endocrinology Memoir 26, 155—177 (1967).

—, and A. AAKVAAG: Progesterone. In: C. H. GRAY and A. L. BACHARACH (eds.): Hormones in blood. 2nd edition London-New York: Academic Press 1967, 221—304.

—, B. RUNNEBAUM, E. E. NISHIZAWA, E. KRISTENSEN, T. KIRSCHBAUM, W. G. WIEST, and K. B. EIK-NES: On the presence of progesterone in blood plasma from normal women. J. clin. Endocr. 25, 170—176 (1965).

—, J. H. VAN DER MAAS, and D. GROEN: Preparation and properties of steroid heptafluorobutyrates. Eur. J. Steroids 2, 119—138 (1967).

—, F. F. G. ROMMERTS, and D. GROEN: Unpublished observation (1966).

NEILL, J. D., E. N. DAY, and G. W. DUNCAN: Gas chromatographic determination of progestins in tissues and blood. Steroids 4, 699—712 (1964).

NELSON, J. P.: Gas chromatography of selected pregnanes and pregnenes. J. Gas Chromatog. 1, 27—29 (1963).

NIENSTEDT, W.: A rapid method for plasma progesterone determination. Acta physiol. scand. 59, Suppl. 213, 110 (1963).

— Studies on defatting of lipophilic steroids for gas-chromatographic determination. Abstract, Meeting on Gas Chromatographic Determination of Hormonal Steroids. Rome. September 1966.

NISHIZAWA, E. E., and K. B. EIK-NES: On the secretion of progesterone and Δ^4-androstene-3,17-dione by the canine ovary in animals stimulated with human chorionic gonadotrophin. Biochim. biophys. Acta 84, 610 to 621 (1964).

OAKS, D. M., E. J. BONELLI, and K. P. DIMICK: Quantitative gas chromatography of urinary steroids using a new liquid phase. J. Gas Chromat. 3, 353—357 (1965).

PATTI, A. A., and A. STEIN: Steroid analysis by gas liquid chromatography. Springfield, Ill.: Charles C. Thomas 1964, 76.

—, P. BONANNO, T. F. FRAWLEY, and A. A. STEIN: Gas-phase chromatography in separation and identification of pregnanediol in urine and blood of pregnant women. Obstet. and Gynec. 21, 302—307 (1963 a).

— — — — Preliminary studies of the application of gas phase chromatography to the separation and identification of steroids in biological fluids. Acta endocr. (Kbh.) 42, Suppl. 77, 1—34 (1963 b).

PEARLMAN, W. H., and E. CERCEO: The estimation of saturated and α,β-unsaturated ketonic compounds in placental extracts. J. biol. Chem. 203, 127—134 (1953).

PODMORE, D. A.: Routine determination of urinary pregnanediol using a gas chromatograph with automatic sample application. J. clin. Pathol. **19**, 619 (1966).

RAISINGHANI, K. H., R. I. DORFMAN, and E. FORCHIELLI: A gas chromatographic method for the estimation of nanogram quantities of progesterone using electron capture detection. Abstract. Meeting on Gas Chromatographic Determination of Hormonal Steroids. Rome, September 1966.

RAMAN, P. B., R. AVRAMOV, M. L. McNIVEN, and R. I. DORFMAN: A method for the determination of pregnanediol, pregnanetriol and pregnanetriolone by gas chromatography. Steroids **6**, 177—193 (1965).

RIONDEL, A., J. F. TAIT, S. A. S. TAIT, M. GUT, and B. LITTLE: Estimation of progesterone in human peripheral blood using ^{35}S-thiosemicarbazide. J. clin. Endocr. **25**, 229—242 (1965).

RIVERA, R., R. I. DORFMAN, and E. FORCHIELLI: A modified method for the analysis of urinary 17-ketosteroids, pregnanediol and pregnanetriol by gas-liquid chromatography in normal subjects and subjects with various endocrine disorders. Acta endocr. (Kbh.) **54**, 37—50 (1967).

ROSENFELD, R. S.: Measurement of urinary steroids by gas chromatography. 3α,17-Dihydroxypregnane-20-one and C_{21}-triols. In: M. B. LIPSETT (ed.): Gas chromatography of steroids in biological fluids. New York: Plenum Press 1965, 127—133.

—, M. C. LEBEAU, R. D. JANDOREK, and T. SALUMAA: Analysis of urinary extracts by gas chromatography. 3α,17-Dihydroxypregnan-20-one, pregnane-3α,17,20α-triol and Δ^5-pregnane-3β,17-20α-triol. J. Chromatog. **8**, 355—358 (1962).

ROTHSCHILD, I.: Intercorrelations between progesterone and the ovary, pituitary and central nervous system in the control of ovulation and the regulation of progesterone secretion. Vitam. and Horm. **23**, 209 to 327 (1965).

RUBIN, M. B.: 17α-20-Ketopregnanes. A review. Steroids **2**, 561—581 (1963).

RÜNNEBAUM, B., H. J. VAN DER MOLEN, and J. ZANDER: Steroids in human peripheral blood of the menstrual cycle. Steroids, Suppl. II, 189—204 (1965).

RUSE, J. L., and S. SOLOMON: The *in vivo* metabolism of 16α-hydroxyprogesterone. Biochemistry **5**, 1065—1071 (1966).

SHEERIN, B. M., and I. F. SOMMERVILLE: Plasma pregnanediol determination by means of thin-layer and gas-liquid chromatography. Abstract. Meeting on Gas Chromatographic Determination of Hormonal Steroids. Rome, September 1966.

SHORT, R. V.: Progesterone in blood. I. The chemical determination of progesterone in peripheral blood. J. Endocr. **16**, 415—425 (1958).

— Progesterone. In: C. H. GRAY and A. L. BACHARACH (eds.): Hormones in blood. London-New York: Academic Press 1961, 379—437.

—, and I. LEVETT: The fluorometric determination of progesterone in human plasma during pregnancy and the menstrual cycle. J. Endocr. **25**, 239 to 244 (1962).

SHORT, R. V., G, WAGNER, A. R. FUCHS, and F. FUCHS: Progesterone concentrations in uterine venous blood after intraamniotic injection of hypertonic saline in midpregnancy. Amer. J. Obstet. Gynec. 91, 132—136 (1964).

SIMMER, H., und I. SIMMER: Progesteron im peripheren Venenblut von Schwangeren mit Spätgestosen. Klin. Wschr. 37, 971 (1959).

SOMMERVILLE, I. F.: Discussions. In: M. B. LIPSETT (ed.): Gas chromatography of steroids in biological fluids. New York: Plenum Press 1966, 177.

— The application of gas liquid radiogaschromatography to the quantitative determination of steroids in human plasma and tissue. In: C. CASSANO (ed.): Research on steroids, Vol. II. Rome: Il pensiero Scientifico 1966,147.

—, and F. DESHPANDE: The quantitative determination of progesterone and pregnanediol in human plasma. J. clin. Endocr. 18, 1223—1236 (1958).

—, and W. P. COLLINS: Steroid gas-liquid radiochromatography. Continuous monitoring of the effluent for carbon-14- and tritium. Steroids, Suppl. II, 223—234 (1965).

—, M. T. PICKETT, W. P. COLLINS, and D. C. DENYER: A modified method for the quantitative determination of progesterone in human plasma. Acta endocr. (Kbh.) 43, 101—109 (1963).

TAIT, J. F.: Discussions. In: M. B. LIPSETT (ed.): Gas chromatography of steroids in biological fluids. New York: Plenum Press 1965, 181.

TALBOT, N. B., R. A. BERMAN, E. A. MACLACHLAN, and J. K. WOLFE: The colorimetric determination of neutral steroids (hormones) in a 24-hour sample of human urine (Pregnanediol; total, alpha and beta alcoholic and nonalcoholic 17-ketosteroids). J. clin. Endocr. 1, 668—673 (1941).

THIJSSEN, J. H. H., and J. ZANDER: Progesterone-4-^{14}C and its metabolites in the blood after intravenous injection into women. Acta endocr. (Kbh.) 51, 563—577 (1966).

TSUDA, K., N. IKEKAWA, Y. SATO, S. TANAKA, and H. HASEGAWA: Steroid studies. XXXV. Gas chromatography of androstane and pregnane derivatives. Chem. and Pharm. Bull. 10, 332—337 (1962).

TURNER, D. A., G. E. JONES, and I. J. SARLOS: Determination of urinary pregnanediol by gas chromatography Anal. Biochem. 5, 99—106 (1963).

VANDENHEUVEL, W. J. A., and E. C. HORNING: A study of retention time relationships in gas chromatography in terms of the structure of steroids. Biochim. biophys. Acta 64, 416—429 (1962).

— — Separation, identification and estimation of steroids. In: H. A. SZYMANSKI (ed.): Biomedical applications of gas chromatography. New York: Plenum Press 1965 a, 89—150.

— — Analyse des stéroïdes par chromatographie en phase gazeuse. Bull. Soc. Chim. Biol. 47, 945—977 (1965 b).

—, B. G. CREECH, and E. C. HORNING: Separation and estimation of the principal human 17-ketosteroids as trimethylsilyl ethers. Anal. Biochem. 4, 191—197 (1962).

VENNING, E. H.: Gravimetric method for the determination of sodium pregnandiol glucuronidate (an excretion product of progesterone). J. Biol. Chem. 119, 473—480 (1937).

VERBOOM, E.: Quantitative determination of pregnane-3α,20α-diol in the urine. Acta endocr. (Kbh.) 24, Suppl. 29, 1—50 (1957).

WALDI, D.: Einfache quantitative Schnellbestimmung von Pregnandiol auf Dünnschichtplatten zum Frühschwangerschaftnachweis und zur Überwachung des Zyklus bei der Frau. Klin. Wschr. 40, 827—830 (1962).

WIEST, W. G., T. KERENYI, and A. I. CSAPO: A double isotope derivative dilution assay for progesterone in biological fluids and tissues. Abstract. Second International Congress on Hormonal Steroids, Milan, 1966. Excerpta Med. Int. Congress Series 111, 114 (1966).

WOOLEVER, G. A., and A. GOLDFIEN: A double isotope derivative method for plasma progesterone assay. Int. J. appl. rad. Isot. 14, 163—171 (1963).

WOTIZ, H. H.: Studies in steroid metabolism. The rapid determination of urinary pregnanediol by gas chromatography. Biochim. biophys. Acta 69, 415—416 (1963).

—, and S. C. CHATTORAJ: Gas chromatographic analysis of urinary pregnanediol: Evaluation and application. Abstract. Meeting on Gas Chromatographic Determination of Hormonal Steroids. Rome, September 1966.

WYMAN, H., and I. F. SOMMERVILLE: The simultaneous determination of progesterone; oestradiol-17β and oestrone in the plasma and other body fluids of human females. Abstracts Second International Congress on Hormonal Steroids, Milan, 1966. Excerpta Med. Int. Congress Series 111, 131 (1966).

YANNONE, M. E., D. B. McCOMAS, and A. GOLDFIEN: The assay of plasma progesterone. J. Gas Chromat. 2, 30—33 (1964).

ZANDER, J.: Progesterone. In: R. I. DORFMAN (ed.): Methods in hormone research, Vol. 1, New York-London: Academic Press 1962, 91—137.

—, und H. SIMMER: Die chemische Bestimmung von Progesteron in organischen Substraten. Klin. Wschr. 32, 529 (1954).

—, W. G. WIEST und K. G. OBER: Klinische, histologische und biochemische Beobachtungen bei polycystischen Ovarien mit gleichzeitiger adenomatöser, atypischer Hyperplasie des Endometriums. Arch. Gynäk. 196, 481 (1962).

ZMIGROD, A., and H. R. LINDNER: Gas chromatographic separation of ketosteroids as ethylene-thioketal derivatives. Steroids. 8, 119—131 (1966).

Chapter 4

Gas Phase Chromatography of Androgens in Biological Samples

K. B. Eik-Nes

I. Introduction

The major androgens in biological fluids are testosterone and androstenedione. Recent investigations have clearly demonstrated that these steroids are interconvertible in body compartments (MAHESH and GREENBLATT, 1962; VANDE WIELE et al., 1963; CAMACHO and MIGEON, 1964), but androstenedione is a much weaker androgen than testosterone. Both hormones can be extracted from human blood plasma with organic solvents of relatively low polarity (OERTEL and EIK-NES, 1959; HORTON, 1965). Non-conjugated testosterone has been isolated and identified in such extracts of plasma from normal subjects (VAN DER MOLEN et al., 1966 b) and of plasma from subjects stimulated with gonadotrophin (OERTEL and EIK-NES, 1959). The technique of gas phase chromatography was used in the isolation of free testosterone from blood plasma of normal men (VAN DER MOLEN et al., 1966). In human urine, testosterone (SCHUBERT and WEHRBERGER, 1960; CAMACHO and MIGEON, 1963) and its 17α-hydroxy epimere (KORENMAN et al., 1964) are present predominately as glucosiduronates and testosterone conjugated with glucosiduronic acid and sulphuric acid has also been found in human blood (HADD and RHAMY, 1965; SAEZ et al., 1967).

Dehydroepiandrosterone (DHEA) can be classified as an androgen (DORFMAN and SHIPLEY, 1956). This steroid can serve as a precursor for androstenedione and testosterone (EIK-NES and HALL, 1965). Conjugated DHEA has been isolated from human plasma (MIGEON and PLAGER, 1954 a). The level of free DHEA in this fluid is extremely low if it exists at all (COHN et al., 1961). It is now well documented

Table 1. *Relative retention time of testosterone on different phases*

Steroid	1% XE-60 * 3 ft 210°	2% XE-60 ** 6 ft 216°	1% SE-30 *** 5 ft 200°	2% SE-30 ** 6 ft 210°	3% QF-1 *** 5 ft 200°	6.8% SE-30 **** 3 ft 240°	3% SE-30 **** 12 ft 220°
19-Nortestosterone, CA	1.00						
Epitestosterone, CA	1.00						
Testosterone, CA	1.18						
Testosterone		3.24	1.00	0.97	1.00	0.57	.52
Epitestosterone		3.00	1.00	0.96	1.06		.51
Testosterone TMSi		1.25		1.18		0.72	
Epitestosterone TMSi		1.00		1.00			
Testosterone TFA		0.35		0.46			
Epitestosterone TFA		0.29		0.41			
Testosterone acetate			1.00		1.00	0.87	.73
Epitestosterone acetate			0.94		1.07		.68

CA: Chloroacetate, TMSi: trimethylsilyl ether, TFA: trifluoroacetoxy derivative.
* Relative to epitestosterone chloroacetate.
** Relative to epitestosterone trimethylsilyl ether.
*** Relative to testosterone.
**** Relative to cholestane.

The heptafluorobutyrate of epitestosterone is "almost completely separated from testosterone heptafluorobutyrate" on a 4 ft, 1% SE-30 column operated at 180° C (EXLEY, 1966). Moreover, some separation of epitestosterone TMSi from testosterone TMSi will occur on a 6 ft, 3% NGS column operated at 225° C (PANICUCCI, 1966).

that the human adrenal gland secretes DHEA sulphate (BAULIEU, 1962), but compared to free DHEA, DHEA sulphate lacks androgenic activity *in vivo* in an animal species like the rat (PEILLON and RACADOT, 1965). Moreover, DHEA sulphate does not show metabolic effects in the human (LIPSETT et al., 1965).

The major metabolites of Δ^4-androstenedione and testosterone are androsterone, etiocholanolone (CALLOW, 1939) and epiandrosterone (DORFMAN, 1941). These steroids are present in blood and urine as conjugates (WEST et al., 1951; MIGEON, 1956; OERTEL and EIK-NES, 1961), and the reduction of androsterone and etiocholanolone to 5α- or 5β-androstanediol respectively appears to be small (SCHILLER et al., 1945). It is quite possible that a metabolic pathway exists for the formation of androstanediols via a direct 17β-hydroxylation of testosterone (BAULIEU and MAUVAIS-JARVIS, 1964 a; BAULIEU and MAUVAIS-JARVIS, 1964 b).

The 11-keto and 11-hydroxy derivatives of etiocholanolone and androsterone are considered to be metabolites of C_{21} adrenal steroids. It should be noted in this respect that 11β-hydroxytestosterone can be found in the urine of male subjects (SCHUBERT et al., 1964) and testes tumors can produce steroids with an oxygen atom at C_{11} (BAGGETT et al., 1957). Thus all of the 11-keto and 11-hydroxy deriv-

Table 2. *Relative retention time (cholestane) of some androgens on different phases*

Steroid	1.5% SE-30 4 ft 225°	3% SE-30 5 ft 230°	3% JXR 3 ft 200°
Δ^4-Androstenedione	0.57		
Testosterone	0.65	0.63	
Testosterone acetate	0.76	0.74	
Testosterone TMSi			0.66
Epitestosterone TMSi			0.57
Testosterone ClCH$_2$Me$_2$Si			1.55
Epitestosterone ClCH$_2$Me$_2$Si			1.31
Epitestosterone		0.70	
Δ^4-Androstenedione		0.54	
Epitestosterone acetate		0.74	
Testosterone HFB		0.58	

TMSi: trimethylsilyl ether, ClCH$_2$Me$_2$Si: chloromethyldimethylsilyl ether, HFB: heptafluorobutyrate (6 ft column, 218° C).

Table 3. *Comparison of relative retention times of equatorial 3-hydroxy-steroids epimeres at C-5*

Steroid structure	Relative retention times	
	3% QF-1 * 237° C	3% NGA ** 225° C
3-Hydroxyandrostan-17-ones		
3α (5β)	1.98	
3α (5β) acetate	2.84	
3α (5β) TMSi		0.98
3β (5α)	2.18	
3β (5α) acetate	3.33	
3β (5α) TMSi		1.22
Androstane-3,17α-diols		
3α (5β)	1.28	
3α (5β) acetate	2.32	
3α (5β) TMSi		0.33
3β (5α)	1.41	
3β (5α) acetate	3.05	
3β (5α) TMSi		0.43
Androstane-3,17β-diols		
3α (5β)	1.36	
3α (5β) acetate	2.81	
3α (5β) TMSi		0.43
3β (5α)	1.49	
3β (5α) acetate	3.25	
3β (5α) TMSi		0.52

* Retention time of cholestane 3.5 min.
** Retention time of cholestane TMSi 11.5 min.
TMSi: trimethylsilyl ether.
Reprinted with the permission of the authors and J. Endocrinol.
The data are from a publication by HEITZMAN and THOMAS (1966).

atives of etiocholanolone and androsterone excreted in the urine may not be of adrenal origin. The major androgens, androstenedione and testosterone, are produced in the gonads, but the production of androstenedione by the human adrenal gland also appears sizeable (CHAPDELAINE et al., 1965).

It was early established that some of the androgens and their most common metabolites could be carried through gas phase chromatography without undergoing structural rearrangements, and columns were found which would separate these compounds from closely

Table 4. *Relative retention time (cholestane) of some 17-ketosteroids on different columns*

Steroid	1% NGS, 6 ft 231°	1% SE-30, 6 ft 195—235°	2.2% SE-30, 6 ft, 5 in programmed *		1% XE-60, 5 ft 200°	3% XE-60, 6 ft 262°		3% QF-1, 6 ft 212°
Androsterone		.34	.38	.37**				2.06—2.12
Etiocholanolone		.37	.34	.35**				2.18
DHEA		.34	.37	.37**				2.07
Androsterone TMSi	.60		.38		.9	1.02	0.94***	1.13
Etiocholanolone TMSi	.73		.39		1.06	1.18	1.14***	1.24
DHEA, TMSi	.84		.46		1.25	1.36	1.30***	1.40
Androsterone, $ClCH_2Me_2Si$					3.05			
Etiocholanolone, $ClCH_2Me_2Si$					3.54			
DHEA $ClCH_2Me_2Si$					4.35			
11β-Hydroxyandrosterone		.61	.47	.63**				3.91—4.0
11-Ketoandrosterone			.63	.43**				3.98—4.0
11β-Hydroxyetiocholanolone		.55	.43	.56**				4.08—4.13
11-Ketoetiocholanolone		.40	.57	.43**				4.20—4.23
11β-Hydroxyandrosterone TMSi	1.87		.48					2.32
11-Ketoandrosterone TMSi			.70					1.78
11β-Hydroxyetiocholanolone TMSi			.49			2.40		2.36
11-Ketoetiocholanolone TMSi	1.36		.75			2.57		2.01
Androsterone HFB						1.07		

Table 4 (continued)

Steroid	1% NGS, 6 ft 231°	1% SE-30, 6 ft .195—235°	2.2% SE-30 6 ft, 5 in programmed *	1% XE-60, 5 ft 200°	3% XE-60, 6 ft 262°	3% QF-1, 6 ft 212°
Etiocholanolone HFB					1.18	
DHEA HFB					1.35	
Androsterone A			.51 **			
Etiocholanolone A			.50 **			
DHEA A			.56 **			
11β-Hydroxyandrosterone A			.84 **			
11-Ketoandrosterone A			.61 **			
11β-Hydroxyetiocholanolone A			.80 **			
11-Ketoetiocholanolone A			.61 **			

TMSi: trimethylsilyl ether
ClCH₂Me₂Si: chloromethyldimethylsilyl ether
HFB: heptafluorobutyrate (6 ft column, 218° C)
A: after acetylation

* For details see VIHKO (1966).
** 12 ft column operated at 220° C
*** Column operated at 218° C.

242   Gas Phase Chromatography of Androgens in Biological Samples

Table 5. *Relative retention time (cholestane) of androgen metabolites on different columns*

Steroid	1% SE-30, 6 ft 215°			1% QF-1, 6 ft 210°			2% CNSi, 6 ft 215°		
	Free	DMH*	HOAC**	Free	DMH	HOAC	Free	DMH	HOAC
5α-Androstan-17-one	.19	.19	.27	.64	.64	.39	.81	.81	.48
5α-Androstane-3,17-dione	.42	.61	.85	4.06	2.0	1.17	6.76	3.48	1.93
3β-Hydroxy-5α-androstan-16-one	.38	.38	.63	2.47	2.47	1.49	5.03	5.03	3.38

* N,N-dimethylhydrazine alone used as reagent. ** Acetic acid used as catalyst in the reaction. (The data are from a publication by VANDEN HEUVEL and HORNING [1963].) Reprinted with the permission of the authors and Biochim. Biophys. Acta.

related steroids. The data from this work have been reviewed by Horning and Vanden Heuvel (1963) and published data on the retention time of androgens and some of their metabolites during gas phase chromatography can be found in Tables 1—5.

In order to understand the dynamics of production and secretion of steroid androgens (Dorfman and Ungar, 1965), methods that will separate and quantify testosterone, androstenedione, DHEA, etiocholanolone and androsterone should give valuable information. The following discussion considers techniques developed over the past 3 or 4 years where steroid separation is achieved by gas phase chromatography and steroid quantification is done by the detector devices of the gas chromatograph. The sensitivity of the latter has often made gas chromatographic techniques methods of choice since the concentration of some of the steroids in question is low in a fluid like blood plasma.

II. Androgens in Blood Plasma

1. Testosterone in Plasma

Few complete GLC methods have thus far been published for the estimation of free plasma testosterone. One of these methods utilizes electron capture for testosterone estimation (Brownie et al., 1964). This detector device has high sensitivity, but in order to differentiate a steroid signal from an unspecific sample signal, it is imperative that all glassware used should be scrupulously clean, that all reagents employed should be in the highest state of purity, and that plasma testosterone should be well separated from other plasma steroids prior to gas phase chromatography (see Chapter 1). This method was developed subsequent to the observation in our laboratory (Brownie et al., 1964) that the chloroacetate of pure steroids (testosterone, 20β-reduced progesterone) would capture electrons and could be determined by electron capture at the nanogram level. This finding has been verified in other laboratories (van der Molen et al., 1965; Nakagawa et al., 1966).

In the method of Brownie et al. (1964), 5 to 10 ml of plasma from normal male subjects will suffice for adequate assay (Resko and Eik-Nes, 1966). When working with plasma from normal women, the use of 20 ml is recommended since the hormone concentration in such plasma is low (HUDSON et al., 1963; RIONDEL et al., 1963; LOBOTSKY et al., 1964). Testosterone in plasma from spermatic venous blood, can be quantified in 1—2 ml (HOLLANDER and HOLLANDER, 1958; EIK-NES, 1967). In order to determine testosterone recovery through this method, testosterone-^{3}H of high specific radioactivity is added to the plasma sample (HUDSON et al., 1963; RIONDEL et al., 1963). The plasma is then made alkaline by the addition of sodium hydroxide. This method originally used by OGATA and HIRANO (1933) for extracting androgens from testicular tissue has found widespread use for the extraction of testosterone (RIONDEL et al., 1963), progesterone (SOMMERVILLE and DESHPANDE, 1958; SHORT, 1958; VAN DER MOLEN and GROEN, 1965) or even estrone (ATTAL et al., 1967) from plasma. The plasma is extracted with ether (the universally used solvent for the extraction of free testosterone) (BRINCK-JOHNSEN and EIK-NES, 1957; SCHUBERT and WEHRBERGER, 1960; OERTEL, 1961; CAMACHO and MIGEON, 1963; HUDSON et al., 1963; RIONDEL et al., 1963; HORTON et al., 1963; FUTTERWEIT et al., 1963; SCHUBERT and FRANKENBERG, 1964; KORENMAN et al., 1964; SANDBERG et al., 1964; ISMAIL and HARKNESS, 1965). The weight of such plasma extracts is low compared to that of plasma extracted at its physiological pH and the use of procedures for removal of extracted plasma fats appears not to be necessary when alkalinized plasma is used for extraction. Following the addition of sodium hydroxide solution, the plasma sample should be extracted immediately.

Preliminary purification is done by thin-layer chromatography (TLC) on glass plates coated with silica gel with the solvent system cyclohexane : ethylacetate (1:1, v/v). Material chromatographing like authentic testosterone on plate is eluted with methanol. In addition to testosterone, this eluate may also contain steroids like pregnanediol, 19-nortestosterone, epitestosterone, 20α- and 20β-hydroxyprogesterone and 17α-hydroxyprogesterone. The eluate is chloroacetylated for 9—12 h (LANDOWNE and LIPSKY, 1963), the sample is extracted with ethylacetate and the extract is washed with hydrochloric acid and water and evaporated to dryness. The residue is purified by TLC with the solvent system benzene : ethylacetate (4:1, v/v) (silica gel plate). Material chromatographing like authentic testosterone chloroacetate (mp. 124—125 °C corr.) is eluted with benzene. Care has to be exercised at this point so that the benzene does not contain particles of silica gel. In addition to testosterone chloroacetate, the eluted plasma sample may contain the chloroacetates of 19-nortestosterone, 17-epitestosterone and 20α- and 20β-progesterone. Following the purification steps of TLC, chloroacetylation and TLC, testosterone in biological samples appears to be in a very high state of purity. When acetate-1-^{14}C is perfused via the artery of the rabbit testis (EWING and EIK-NES, 1966), testosterone-^{14}C in the venous blood of the perfused organ, purified as outlined, can be crystallized to constant specific radioactivity following the addition of authentic testosterone chloroacetate (Table 6). It should be noted that 17-epitestosterone has been found in bovine spermatic venous blood (LINDNER, 1959).

Table 6. *Crystallization of biosynthesized radioactive testosterone*

Solvent	Crystallization Number	Specific radioactivity dpm/μg
Benzene : hexane	1	60
Acetone : hexane	2	66
Ethylacetate : hexane	3	65
Aqueous methanol	4	64

Acetate-1-^{14}C was perfused via the artery of the rabbit testis and testosterone (chloroacetate) isolated in the venous blood of the perfused organ by the method of BROWNIE et al. (1964). From EWING and EIK-NES (1966). Reprinted with the permission of Canad. J. Biochem.

Following the last TLC purification step, a known amount of an internal standard (20 nanograms of 20β-hydroxyprogesterone chloroacetate) is added to the sample and a 1/10 aliquot of this mixture is removed for the estimation of recovery of added testosterone-^{3}H. The average recovery of testosterone up to this step varies between 40—75%. With experience in the use of the method, the mean recovery is 65%$\pm$2.7% (one standard deviation in 815 experiments). The major loss occurs between chloroacetylation and the second TLC.

The sample is then subjected to GLC analysis with a 3 ft $\times$ 0.4 cm U shaped glass column. The stationary phase is 1% XE-60, the column temperature 210° C, detector temperature 220° C and flash heater temperature 250° C. High purity nitrogen led through a tube filled with molecular sieve (type 13X, Linde) is used as the carrier gas phase (gas pressure is 40 psi). The gas chromatograph is equipped with an Aerograph electron capture detector. Instead of direct voltage which tends to give a relatively high noise level, and thus decreases sensitivity and reproducibility of detection markedly, pulsating voltage is applied to the electron capture cell. For maximal sensitivity with testosterone chloroacetate, 50 volts having a pulse width of 10 μsec, a pulse position of 100 μsec with an internal repetition rate of 10 KC, are applied to the electron capture cell. The impedance is 50 ohms. The output of the electron capture detector is directed to the electrometer of the gas chromatograph.

Quantitative evaluation of the peak areas on the gas chromatography tracing is done by triangulation and the amount of testosterone in the sample is calculated by the following equation:

$$S(\mu g) = \frac{X_s}{10 X_p} \times \frac{C_s}{C_x} \times \frac{T_x}{T_s} \times \frac{288.4}{364.5} \times 0.01 - M$$

X_s = cpm of testosterone-^{3}H initially added to the plasma.
X_p = cpm of ^{3}H in the aliquot removed prior to gas chromatography.
C_s = area (cm²) of 20 nanograms of 20β-hydroxyprogesterone chloroacetate.
C_x = area (cm²) of 20β-hydroxyprogesterone chloroacetate from the sample.
T_s = area (cm²) of 0.01 μg testosterone chloroacetate.
T_x = area (cm²) of testosterone chloroacetate from the sample.
288.4 = molecular weight of testosterone.
364.5 = molecular weight of testosterone chloroacetate.
M = mass (μg) of testosterone-^{3}H added to the plasma.

One nanogram of pure testosterone chloroacetate can be detected with some precision (13%) by electron capture. The calibration curve (cm² peak area versus μg) for pure testosterone chloroacetate is linear from 0.001 to 0.03 μg and over this range of testosterone chloroacetate concentration the quantification of a single peak has a standard deviation of 5%. The accuracy of the method is about 0.005 μg testosterone chloroacetate but at a plasma concentration of 0.010 μg testosterone/100 ml, the accuracy is only about 40%. At higher plasma concentrations of the hormone like those found in spermatic venous blood (EIK-NES, 1967), the accuracy of estimation is about 5%. This might be due to inherent inaccuracies in the gas chromatographic quantification alone (Table 7). Samples of 10 ml of plasma obtained from sixteen different human subjects and containing from 0.13 to 0.73 μg testosterone/100 ml were divided and individual testosterone

Table 7. *Levels of testosterone in spermatic venous blood plasma of an anesthetized dog. All estimations were done in triplicate and the data are expressed as µg of testosterone secreted in 60 sec*

Sample	µg secreted in 60 sec.		
1	0.234	0.229	0.236
2	0.230	0.234	0.235
3	0.221	0.225	0.219
4	0.216	0.222	0.224
5	0.217	0.214	0.222
6	0.215	0.213	0.219
7	0.210	0.207	0.215
8	0.207	0.210	0.213
9	0.201	0.208	0.205
10	0.198	0.197	0.200
11	0.196	0.191	0.200
12	0.201	0.198	0.200
13	0.190	0.193	0.203
14	0.187	0.190	0.198
15	0.185	0.190	0.173
16	0.172	0.181	0.194
17	0.180	0.204	0.186

Seventeen sequential, 60 sec. samples of spermatic venous blood were collected (EIK-NES, 1967) and the blood plasma was extracted with ether. The extract was divided in three equal portions and each portion was processed for testosterone by the method of BROWNIE et al. (1964).

assays were carried out on the 32 samples of 5 ml plasma. PEARSON's r for the testosterone concentration in these samples was 0.962 and the SPEARMAN's rank correlation coefficient was 0.866. The mean discrepancy between duplicate estimation was 0.027 µg/100 ml plasma. This mean discrepancy does not differ significantly from zero (RESKO and EIK-NES, 1966).

When 10 or 20 ml of water is processed by this method, the gas chromatographic tracings of such samples are straight or slightly convex lines (Fig. 1). This is also the case if 10 ml plasma samples from ovariectomized-adrenalectomized women are carried through the method (Fig. 1). The fact that no detectable testosterone can be found in blood plasma from this category of patients might be due to the insensitivity of the method at low concentrations of testosterone.

The problem of interference by epitestosterone when using this method for plasma testosterone estimation has, however, not been solved (Table 1). Testosterone chloroacetate and epitestosterone chloro-acetate have about the same retention time on the gas chromatography column used, but one can observe two peaks from a mixture of 0.010 μm pure testosterone chloroacetate and 0.001 μg pure epitestosterone chloroacetate. If a double peak is seen in the testosterone region following gas phase chromatography of a plasma sample, it is recommended that the assay be repeated chromatograph-

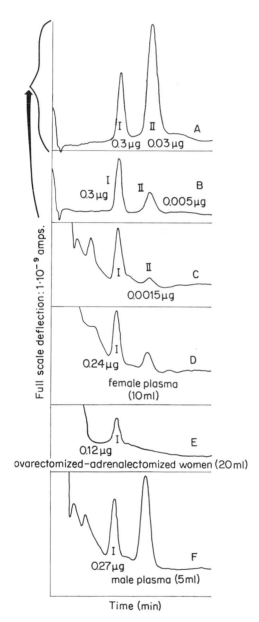

Fig. 1. Gas chromatograms of steroids of human plasma processed by the method of BROWNIE et al. (1964). A. Pure cholesterol chloracetate (I) and pure testosterone chloracetate. B. Pure cholesterol chloracetate (I) and pure testosterone chloracetate. C. 2500 cpm testosterone-³H (specific activity 2.72 μc/μg added to water and processed by the method. D. 10 ml of blood plasma from a normal woman processed by the method. E. 20 ml of blood plasma from an adrenalectomized and ovariectomized woman processed by the method. F. 5 ml of blood plasma from a normal male processed by the method. In all of these experiments, the chloracetate of cholesterol was used as internal standard. Reprinted with the permission of J. clin. Endocr. 1964.

ing the plasma extract on paper in a Bush A_2 system (KORENMAN et al., 1963) before chloroacetylation. We have hitherto failed to see a double peak in the testosterone chloroacetate region in 250 different samples of 10 ml human plasma and in 1500 different samples of from 0.1—1 ml spermatic venous blood from the dog (Fig. 2).

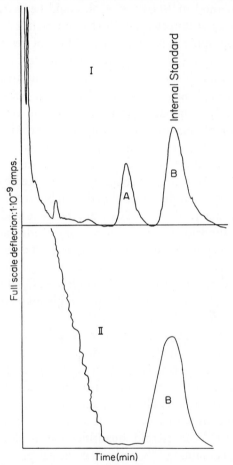

Time(min)

Fig. 2. Gas chromatograms of steroids of spermatic venous blood plasma samples processed by the method of BROWNIE et al. (1964). I. Spermatic venous blood plasma collected in 3 sec from a normal dog. A. Identical retention time to pure testosterone chloroacetate. B. Internal standard (chloroacetate of 20β-reduced progesterone). II. Spermatic venous blood plasma collected for 10 min from a 6 week hypophysectomized dog. B) Internal standard (chloroacetate of 20β-reduced progesterone). For details on collecting spermatic venous blood in the dog, see EIK-NES (1967)

The few data on concentration of plasma testosterone in men and women obtained by this method agree with the data obtained by other methods (HUDSON et al., 1963; RIONDEL et al., 1963), though these methods may be more suitable for the estimation of the low testosterone levels in blood of normal women. Admittedly, the sensitivity of the method of BROWNIE et al. could be increased by using another derivative of testosterone. CLARK and WOTIZ (1963) published a gas chromatographic tracing from 0.001 µg of testosterone-heptafluorobutyrate. Exley (1966) used this derivative for the estimation of testosterone though no data on hormone concentrations in blood plasma from normal men and women have been published using the method. In the "preliminary technique", 0.2 Mµc testosterone-^{3}H is added to 1 ml of plasma and the mixture is extracted with ether. The extract is evaporated to dryness. The residue is chromatographed (TLC) using silica gel H_{254} and the solvent system benzene:ethylacetate (1:1, v/v). Testosterone standards are located by UV scanning and material on the sample lane is eluted with benzene. After evaporation of this extract to dryness, 50 µl dry benzene and 100 µl heptafluorobutyric anhydride are added to the dry residue and the mixture kept at 70° for 30 min. Excess reagent is then blown off with nitrogen. The yield of esterified product is better than 75%. The residue after evaporation is chromatographed on cellulose C.C. 41 in the solvent system acetone:water (3:1, v/v). Again sample material is located by UV scanning of standards of testosterone heptafluorobutyrate and eluted with acetone. High speed centrifugation is required at this step. An aliquot of the eluate is used for recovery calculations, but no data are available on hormone recovery up to this step. To the rest of the sample is added 1 nanogram of estriol triheptafluorobutyrate. The mixture is applied to a small steel gauze, and gas phase chromatography is carried out with a 4 ft 1% SE-30 column operated at 180° C (flash heater, 190° C). Steroid quantification is done by electron capture. Argon containing 5% methane is the gas phase and the pulse-sampling technique is applied to the electron capture cell.

As little as 2.5×10^{-11} gram of pure testosterone can be quantified by the detector device, but no data have been published on accuracy and reproducibility of hormone detection at this level. In a few experiments, measurement of specific radioactivity of radioactive testosterone, processed by the method, gave data within 3—4% of the expected values. The specificity of the method is unknown, but the author states that "the heptafluorobutyrate of epitestosterone is almost completely separated from testosterone heptafluorobutyrate on 1% SE-30" (EXLEY, 1966).

To the best of our knowledge, this is the first attempt to utilize CLARK and WOTIZ' (1963) interesting observation on steroid hepta-fluorobutyrates in a micro method for testosterone estimation. If this method can be applied to adequate, reproducible estimations of testo-sterone in blood plasma, it is not unduly optimistic to expect that testosterone in physiological samples of blood plasma from normal women could be measured by the same accuracy as with the isotope method developed by the research group of Dr. J. F. TAIT. It is, however, much too early to predict the applicability of EXLEY's method to the problem of testosterone estimation in low titre human blood samples though the preliminary data of VAN DER MOLEN look promising (Fig. 3).

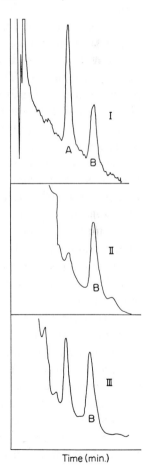

Fig. 3. Gas phase chromatography of: I. 0.0004 pure testosterone heptafluorobutyrate (A) and 0.0004 µg 20β-hydroxyprogesterone hepta-fluorobutyrate (B). Attenuation: 1/32. II. 3.3 ml blood plasma from a woman. B is the tracing of the internal standard (pure 20β-hydroxyprogesterone heptafluorobutyrate). At-tenuation: 10/16. III. 0.8 ml blood plasma from a man. B is the tracing of the internal standard (pure 20β-hydroxyprogesterone hepta-fluorobutyrate). Attenuation: 10/16. The plas-ma samples were processed by the method of BROWNIE et al. (1964), but after first TLC, sample testosterone was reacted with 0.5 ml tetrahydrofurane containing 0.015 ml hepta-fluorobutyric acid for 15 min at room temper-ature. The sample was then evaporated to dryness and the residue chromatographed (TLC, silica gel, benzene : ethylacetate (9 : 1)). Sample material behaving like authentic testosterone heptafluorobutyrate was eluted. The eluate was evaporated to dryness and a known amount of the internal standard added. The sample was then processed as discussed on page 244. Re-covery of testosterone-^{3}H to the stage of GLC was 20% in both experiment II and III. (Data kindly provided by H. J. VAN DER MOLEN.)

Time (min.)

Of all methods published for the estimation of plasma testosterone, the technique of Riondel et al. (1963) appears to have the best precision and accuracy at low concentrations of plasma testosterone. Water blanks carried through this method give very low values and in blood from ovariectomized-adrenalectomized women the mean testosterone concentration is 0.013 µg/100 ml $\pm$ 0.004 (one standard deviation). At plasma concentrations of 0.02 µg, 0.03 µg and 0.07 µg testosterone per 100 ml, the precision of estimation is 30, 15 and 6% respectively. Finally, when 0.0113, 0.0226, 0.0452 and 0.0904 µg of testosterone is added to 10 ml of plasma from ovariectomized-adrenalectomized women, the mean per cent of divergence between the amount of testosterone added and the amount of testosterone found is 5%.

In the method of Guerra-Garcia et al. (1963), testosterone-^{3}H is added to 15 ml of male plasma and the sample is extracted with ether. The extract is washed with 1 N sodium hydroxide and 2% sodium bicarbonate solution. The ether extract is evaporated to dryness. The residue is dissolved in 70% methanol and left in the cold for 12 h. This latter procedure is used to precipitate fat; it has been successfully employed for this purpose in methods for the estimation of plasma progesterone (Zander, 1962). The methanol is extracted with petroleum ether and the alcohol is reduced to $^1/_3$ of its volume. Testosterone is then extracted from this solution with benzene. The residue of the benzene extract is chromatographed (TLC, silica gel) in the solvent system benzene:methanol (85:15, v/v). Material in the plasma extract behaving like authentic testosterone is eluted. Tritium is determined in an aliquot of the eluate. The recovery of testosterone-^{3}H added to water and processed as described is 65%. When testosterone-^{3}H is added to plasma, the recovery of tritium is, however, much lower-about 40%.

The purified testosterone sample is separated with a 6 ft $\times$ $^1/_6$ in. stainless steel column filled with 3% SE-30. Column and flash heater temperatures are maintained at 250° C, and the gas chromatograph is equipped with a flame ionization detector. The retention time for testosterone is about 8 min in this system, but the testosterone plasma peak appears to come too close to the front on the gas chromatographic tracings. A sample of 0.01 µg pure testosterone gives 8—10% of full scale recorder deflection. The sensitivity for adequate testosterone detection by this method is about 0.05 µg. With a recovery of

40% of plasma testosterone, volumes of male plasma larger than 15 ml are recommended. The few levels of testosterone in normal male plasma estimated by this method are in the range of levels found by other methods (HUDSON et al., 1963; RIONDEL et al., 1963; BROWNIE et al., 1964). The precision of the method of GUERRA-GARCIA et al. is not known and it appears unlikely that this method can be used for the estimation of testosterone in physiological amounts of plasma from normal women. Whether or not epitestosterone interferes with testosterone estimation in this method is, moreover, unknown.

SURACE et al. (1966) report on the estimation of testosterone in human blood obtained from both sexes. The plasma (exact volume not given) is processed much in the same way as in the method of GUERRA-GARCIA et al. (1963), but the defatted extract is fractionated by horizontal TLC in the solvent system benzene:ethylacetate (6:4, v/v). Silica gel G or silica gel HF_{254} containing a fluorescent indicator were used. After chromatography for 90 min in this system (R_f testosterone 0.44±0.02 (one standard deviation), R_f epitestosterone 0.47±0.03 (one standard deviation), material in the plasma sample chromatographing like authentic testosterone is eluted with ethanol. The ethanol solution is evaporated to dryness. The recovery of testosterone-^{14}C (added to 10 ml of plasma) to this step is 72—82%.

The residue is acetylated and the sample is then chromatographed on an 80 cm × 0.2 cm GLC column filled either with 3% SE-30 or with 1% QF-1. The column is operated at 240° C and the gas chromatograph is equipped with a double flame ionization detector.

At testosterone concentrations between 0.11—0.33 µg/100 ml of plasma, the average deviation between duplicates is 7.8%±2.8. The range of testosterone levels in the plasma of normal male subjects is about the same as that found when such samples are assayed by other testosterone methods. The mean plasma concentration of 0.11 µg per 100 ml observed for normal women is high (Table 8). The specificity of this method is probably the same as for the technique of GUERRA-GARCIA et al. (1963).

GOLDFIEN et al. (1965) published a technique for the simultaneous estimation of testosterone, androstenedione and free DHEA in blood plasma. About 40—60 ml plasma from the normal woman is needed in order to find detectable levels of testosterone. After the addition of tritiated reference steroids to the plasma, it is extracted with methylenedichloride. The extract is washed with sodium hydroxide solution,

Table 8. *Mean levels of testosterone in blood plasma from normal, adult women*

Authors	Final analysis	µg/100 ml
BROWNIE et al. (1964)	Electron capture	0.060 ± 0.03
SURACE et al. (1966)	Hydrogen flame	0.11 ± 0.06 (0.04 − 0.24)
GOLDFIEN et al. (1965)	Hydrogen flame	0.017 ± 0.009 (0 − 0.35)
VAN DER MOLEN et al. (1966 a)	Electron capture	0.036 (0.02 − 0.08)
HUDSON et al. (1963)	Double isotope	0.12 (0 − 0.35)
HUDSON et al. (1964)	Double isotope	0.083 ± 0.007
RIONDEL et al. (1963)	Double isotope	0.059 ± 0.079
LOBOTZKY et al. (1964)	Double isotope	0.054 ± 0.015 (0.0033 − 0.10)
BURGER et al. (1964)	Double isotope	0.18 (0.06 − 0.31)
KIRSCHNER et al. (1965)	Double isotope	0.07 (0.02 − 0.12)
COPPAGE and COONER (1965)	Double isotope	0.12 (0.012 − 0.20)
SAROFF et al. (1966)	Double isotope	0.08 (0.03 − 0.22)
HORTON and MANN (1966)	Double isotope	0.042 ± 0.005
RIVAROLA and MIGEON (1966)	Double isotope	0.054 ± 0.015 (0.034 − 0.077)
KLIMAN and BRIEFER (1967)	Double isotope	0.04 ± 0.03
FORCHIELLI et al. (1963)	Fluorescence	0.12 (0.02 − 0.26)
LAMB et al. (1964)	Fluorescence	0.11 (0.05 − 0.29)

It should be noted that the plasma concentration of testosterone in normal women varies during the menstrual cycle. A mean concentration of 0.047 µg/100 ml ± 0.010 and 0.061 µg/100 ml ± 0.018 has been reported during menstruation and during the time of ovulation respectively (LOBOTZKY et al., 1964).

Range of values and one standard deviation of the mean value are given in some instances.

acetic acid, water and defatted in the cold (ZANDER, 1962). The fat-free extract is chromatographed on paper in the solvent system cyclohexane: methanol: water (100: 100: 1). The three steroids are separated in 15 h. Each steroid is eluted individually and carried through gas phase chromatography on a 2 ft 8 in. 1% XE-60 column operated at 180° C.

When a pool of male plasma was assayed for testosterone by this method, a mean concentration of 0.55 μg/100 ml ± 0.05 (standard deviation) was found for seven samples. After paper chromatography, the testosterone area in 10 ml samples from this pool was converted by chromic acid oxidation to $\varDelta^4$-androstenedione. This derivative was purified by paper chromatography in the same solvent system. The $\varDelta^4$-androstenedione was quantified by a hydrogen flame detector after gas phase chromatography. A mean hormone concentration of 0.55 μg/100 ml was recorded (standard deviation 0.06, 6 experiments).

The recovery of tritiated testosterone varies from 27—48%. The specificity of the method appears to be adequate. Of interest is the low concentration of testosterone found in blood plasma from normal women (Table 8). Since a large volume of plasma (40—69 ml) is needed for the estimation of testosterone in blood from normal women and since prior to gas phase chromatography only one paper chromatographic separation is used for sample purification and steroid isolation, there is some evidence to suggest that a small amount of testosterone may be lost in non-steroidal "front" material during gas phase chromatography. Such gas chromatograms are difficult to quantify. Also, if relatively large amounts of non-steroidal material are eluted from the column before testosterone, the sensitivity of assay may decrease due to altered detector characteristicis.

In spite of the fact that testosterone conjugated with glucosiduronic acid is present in human blood (HADD and RHAMY, 1965), only two methods (PANICUCCI, 1965; VAN DER MOLEN et al., 1966 a) have been aimed at the estimate of conjugated testosterone in blood. Both methods employ gas phase chromatography. VAN DER MOLEN and co-workers first remove free testosterone from the plasma by ether extraction. The conjugated testosterone is extracted with ethanol (OERTEL and EIK-NES, 1959). The conjugated hormone contained in this extract is hydrolyzed with β-glucuronidase for 48 h, testosterone-³H is added to the hydrolysate and the mixture is extracted with ether. If the ether extract appears rich in fat, it is evaporated to dryness and the residue is partitioned between hexane and 70% methanol. The purified extract is processed by the method of BROWNIE et al. (1964). As expected, the concentration of testosterone glucosiduronate in plasma from normal men is higher (range 0.09—0.59 μg/100 ml) than in plasma from normal women (range 0.02—0.22 μg/100 ml), but the difference observed is much smaller than for free plasma testosterone. This preliminary finding warrants further exploration in light of a mean concentration of testosterone glucosiduronate of 0.11 μg/100 ml plasma from normal women (12 subjects) which is at least twice as high as the concentration of free testosterone found in the same plasma samples.

In the method of PANICUCCI (1966), free plasma testosterone appears not to be removed prior to β-glucuronidase hydrolysis followed by solvolysis, but a recovery standard of testosterone-³H is added to the sample before hydrolysis. The hydrolysate is extracted with ether, fat and phenolic steroids are removed by solvent partitions, and the purified extract is chromatographed (TLC, silica gel HF_{254}) in the solvent system benzene:methanol 85:15. Sample material chromatographing like authentic testosterone is eluted, and the TMSi derivative is prepared. This is chromatographed on a 6 ft 3% NGS column operated at 225° C. Steroid quantification is done by an argon ionization detector which would detect 0.01 μg of the TMSi derivative of testosterone. It is surprising to note that the range of testosterone in blood of normal men was found to be 0.20—0.90 μg/100 ml since the technique should measure the sum of free and conjugated testosterone (SAEZ et al., 1967). The TMSi ethers of testosterone and epitestosterone are separated in the GLC step (see Chapter 1).

Conclusion

In summary, GLC methods are available for the estimation of free testosterone in male blood. When the equipment is at hand, the cost per analysis of testosterone is less than that using other methods (HUDSON et al., 1963; RIONDEL et al., 1963; LIM AND BROOKS, 1965). Thus, a wider scale investigation of clinical problems involving testosterone secretion in the male is possible by gas phase chromatography methods. Also, for diagnostic purposes, the time involved in plasma testosterone estimation by the gas chromatographic methods is shorter than by radioisotope methods. This may occasionally be an important factor, but precision should never be sacrificed for speed. It can therefore be questioned whether or not the gas chromatograph has advanced knowledge on testosterone in plasma since methods not

Table 9. *Lower operational limit for quantification of pure testosterone*

Principle	Sensitivity (µg)	Authors
Isotope labeling with thiose-micarbazide-^{35}S	0.001—0.002	RIONDEL et al., 1963
Isotope labeling with acetic anhydride-^{3}H	0.005—0.05	HUDSON et al., 1963; BURGER et al., 1964
Argon ionization detection	0.02—0.05	KORENMAN et al., 1963; KORENMAN et al., 1964a; BROOKS, 1964; SANDBERG et al., 1964
Flame ionization detection	0.01—0.02	FUTTERWEIT et al., 1963; GUERRA-GARCIA et al., 1963; IBAYASHI et al., 1964
Electron capture of chloroacetate	0.001—0.002	BROWNIE et al., 1964; RESKO and EIK-NES, 1966; VAN DER MOLEN et al., 1966a
Electron capture of hepta-fluorobutyrate	0.0001	CLARK and WOTIZ, 1963; EXLEY, 1966
Absorption: sulfuric acid chromogen (λ max: 299 mµ)	1.0—2.0	BURNSTEIN and LENHARD, 1953; CAMACHO and MIGEON, 1963
Absorption: anisaldehyde-ethanol-sulfuric acid chromogen (λ max: 510 mµ, $\varepsilon = 50\,000$)	0.1—0.2	OERTEL and EIK-NES, 1959
Absorption: sulfuric acid-ethanol/thiocol-cupri sulfate chromogen (λ max: 635 mµ)	0.2—0.4	KOENIG et al., 1941; MARTIN, 1962
Absorption: sulfuric acid-$(NH_4)_2Fe(SO_4)_2$-KM_nO_4 chromogen (λ max: 630, $\varepsilon = 14\,000$)	0.5—1	SACHS, 1964
Fluorescence: sulfuric acid-ethanol chromogen	0.01—0.05	WILSON, 1960; KORENMAN et al., 1963; KORENMAN et al., 1964a; SACHS, 1964; GERDES and STAIN, 1965
Conversion to estradiol and fluorescence in phosphoric acid	0.005—0.010	FINKELSTEIN et al., 1947; FINKELSTEIN, 1952; FINKELSTEIN et al., 1961

Table 9 (continued)

Principle	Sensitivity (µg)	Authors
Conversion to Δ^4-androstenedione and absorption of Zimmermann chromogen	1.5—2.5	HORTON et al., 1963; VERMEULEN and VERPLANCKE, 1963
Ultraviolet absorption (λ max: 240 mµ, $\varepsilon = 17\,000$)	0.5—1.0	DORFMAN, 1953; SCHUBERT and WEHRBERGER, 1960; CAMACHO and MIGEON, 1963
Absorption: dinitrophenylhydrazone derivative (λ max: 380 mµ, $\varepsilon = 27\,000$)	0.1—0.2	MADIGAN et al., 1951; REICH et al., 1953; LUCAS et al., 1957
Absorption: isonicotinic acid hydrazone derivative (λ max: 380 mµ, $\varepsilon = 11\,000$)	1.0—2.0	UMBERGER, 1955; TAMM et al., 1963
Absorption: thiosemicarbazone derivative (λ max: 308 mµ, $\varepsilon = 35\,600$)	0.1—0.3	PEARLMAN and CERCEO, 1953; BUSH, 1953 UMBERGER, 1955; RIONDEL et al., 1963
Absorption: p-nitrophenylhydrazone derivative (λ max: 540 mµ, $\varepsilon = 32\,000$)	0.1—0.3	NISHINA et al., 1964

employing this instrument appear more applicable for low plasma concentration of the hormone (HUDSON et al., 1963; RIONDEL et al., 1963; LIM AND BROOKS, 1965) (Table 9). The combined techniques of double isotope dilution and gas phase chromatography may, however, in the future comprise a powerful method for the estimation of small amounts of testosterone in biological fluids (KLIMAN and BRIEFER, 1967). Finally, measurement of plasma testosterone by competitive protein binding analysis (FRITZ and KNOBIL, 1967) may suspend further attempts to use gas phase chromatography or isotope dilution as methods for the estimation of testosterone in human blood.

The radioisotope techniques employ isotope of different energy spectra for steroid estimation. It is difficult to use such techniques for steroid quantitation when the steroid is biosynthetized from radioactive precursors (TAIT, 1966, personal communication). An example is given in Fig. 4 and 5 of the usefulness of gas phase chromatography with electron capture detection for specific radioactivity estimation of spermatic venous blood testosterone. In this particular experiment, a mixture of acetate-1-^{14}C and cholesterol-7α-^{3}H was infused via the spermatic artery of the rabbit testis. The concentration of testosterone

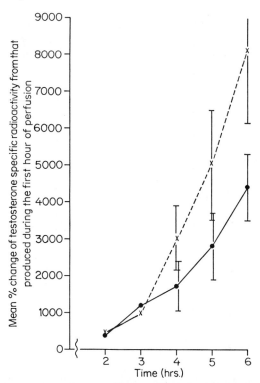

Fig. 4. Effect of interstitial cell stimulating hormone (ICSH) on mean specific radioactivity of testosterone-^{14}C produced by rabbit testes perfused with a mixture of acetate-1-^{14}C and cholesterol-7α-^{3}H via the spermatic artery. The data are from 4 control testes and 8 testes also perfused with ICSH. When used, ICSH was perfused at a constant rate from the 3rd—6th h of experiment. Spermatic venous blood testosterone was determined by the method of BROWNIE et al. (1964).
$\top$ One standard error of the mean. (From EWING and EIK-NES, 1966.) Reprinted with the permission of Canad. J. Biochem.

in these samples was much too low to be determined by the available spectrophotometric or fluorometric methods for quantitative estimation of the hormone (EIK-NES et al., 1967) (Table 9). Through the use of gas phase chromatography with sensitive detection, valuable data were obtained relating to metabolic disposal of acetate and cholesterol in the testis (EWING and EIK-NES, 1966). It is in this specific field of endocrine research that gas phase chromatography with sensitive detectors may give significant information.

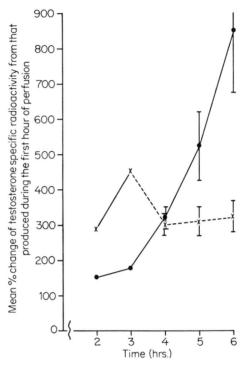

Fig. 5. Effect of ICSH on mean specific radioactivity of testosterone-³H produced by rabbit testes perfused with a mixture of acetate-1-¹⁴C and cholesterol-7α-³H via the spermatic artery. The data are from 4 control testes and 8 testes also perfused with ICSH. When used, ICSH was perfused at a constant rate from the 3rd—6th h of experiment. Spermatic venous blood testosterone was determined by the method of BROWNIE et al. (1964).
$\underline{\text{I}}$ One standard error of the mean. (From EWING and EIK-NES, 1966.) Reprinted with the permission of Canad. J. Biochem.

2. Δ⁴-Androstenedione in Plasma

Methods using gas phase chromatography for the determination of this hormone in plasma were first developed for the estimation of Δ⁴-androstenedione in ovarian and testicular venous blood (NISHIZAWA and EIK-NES, 1964; AAKVAAG and EIK-NES, 1965; VAN DER MOLEN and EIK-NES, 1967, VAN DER MOLEN and GROEN, 1967). NISHIZAWA and EIK-NES (1964) extract plasma from canine ovarian vein blood with methylenedichloride after addition of androstenedione-^{14}C. Following removal of estrogens, the extract is evaporated and the residue is dissolved in ligroin which is then extracted with 70% methanol. The methanol is evaporated and the aqueous residue is extracted with ether. After evaporation of the ether extract, the residue is chromatographed on paper in the solvent system methylcyclohexane: propylene glycol for 11 h. Material chromatographing like authentic Δ^4-androstenedione is eluted and applied to a 6 ft 0.75% SE-30 column operated at 213° C.

The recovery of Δ^4-androstenedione-^{14}C through the method including gas chromatography is 27% ± 1.6 (one standard deviation in 32 experiments). No data are given for accuracy or sensitivity of this method, but samples containing less than 0.2 µg of the steroid cannot be detected with any degree of precision. There appears to be good correlation between plasma concentration of Δ^4-androstenedione determined by ultraviolet spectrophotometry after elution from the paper chromatogram and those determined by the argon detector after gas phase chromatography. Moreover, when plasma from animals receiving acetate-1-^{14}C via the ovarian artery was assayed by this method, Δ^4-androstenedione-^{14}C could be collected from the gas chromatographic column in a high state of radiochemical purity. AAKVAAG and EIK-NES (1965) use this method for quantitation of Δ^4-androstenedione in ovarian venous blood, but after the paper chromatographic step, plasma Δ^4-androstenedione is chromatographed (TLC, silica gel) in the solvent system benzene:ethylacetate (3:1, v/v). Material in the plasma sample chromatographing like authentic hormone is eluted and then chromatographed on a 3 ft 2% SE-30 column. Progesterone is used as an internal standard. This modification of the original method is preferred when working with ovarian vein blood. Sensitivity is about 0.15 µg of hormone per sample. At plasma concentrations of 2, 4 and 8 µg of Δ^4-androstenedione, the accuracy of estimation is 12%, 7% and 5% respectively.

VAN DER MOLEN and EIK-NES (1966) employ gas phase chromatography for the estimation of Δ^4-androstenedione in spermatic venous blood of the dog. The pH of the plasma is adjusted to 9. with sodium hydroxide solution, Δ^4-androstenedione-^{3}H added to the plasma which is then extracted with ether (BROWNIE et al., 1964). The extract is evaporated and the residue chromatographed on paper in the solvent system methylcyclohexane : propyleneglycol. In this system the steroids in the spermatic venous blood of the dog chromatograph as follows:

Area A: 0—7 cm from the application line: androstenediol, 17α-hydroxypregnenolone, 17α-hydroxyprogesterone and testosterone.

Area B: 7—12 cm from the application line: dehydroepiandrosterone.

Area C: 15—22 cm from the application line: Δ^4-androstenedione and Δ^5-pregnenolone.

Area D: 26—30 cm from the application line: progesterone.

Area C is eluted and rechromatographed in 70% methanol : ligroin for 8—9 h (Bush A system). The R_fs of Δ^4-androstenedione and Δ^5-pregnenolone in this system are 0.40 and 0.50 respectively. The material in plasma behaving chromatographically like authentic Δ^4-androstenedione is eluted, acetylated and chromatographed (TLC, silica gel) in benzene : ethylacetate (2 : 1, v/v). This latter step will avoid possible contamination of Δ^4-androstenedione with Δ^5-pregnenolone and DHEA. Δ^4-Androstenedione (R_f 0.50) is eluted, testosterone added as an internal standard, and an aliquot of the eluate is removed for recovery estimation. The rest of the mixture is chromatographed on a 6 ft 1% XE-60 glass column. Steroid quantification is done with a flame ionization detector.

The recovery before gas chromatography is about 50% in this method. When the concentration of Δ^4-androstenedione in the final sample for gas chromatography analysis varies between 0.06—3.0 μg, the precision of assay is 4.6% (VAN DER MOLEN and GROEN, 1967). This method has been applied to the measurement of specific radioactivity of spermatic venous blood Δ^4-androstenedione following infusion of Δ^5-pregnenolone-^{14}C via the spermatic artery (VAN DER MOLEN and EIK-NES, 1966).

In their study of the effect of gonadotrophins on ovarian biosynthesis of steroids, McKERNS and NORDSTRAND (1965) employed a gas chromatographic method for purification and quantification of Δ^4-androstenedione in ovarian tissue homogenates. The homogenate is extracted with methylenedichloride : methanol (2 : 1, v/v). The extract is evaporated and the residue is dissolved in methylenedichloride. After washing with water, TMSi ethers are made of the steroids contained in the methylenedichloride solution. Fat is then removed by the addition of silica gel G to the methylenedichloride solution and the defatted mixture of TMSi derivatives of ovarian steroids is separated by gas phase chromatography. Under the conditions of this experiment, a hybrid column (6 ft × 0.4 cm) containing a mixture of 3% XE-60 and 3% SE-30 (1 : 1, w/w) and operated at 235° C gave the best separation of Δ^4-androstenedione from the other ovarian steroids contained in the purified extract. It should be noted that with continuous use the hybrid column loses polarity (this is probably due to bleeding of the XE-60 phase). The recovery of known amounts of steroids (no data given for Δ^4-androstenedione, however) added to ovarian homogenates and processed as described is adequate. The TMSi derivatives of 20α- and 20β-hydroxyprogesterone will, however, interfere seriously with accurate measurement of ovarian tissue Δ^4-androstenedione on the hybrid column. This problem is circumvented by chromatographing a part of the extract on a 3.8% SE-30 column (4 ft × 0.3 cm). For investigations of Δ^4-androstenedione formation by the ovary in *in vitro* systems, this method offers great promise. Purification by paper or thin-layer chromatography before derivative formation should be done, however, to remove the danger of 20α- and 20β-hydroxyprogesterone interfering in Δ^4-androstenedione isolation and quantification following gas phase chromatography on the hybrid column.

By the method of GOLDFIEN et al. (1965), plasma levels of Δ^4-androstenedione can be measured in blood from normal men and women. After paper chromatography (see page 254), plasma Δ^4-androstenedione is chromatographed under the same conditions as plasma testosterone. The recovery before gas phase chromatography of the radioactive standard is between 20—55% and in a sample of pooled plasma from male subjects, 0.15 ± 0.04 µg Δ^4-androstenedione could be determined (8 experiments). The mean level of Δ^4-androstenedione in blood from normal women (Table 10) checks well with the values observed by HORTON (1965).

VAN DER MOLEN and his co-workers (1966 a) add radioactive Δ^4-androstenedione of high specific activity to 10 ml of plasma and the sample is processed as it is in the testosterone method of BROWNIE et al. (1964) (see page 244) with the following exceptions: thin-layer chromatography is carried out in the solvent system benzene : ethylacetate 2 : 1, thus enabling separation of Δ^4-androstenedione from plasma progesterone. Plasma Δ^4-androstenedione is then eluted and

Table 10. *Mean levels of Δ⁴-androstenedione in blood plasma from normal adult women and men*

Authors	No. of sub-jects	Sex	Endpoint of analysis	µg/100 ml
GOLDFIEN et al., 1965	21	F	Flame ionization	0.163 ± 0.096 (0.023 − 0.410)
VAN DER MOLEN et al., 1966 a	7	F	Electron capture	0.28 (< 0.10 − 0.40)
VAN DER MOLEN et al., 1966 a	9	M	Electron capture	0.20 (< 0.10 − 0.25)
HORTON, 1965	10	F *	Double isotope	0.145 ± 0.044
HORTON, 1965	10	F **	Double isotope	0.160 ± 0.029
HORTON, 1965	12	M	Double isotope	0.075 ± 0.014
GANDY and PETERSON, 1964	6	F	Double isotope	0.15 − 1.90
GANDY and PETERSON, 1964	14	M	Double isotope	0.20 − 0.91
RIVAROLA and MIGEON, 1966	9	F	Double isotope	0.197 ± 0.054 (0.124 − 0.301)
RIVAROLA and MIGEON, 1966	10	M	Double isotope	0.114 ± 0.022
SAROFF et al., 1966	4	M	Double isotope	0.10 − 0.22
HORTON and MANN, 1966	8	F	Double isotope	0.139 ± 0.006
HORTON and MANN, 1966	4	M	Double isotope	0.077
LIM and BROOKS, 1966	10	F	Double isotope	0.095 (0.022 − 0.144)
LIM and BROOKS, 1966	10	M	Double isotope	0.060 (0.024 − 0.093)

* Plasma obtained from women during the follicular state.
** Plasma obtained from women during the luteal state.
Range of values and one standard deviation of the mean value are given in some instances.

reduced with borohydride to testosterone, although the yield of this reaction at the submicrogram level is poor. The formed testosterone is then chloroacetylated and the derivative processed like testosterone-chloroacetate in the method of BROWNIE et al. (1964). Concentrations of less than 0.1 µg Δ^4-androstenedione/100 ml plasma cannot be distinguished from zero concentrations of the hormone. When 0.040 µg Δ^4-androstenedione is added to water and processed by this method, a mean concentration of 0.042 µg is recorded with a precision of assay of 10%. This method should have a high specificity but the concentrations found in plasma from normal male and female subjects are high (Table 10).

Since the techniques for estimating Δ^4-androstenedione in human plasma are still in their infancy, not too much emphasis should be placed on the rather preliminary data recorded in Table 10. Regardless of the analytical method, there is considerable disagreement about the circulating levels of the hormone in normal subjects. HORTON (1965) published data on the validity of his double isotope method showing that the precision of assay for high plasma concentrations of Δ^4-androstenedione is 4.3%. The method should be applicable to the estimation of 0.020 µg hormone/100 ml plasma. In plasma from 3 ovariectomized-adrenalectomized patients, 0.0012, 0.0012 and 0.0013 µg Δ^4-androstenedione were found per 100 ml. These values are not significantly different from the values obtained when samples of water were processed by this method.

Conclusion

At the current stage of development gas phase chromatography has contributed little to the technology of Δ^4-androstenedione estimation in physiological amounts of human plasma. Admittedly, the method of HORTON (1965) is laborious and operates with an extremely low recovery. In the method of GOLDFIEN et al. (1965), less time is involved per assay, the recovery of added reference steroid is high, but large amounts of blood are needed. Moreover, further data on the specificity, accuracy, sensitivity and precision of this method must be published. It is difficult to understand the rather high plasma levels of Δ^4-androstenedione found by the method of VAN DER MOLEN et al. (1966 a). Analytical trouble was encountered in the conversion of Δ^4-androstenedione to testosterone.

Since the concentration of the hormone in human blood is low (Table 10), a sensitive estimation procedure must be used. During the last year our laboratory has converted purified plasma Δ^4-androstenedione to testosterone by a 17β-hydroxy steroid dehydrogenase obtained from placental tissue. The enzymic conversion to testosterone is high (better than 85%). Testosterone is then chloroacetylated and estimated by electron capture (BROWNIE, 1964). Chromatographic tracings from analysis of Δ^4-androstenedione in peripheral and spermatic venous blood of the stallion are presented in Fig. 6. The recovery of Δ^4-androstenedione through the method is rather low, about 20%. The precision and sensitivity of testosterone quantification are as published by our laboratory (BROWNIE et al., 1964).

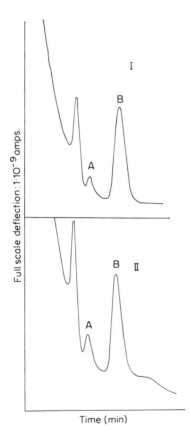

Fig. 6. Gas phase chromatography of: I. 5.7 ml peripheral blood plasma from a stallion. Peak A has the same retention time as pure testosterne chloroacetate. B is the tracing of the internal standard (pure 20β-hydroxyprogesterone chloracetate). II. 0.9 ml plasma from spermatic venous blood of the stallion used in Experiment I. The plasma was extracted with methylene dichloride after the addition of a trace amount of Δ^4-androstenedione-^{3}H. The extract was evaporated to dryness and the residue dissolved in toluene. The toluene was extracted with 1 N sodium hydroxide solution to remove phenolic compounds and the toluene was then evaporated to dryness. The residue was chromatographed (TLC, silica gel) in the solvent system cyclohexane: ethylacetate 1 : 1, material in the plasma sample chromatographing like authentic Δ^4-androstenedione removed and converted to testosterone by a placental 17β-hydroxysteroid dehydrogenase. The product of this reaction was chromatographed (TLC, silica gel) in the same solvent system as used in the first TLC and material chromatographing like authentic testosterone eluted and the eluate evaporated to dryness. The residue was then processed as described by our laboratory (BROWNIE et al., 1964), except that the chloracetate of 20β-hydroxyprogesterone was used as internal standard (G. M. CONNELL and K. B. EIK-NES. Unpublished, 1967)

3. 17-Ketosteroids (17-KS) in Plasma

The concentration of the two predominant 17-ketosteroids of human plasma, DHEA and androsterone, is relatively high (MIGEON and PLAGER, 1954 b; MIGEON, 1956) and the sensitive detector devices of the gas chromatograph offer little improvement in methodology. Precise assay for these steroids can be made on physiological amounts of plasma by techniques using spectrophotometry (GARDNER, 1953; MIGEON and PLAGER, 1954 b; CLAYTON et al., 1955; TAMM et al., 1957; OERTEL and EIK-NES, 1958, CERESA and CRAVETTO, 1958; SAIER et al., 1959; EIK-NES et al., 1959; SIMMER et al., 1959; HUDSON and OERTEL, 1961).

Androsterone and DHEA circulate in human plasma as conjugates. Since it is preferable to work with the free steroids, the steroid conjugates must be hydrolyzed prior to purification. It will serve no purpose to review data supporting artefact formation of conjugated 17-ketosteroids following acid hydrolysis. These artefacts are probably products of dehydration, halogenation and other rearrangements (DORFMAN and SHIPLEY, 1956). The gas chromatographic evidence presented by COOPER and CREECH (1961) on artefact formation of DHEA following acid hydrolysis at elevated temperature is no great surprise.

Besides the use of enzymes for cleavage of conjugated 17-ketosteroids, several non-enzymic methods have been introduced for this hydrolysis (BURSTEIN and LIEBERMAN, 1958; JACOBSOHN and LIEBERMAN, 1962, EBERLEIN, 1963; DePAOLI et al., 1963). These methods are certainly to be preferred over acid hydrolysis though specific enzymic hydrolysis appears to be the method of choice (DePAOLI et al., 1963; CAWLEY et al., 1965). It should, however, be realized that even such methods may give false values since urine and probably also blood plasma contain substances which will inhibit the enzyme β-glucuronidase (LEVVY, 1956). This area of methodology is at best ill explored.

Whether free DHEA exists in human plasma has been debated (TAMM et al., 1957; COHN et al., 1961). In light of the reports that DHEA sulphate has no biological activity (LIPSETT et al., 1965) and that free DHEA has some androgenic effect (PEILLON and RACADOT, 1965), estimation of "free" plasma DHEA may be of significance. Free plasma DHEA can be measured by the method of GOLDFIEN et al. (1965). After paper chromatography (see page 254), plasma DHEA is eluted and carried through gas phase chromatography on a 2 ft 8 in 1% XE-60 column. The recovery of labeled DHEA, added to the plasma before extraction and carried through the paper chromatographic step, is about 35%. When samples of from 40—60 ml of plasma from twenty two individual normal women were processed by this method, a mean concentration of 0.720 µg ± 0.432 DHEA per 100 ml was found with values as low as 0.180 and as high as 1.92 µg/100 ml of plasma. Concentrations at this level could not have been determined with any degree of accuracy by colorimetric technique; gas phase chromatography with sensitive detection may therefore offer methodological improvement in this field. Experiments are, however, needed to demonstrate that "free" DHEA is not produced in the process of sample handling (BAULIEU, 1962). It is of interest to note that SAROFF et al. (1966) and GANDY and PETERSON (1964) using isotope techniques find levels of free DHEA in plasma of normal women in much the same range as those reported by GOLDFIEN et al. (1966).

Conjugated 17-KS in human plasma have been estimated following gas phase chromatography and as in most blood plasma assays, considerable time must be spent on sample purification.

SJÖVALL and VIHKO (1965) extract 5—10 ml serum with acetone : ethanol (1 : 1, v/v) for 12—16 h at 39° C (VIHKO, 1966). Care is also exercised to reextract the precipitated protein (OERTEL and EIK-NES, 1958, EIK-NES et al., 1959). The combined extract is then chromatographed on methylated Sephadex-G 25 in order to separate conjugated steroids from phospholipids, triglycerides, cholesterol and its esters. The conjugated steroids are then subjected to solvolysis (BURSTEIN and LIEBERMAN, 1958), and cholesterol is removed from the free steroids by column chromatography on silicic acid. To the C_{19} steroid fraction from this column is added epicoprostanol as an internal standard, and the TMSi ethers of this mixture are formed. The ethers are chromatographed either on 3% QF-1 (glass column 1.8 m × 0.4 cm, column temperature 190° C) or on 2.2% SE-30 (glass column 2 m × 0.35 cm, column temperature 220° C for 6 min, then programmed at a rate of 2°/min to 255° C). Since the values of serum androsterone are 30% higher when determined with a QF-1 than with an SE-30 column, the former is used for purification of serum DHEA and the latter for serum androsterone. Serum androsterone of extremely high purity can be detected following gas phase chromatography on a

2.5 m × 0.35 cm glass column containing hexamethyldisilazane treated QF-1. This column is operated at 220° C. On the QF-1 column the TMSi ethers of DHEA, androsterone and 3β,17β-dihydroxyandrost-5-ene are well separated (SJÖVALL and VIHKO, 1966). If the DHEA serum peak in this separation has an extra elevation with slightly longer retention time than DHEA (TMSi), it is probably due to contamination with serum epiandrosterone (SJÖVALL and VIHKO, 1966). The SE-30 column separates the TMSi ethers of DHEA and androsterone from the TMSi ether of 3β,20α-dihydroxypregn-5-ene (SJÖVALL and VIHKO, 1966).

In an extension of this work, VIHKO (1966) has demonstrated the validity of the original SJÖVALL-VIHKO (1963) method. When the sulphates of androstenediol, androsterone, dehydroepiandrosterone, epiandrosterone and etiocholanolone were added to serum and processed by the method, they were recovered in yields better than 75%. The precision of the method is high and similar for androstenediol, androsterone, dehydroepiandrosterone and epiandrosterone. Moreover, as little as about 2 μg of any of these steroids in 100 ml of serum can be quantified. The serum levels of DHEA and androsterone found by this method in normal subjects are high, though not out of range with those published for dehydroepiandrosterone sulphate and for androsterone sulphate by other workers (HUDSON and OERTEL, 1961; OERTEL and KAISER, 1962; McKENNA and RIPPON, 1965; CONRAD et al., 1965). VIHKO (1966) records the absence of etiocholanolone sulphate in serum from normal subjects.

The plasma 17-ketosteroid method of MIGEON and PLAGER (1954 b) is the basis for the gas chromatographic technique of SANDBERG and co-workers for the routine estimation of androsterone and DHEA in 5 ml of plasma (SANDBERG et al., 1965 b). After the addition of 7α-DHEA-^{3}H sulphate to the plasma, conjugated 17-ketosteroids are extracted with warm ethanol. The alcohol is evaporated to dryness, the residue is dissolved in water containing sulphuric acid (pH 0.8) and the solution is extracted continuously with ether for 48 h. After washing the ether extract with sodium bicarbonate solution and water, the ether is evaporated to dryness and the residue is chromatographed on an alumina column. The steroids under investigation are eluted from the column in 0.5% ethanol in benzene. This eluate is chromatographed (TLC, silica gel) in the solvent system ligroin : ethylacetate (1 : 1, v/v). The R$_f$ of authentic DHEA and androsterone in this system is 0.53—0.56 while that of etiocholanolone is 0.42. Plasma material with these R_f values is eluted from the plate and ^3H is measured in an aliquot of the plasma DHEA sample. To the rest of the plasma samples is added a known amount of epitestosterone and TMSi ethers are formed. The steroid TMSi ethers are then separated by gas phase chromatography on a 6 ft glass column packed with 2% XE-60. This column is operated at 216° C and steroid quantification is done by an argon ionization detector. If material behaving chromatographically like the TMSi ether of authentic etiocholanolone is found in an aliquot of the plasma sample, the rest of the plasma etiocholanolone sample is converted to its trifluoroacetoxy derivative (VANDEN HEUVEL et al., 1961) and chromatographed on an XE-60 column.

The mean recovery of DHEA-^3H sulphate assayed by the method is 72% with a recovery range of from 46—95%. The major loss of radioactivity occurs during the TLC purification. The precision of measurement using purified plasma steroids is about the same in the range of from 29—47 μg of androsterone and in the range of from 84—104 μg DHEA/100 ml with a standard deviation varying from 0.9—2.1 for androsterone and from 2.2—3.1 for DHEA. At plasma concentrations of androsterone from 16—36 μg per 100 ml, the precision of estimate ranges from 0.3—5 μg. For DHEA this precision varies from 1.3—17 at plasma concentrations of DHEA varying from 49—128 μg/100 ml. Concentrations of less than 2 μg etiocholanolone/100 ml of plasma cannot be measured adequately by the technique of SANDBERG et al. Since there is no agreement between investigators as to whether etiocholanolone is present (BAULIEU, 1960; OERTEL and EIK-NES, 1961; DRAY and ADAM, 1962; EBERLEIN, 1963; DENEVE and VERMEULEN, 1965) or absent (CLAYTON et al., 1955; CONRAD et al., 1961; VIHKO, 1966) in normal human plasma, gas chromatography with sensitive detection of an etiocholanolone derivative (CLARK and WOTIZ, 1963; BROWNIE et al., 1964; NAKAGAWA et al., 1966; THOMAS, 1966) should be used to settle this somewhat thorny problem.

In the preceding methods for the measurement of plasma 17-KS, these compounds have been extracted as conjugates with an alcohol. Such extractions may occasionally give emulsion trouble, a problem circumvented in the method of SJÖVALL et al. (1966) where plasma or serum DHEA sulphate is adsorbed on a strong ion exchanger by direct application to an Amberlyst XN 1006 column (SANDBERG et al., 1965 a). Conjugated DHEA is eluted from the Amberlyst XN 1006 column with 80% ethanol-water containing ammonium carbonate and p-toluenesulfonic acid, and after the addition of epicoprostanol as an internal standard to this eluate, conjugated DHEA is hydrolyzed either by the method of VESTERGAARD and CLAUSSEN (1962) or by the method of BURSTEIN and LIEBERMAN (1958). Following extractions of free steroid from the hydrolysate and TMSi ether formation, the DHEA derivative is chromatographed on 6 or 12 ft × 0.4 cm columns of 1—2% QF-1 or 1—1.5% NGS. These columns are maintained at 190—215° C and quantification following gas phase chromatography is done either with an argon or a flame ionization detector.

The recovery of a total of 3.9 µg of DHEA sulphate added to plasma and serum and processed by this method varies between 80 to 98% and the specificity of the method is most adequate since the DHEA-TMSi ether in purified blood samples could be identified by mass spectrometric examination in a gas chromatography-mass spectrometry combination instrument (see Chapter 1). This method appears to have the same specificity as the method of SJÖVALL and VIHKO (1965) although with increased adrenal activity like that seen following ACTH administration the more time-consuming method of SJÖVALL and VIHKO (1965) is probably the preferred one. In the method of SJÖVALL et al. (1966), material interfering with the accurate estimation of DHEA is present in plasma of subjects treated with ACTH.

DEMOOR and HEYNS (1966) remove free DHEA and androsterone from plasma prior to solvolysis. The solvolysate is extracted with petroleum ether, purified by chromatography on a small alumina column, and the TMSi ethers of DHEA and androsterone formed. Gas phase chromatography of these ethers is then performed on a 6 ft column packed with 0.60% XE-60 and 0.35% SE-30. The column is operated at 210° C and steroid quantification is done by a flame ionization detector. The recovery through the method is better than 90% for DHEA sulphate, and at plasma levels of 61 µg DHEA and of 27 µg androsterone/100 ml, the standard deviation in duplicate estimations is 6.9 µg for DHEA and 3.5 µg/100 ml for androsterone. No diurnal variation of DHEA sulphate levels in normal subjects could be found. This is also the observation of LAMB et al. (1964) assaying DHEA by a technique not involving gas phase chromatography. Migeon et al. (1957), Eik-Nes et al. (1959), Fotherby and Strong (1960) and Kirschner et al. (1965) all found diurnal variation of conjugated DHEA in plasma of normal subjects. One notes with interest that DeMoor and Heyns (1966) fail to find increments in plasma concentrations of DHEA sulphate in normal subjects following the administration of ACTH. Administration of this trophin resulted, however, in a threefold increase in excretion of total DHEA in the urine. These data suggest that further exploration of the ratio between DHEA sulphate and DHEA glucosiduronate in blood plasma of normal men and women are warranted both during a 24 h day and during administration of ACTH. The sensitive detectors of the gas chromatograph should permit accurate measurements of the small amounts of DHEA glucosiduronate present in human plasma (Migeon, 1960).

In spermatic venous blood of the dog (Eik-Nes and Hall, 1962; Ibayashi et al., 1965), DHEA exists predominately as a free compound and both Ibayashi et al. (1965) and van der Molen and Eik-Nes (1967) use gas phase chromatography for purification and measurement of DHEA in this blood source. Ibayashi et al. (1965) extract spermatic venous blood with ether : chloroform (4 : 1) and after washing the extract in the standard fashion with 0.1 N sodium hydroxide solution and water, the ether chloroform extract is evaporated to dryness. The residue is chromatographed on paper in the solvent mixture petroleum ether (100) : methanol (85) : water (15) for 5 h. In this system of paper chromatography, DHEA and Δ^4-androstenedione do not separate too well. The combined DHEA and Δ^4-androstenedione area is eluted and chromatographed on a 1.4 m 1% SE-30 column. The gas chromatograph is equipped with an argon ionization detector and chromatography is done at 225° C. The relative retention time (cholestane) of DHEA and Δ^4-androstenedione with this column is 0.41 and 0.57 respectively. The levels of DHEA in spermatic venous blood of dogs stimulated with gonadotrophins are much higher by the method of Ibayashi et al. (1965) than those reported by van der Molen and Eik-Nes (1967). Moreover, van der Molen and Eik-Nes (1967) find Δ^4-androstenedione in spermatic venous blood of the normal dog and Ibayashi and co-workers have difficulties in detecting this hormone in the spermatic venous blood of dogs not treated with gonadotrophins. The reasons for these discrepancies are currently not known.

The technique used by VAN DER MOLEN and EIK-NES in the latter investigation has already been discussed (see page 262). Plasma DHEA is eluted from the first paper chromatogram (Area B, page 262), purified by TLC in the solvent system benzene : ethylacetate (2 : 1, v/v) and chromatographed on a 6 ft × 0.4 cm 1% XE-60 column. A flame ionization detector is used for steroid quantification. When the concentration of DHEA in the final sample for gas chromatography analysis varies between 0.03—3.5 µg, the precision of assay is 3.8%. Recovery of DHEA from plasma up to the step of gas chromatography is about 50%.

•Finally, in the gas chromatographic method of McKERNS and NORDSTRAND (1965), free DHEA can be isolated from a homogenate of ovarian tissue. A 3% SE-30 column operated at 210—225° C appears best for the separation of DHEA from other steroids present in ovarian tissue. In this system of chromatography the following steroid TMSi derivatives may interfere with adequate DHEA TMSi isolation: Δ^4-androstenedione, estrone and 19-nortestosterone. The two latter compounds could be separated from DHEA by a toluene sodium hydroxide partition of the original extract. Since these authors chromatograph their biological sample on different columns, separation of the DHEA derivative can be achieved, but the method requires repeated chromatography of the same sample and at low DHEA concentrations in the original extract the application of the method may be somewhat limited.

Conclusion

Methods for the estimation of plasma 17-ketosteroids by the technique of gas phase chromatography indeed exist. Whether for total 17-ketosteroids these methods offer a distinct advantage over colorimetric methods is doubtful since hydrolysis of plasma also liberates conjugated plasma material of non-steroidal nature and extensive purification of the plasma extract is required before adequate measurement of plasma 17-KS can be made regardless of the final method of analysis that is employed. The ease of separating individual plasma 17-ketosteroids is, however, a distinct feature of adequately designed gas chromatographic methods. Moreover, the scholarly exploration of VIHKO (1966) clearly demonstrates the usefulness of gas phase chromatography for the estimation of circulating levels of epiandrosterone and androsterone in man. The importance of estimations of individual 17-ketosteroids is beyond the scope of this discussion, but the clinical and experimental value of the observations is greatly enhanced by adequate steroid separation.

The detector devices of the gas chromatograph may also lead to better precision for 17-KS estimation than by colorimetric assays, but in one of the better of these latter methods, precision of assay below 75 µg 17-ketosteroids/100 ml was 3.8 µg/100 ml (DeNeve and Vermeulen, 1965). Such precision should be sufficient for the clinical laboratory. Further work in the field of gas chromatography of plasma 17-ketosteroids should therefore concentrate on the estimation of plasma 17-ketosteroids existing in concentrations below the detection limit of colorimetric analysis (Oertel and Kaiser, 1962). Such work appears fortunately to be under way (Sjövall and Vihko, 1966; Vihko, 1966).

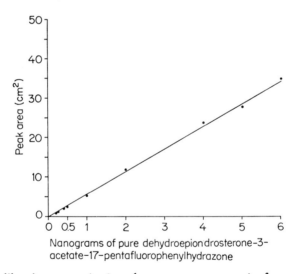

Fig. 7. Calibration curve (cm² peak area vs. nanograms) of pure dehydro-epiandrosterone-3-acetate-17-pentafluorophenylhydrazone. GLC was done on a 2 ft 1% XE-60 column operated at 206° C. Conditions of GLC are described in a publication by Brownie et al. (1964). (From G. F. Wassermann and K. B. Eik-Nes. Unpublished, 1967)

It has been pointed out that the estimation of free plasma DHEA may be of importance. Attal et al. (1967) have published that steroid pentafluorophenylhydrazones will capture electrons and can be determined with high sensitivity following gas phase chromatography. We have used this derivative for the quantification of free DHEA in peripheral blood plasma, in adrenal venous and in spermatic venous blood plasma of the dog (WASSERMANN and EIK-NES, 1967). The

Fig. 8. Gas phase chromatography of: I. 9.7 ml adrenal venous blood plasma from a dog. Peak A has the same retention time as the pure 3-acetate-17-pentafluorphenylhydrazone of dehydroepiandrosterone. B is the tracing of the internal standard (21-acetate of pure deoxycorticosterone). II. 7.4 ml peripheral blood plasma from the dog used in Etperiment I. The plasma (pH 10) was extracted with ethylether after the addition of a trace amount of dehydroepiandrosterone-^{3}H. The extract was washed with water and evaporated to dryness. The residue was chromatographed on paper in the solvent system methylcyclohexane : propylene glycol for 12 h. Material in the plasma samples chromatographing like authentic dehydroepiandrosterone was eluted and the eluate evaporated to dryness. The residue was reacted with pentafluorophenylhydrazine (see Chapter 2, p. 85) and the products chromatographed (TLC, silica gel, benzene : ethylacetate 7 : 1). Material in the plasma samples chromatographing like authentic dehydroepiandrosterone-17-pentafluorophenylhydrazone was eluted and evaporated to

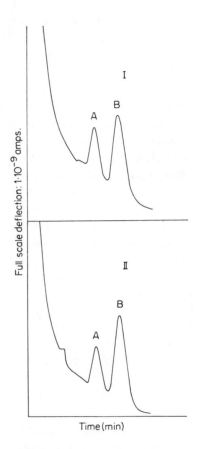

dryness. The residue was acetylated (see Chapter 2, p. 81) and the products chromatographed (TLC, silica gel, benzene : ethylacetate 49 : 1). Material in the plasma samples chromatographing like authentic 3-acetate-17-pentofluorophenylhydrazone of dehydroepiandrosterone was eluted and an aliquot of the eluate removed for estimation of radioactivity. The recovery of the added dehydroepiandrosterone-H^3 was 18% in Experiment I and 16% in Experiment II. To the rest of the eluate was added 15 nanograms of pure deoxycorticosterone acetate. GLC was done as stated in the legend of Fig. 7 (see also BROWNIE et al., 1964). (From G. F. WASSERMANN and K. B. EIK-NES. Unpublished, 1967)

results obtained so far are promising (Figs. 7 and 8). Needless to state that "plasma DHEA" must be purified extensively prior to gas phase chromatography.

III. Androgens in Urine

1. Testosterone in Urine

Since the isolation of testosterone from human urine (SCHUBERT, 1960; CAMACHO and MIGEON, 1963), considerable work has been devoted to the development of adequate methods for the quantification of the hormone in this biological source. Several of these methods use gas phase chromatography for steroid purification but, again, unless extreme analytical care is exercised, urinary epitestosterone will chromatograph with urinary testosterone (see Chapter 1). Moreover, better than 98% of all the testosterone in urine is conjugated probably at C_{17} of the steroid nucleus, and in most methods for testosterone estimation, these hormone conjugates are cleaved by some type of hydrolysis prior to purification and quantification. Completeness of hydrolysis and degree of hormone destruction during hydrolysis are therefore of paramount importance for evaluating level of the hormone in urine by any given method. Unfortunately, these two factors are not too well controlled in current methods for the measurement of urinary testosterone. This lack of control is, however, not characteristic only for methods using gas phase chromatography. Finally, the presence of epitestosterone in human urine (BROOKS and GIULIANI, 1964; KORENMAN et al., 1964; DRAY and LEDRU, 1966) has created an analytical problem in very many methods claiming to be specific for the estimation of testosterone.

The excretion of free testosterone in human urine is small, but it can be estimated either by isotope dilution (DULMANIS et al., 1964), or by electron capture following gas phase chromatography (VAN DER MOLEN et al., 1966 a).

As an introduction to the problems encountered when trying to estimate testosterone in urine by the techniques of gas phase chromatography, Tables 11 and 12 may well serve as an object lesson. Whichever way we look at it, this method is laborious and time-consuming and it is possible that VAN DER MOLEN and his co-workers feared

Table 11. *Extraction of testosterone fractions from human urine* (VAN DER MOLEN et al., 1966 a)

Urine:
1. Add labeled testosterone
2. Ether extraction ⎯⎯⎯⎯⎯⎯⎯⎯⎯⎯⎯→ "Free" testosterone

Remaining urine:
1. Adjust pH to 5.4
2. Add 1/10 vol acetate buffer (pH 5.4)
3. Incubate (48 h, 37° C) with β-glucuronidase
4. Add labeled testosterone
5. Ether extraction ⎯⎯⎯⎯⎯⎯⎯⎯⎯→ "Testosterone glucosiduronate"

Remaining urine:
1. Adjust pH to 1
2. Incubate (48 h, 37° C)
3. Add labeled testosterone
4. Ether extraction ⎯⎯⎯⎯⎯⎯⎯⎯⎯→ "pH 1 hydrolyzed testosterone"

Table 12. *Purification and estimation of testosterone in ether extracts of urine* (VAN DER MOLEN et al., 1966 a)

---

1. TLC in benzene : ethylacetate (1 : 1).
2. Paper chromatography in methylcyclohexane/propyleneglycol.
3. Acetylation of sample testosterone followed by TLC in benzene : ethylacetate (4 : 1)
4. Saponification of acetate.
5. Paper chromatography in ligroin : methanol : water (50 : 35 : 15).
6. TLC in benzene : ethylacetate (1 : 1).
7. Addition of Δ^4-androstenedione as internal standard for GLC.
8. Sampling for counting of radioactivity.
9. GLC, 6 ft 1% XE-60 column, 220° C, flame ionization detection.
⎯⎯⎯→ At low testosterone concentrations
    a) Chloroacetylation (BROWNIE et al., 1964).
    b) TLC in benzene : ethylacetate (7 : 1).
    c) Addition of 20β-chloroacetoxypregn-4-en-3-one as internal standard for GLC.
    d) Sample processed *ad modum* BROWNIE et al. (1964). See page 244.

contaminating sample testosterone with epitestosterone too much. It was observed during this work, however, that if Step 6 in Table 12 were omitted, material was still present in the extract (after purification by two TLC steps and the use of paper chromatographic systems) which would interfere seriously with adequate quantification of testosterone during gas phase chromatography. Thus, excessive use of different systems of chromatography prior to gas phase chromatography may be justified when estimating testosterone in human urine. This is also the experience of VESTERGAARD et al. (1966).

FUTTERWEIT et al. (1963) reported on the first method for the estimation of urinary testosterone using gas phase chromatography. This method has been modified (FUTTERWEIT et al., 1964; FUTTERWEIT et al., 1965 a) and in its current form it will measure the combined excretion (FUTTERWEIT et al., 1965 b) of free and conjugated testosterone and epitestosterone glucosiduronates.

Individual assay by this method is done on a 100 ml portion of a 24 h collection of urine. To this sample is added testosterone-1,2-³H; the pH is adjusted to 5 with sulphuric acid and 60,000 FISHMAN units of liver β-glucuronidase and 5 ml 0.1 M acetate buffer is added to the urine. The mixture is then incubated for 96 h at 37° C. Following hydrolysis the sample is extracted with ether, the ether extract is washed with sodium hydroxide solution and water, and the washed ether is evaporated to dryness. A Girard "T" separation is then performed on this residue and the neutral ketonic fraction is subjected to TLC on glass plates with silica gel G in the solvent system benzene : ethylacetate (3 : 2). Material in the sample behaving chromatographically like authentic testosterone is eluted and radioactivity is counted in 1/10 of this eluate. The recovery of testosterone-³H thus far varies between 55—80%. The rest of the eluate is carried through GLC with a 3—4 ft × 0.19 cm stainless steel column containing 4 to 6.8% SE-30 Anakrom ABS. Solid injection of the sample is used with a column temperature of 240° C and vaporizer temperature of 310 to 325° C. Steroid quantification is done with a hydrogen flame ionization detector.

The reproducibility of this method for normal excretion levels of testosterone is ±7% and the method can detect between 2—4 µg testosterone per 24 h urine volume (FORCHIELLI et al., 1965; FUTTERWEIT et al., 1965 a; FUTTERWEIT et al., 1965 b; GIBREE et al., 1965; POCHI et al., 1965).

Testosterone samples processed by this method were subjected to acetylation or to the formation of TMSi ether derivatives and then exposed to gas phase chromatography. If the urinary material with the same retention time as authentic testosterone acetate or testosterone TMSi was collected, the infrared spectra of such samples were similar to those of authentic testosterone derivatives chromatographed on the same column. Some compound rearrangement appears to take place during gas phase chromatography (FUTTERWEIT et al., 1965 a).

The method will determine losses by destruction of free testosterone during the hydrolysis step, but it will not indicate completeness of hydrolysis of testosterone and epitestosterone glucosiduronates. Human urine contains unknown substances which will inhibit the enzyme β-glucuronidase (EIK-NES, 1968), and the amount of such substances in the urine differs from subject to subject. The method will not determine testosterone sulphates and some evidence has been presented that androgen sulphates are produced in man (DIXON et al., 1965; DESSYPRIS et al., 1966). The recovery of testosterone and the precision of assay of the hormone by this method compare favorably with other methods for urinary testosterone not using gas phase chromatography and requiring more time per assay (COMACHO and MIGEON, 1963; VERMEULEN and VERPLANCKE, 1963; DULMANIS et al., 1964; SCHUBERT and FRANKENBERG, 1964; VOIGT et al., 1964; LIM and DINGMAN, 1965; ZURBRÜGG et al., 1965; HORN et al., 1966; ROSNER and CONTE, 1966). The major drawback with this method is that testosterone and epitestosterone are not separated by the different systems of chromatography (BROOKS and GIULIANI, 1964). Since the excretion of epitestosterone in human urine is rather high (BROOKS, 1964), and since we have no clear view of the metabolic relationship between testosterone and epitestosterone (KORENMAN et al., 1963; BROOKS, 1964; KORENMAN et al., 1964 b; ACEVEDO and CORRAL-GALLARDO, 1965) — if such a relationship exists — a method measuring the combined concentration of these two steroids in the same sample may not always be a desirable one for the endocrine laboratory. This method will, however, distinguish low and high excretors of testosterone plus epitestosterone (GIBREE et al., 1965; POCHI et al., 1965), and thus aid considerably in endocrine diagnosis involving androgen production. Data on excretion of testosterone (+epitestosterone) in normal subjects obtained by this method fall within the range of data obtained by other methods (Table 13). It is somewhat premature to compare the different published methods for the estimation of urinary testosterone with each other, particularly with respect to the biological data which have been reported. The use of biological criteria for assessment of methodology specificity may not always be sound. If testosterone can be found in the urine of an ovariectomized-adrenalectomized woman,

Table 13. *Range of excretion of "testosterone" in normal adult subjects* ($\mu g/24\ h$)

Authors	Method of analysis	Epitesto-sterone separated from testo-sterone?	Men	Women
Camacho and Migeon, 1963	Spectro-photometry	No	46—106	<8
Vermeulen and Verplancke, 1963	Spectro-photometry	No	15—90	5—12
Horton et al., 1963	Spectro-photometry	No	50—93	2—8
Schubert and Frankenberg, 1964	Spectro-photometry	Yes	10—75	<5—25
Voigt et al., 1964	Spectro-photometry	No	32—63	3—18
Rosner et al., 1965	Spectro-photometry	Yes	27—143	6—57
Zurbrügg et al., 1965	Spectro-photometry	No	42—79	0—6
Lim and Dingman, 1965	Spectro-photometry	Yes	30—86	4—10
Horn et al., 1966	Spectro-photometry	Yes	5—79	<1—4
Rosner and Conte, 1966	Spectro-photometry	Yes	25—95	
Dulmanis et al., 1964	Double isotope	Yes	39—383	26—139
Futterweit et al., 1964	Ionization detector	No	38—332	2—8
Ibayashi et al., 1964	Ionization detector	No	19—200	<5
Brooks, 1964	Ionization detector	Yes	30—120	7—18
Sandberg, 1964	Ionization detector	Yes	20—180	
van der Molen et al., 1966 a	Ionization detector	Yes	23—167	2.5—9.2
Vermeulen, 1966	Ionization detector	Yes	30—351	2.9—12.1
de Nicola et al., 1966	Ionization detector	Yes	10—173	1.5—13.0
Panicucci, 1966	Ionization detector	Yes	25—95	

this may be due to inferior methodology, but could also arise from incomplete surgical removal of the glands. Since testosterone excretion varies grossly between the sexes and is affected by factors like age (MORER-FARGAS and NOWAKOWSKI, 1965, VERMEULEN, 1966), perhaps even by ovarian activity (LOBOTSKY et al., 1964), time of day (RESKO and EIK-NES, 1966), and certainly undergoes spontaneous variations as seen in normal male subjects (ISMAIL and HARKNESS, 1965), inspection of the data of Table 13 may not be of much help in selecting an adequate method for the estimation of testosterone excretion in man. Moreover, the methods listed in Table 13 differ with regard to use of an internal standard and with regard to the incorporation of the "free" testosterone fraction with the testosterone "glucosiduronate" fraction.

Many of the criticisms which can be leveled against the method of FUTTERWEIT and his co-workers are also applicable to the testosterone method of IBAYASHI et al. (1964). With only small modifications, the steps of sample preparation, hydrolysis of testosterone glucosiduronate, extraction of the hydrolysate and purification of ether extract are the same in both methods, but no Girard "T" separation is done in the method of IBAYASHI et al. The production of a neutral ketonic fraction by Girard separation has been found helpful when estimating testosterone in the urine from children (BROOKS, 1964).

IBAYASHI et al. chromatograph the urinary extract on glass plates coated with Kieselgel HF_{254} in the solvent system benzene : ethylacetate 1 : 1, and material chromatographing like authentic testosterone is eluted, evaporated and the residue acetylated. This derivative is chromatographed on glass plates coated with Kieselgel HF_{254} in the solvent system benzene : ethylacetate (3 : 1). The material with the chromatographic mobility of synthetic testosterone acetate is eluted. Part of the eluate is examined for radioactivity, and the rest is separated with a 1.5 m × .4 cm stainless steel column filled with 1.5% SE-30 on Anakrom A. The column is maintained at 216° C with detector and flash heater temperatures of 240° C. Less than 5 µg of testosterone in a 24 h urine cannot be detected by this method and the recovery of the radioactive standard is 54.8% ± 0.49 (one standard deviation).

Neither the solvent systems used for TLC or the column used for gas phase chromatography in the method of IBAYASHI et al. will separate the acetates of testosterone and epitestosterone (BROOKS and

Giuliani, 1964). Therefore, unless Kieselgel HF$_{254}$ has a better ability to separate the two steroids than silica gel G, the two compounds will be estimated together. The range of "testosterone" excretion values estimated by the method in male subjects varying in age from 19—25 years (18 subjects), show a more narrow limit (Guerra-Garcia and Whittembury, 1965) than by method of Futterweit et al., though as already stated it is much too early to compare the different published methods for estimation of urinary testosterone with each other on the basis of biological data.

Brooks (1964) assays testosterone and epitestosterone glucosiduronates separately in the same sample of human urine. Hydrolysis is done with limpet β-glucuronidase. After the addition of testosterone-^{14}C to the hydrolysate, it is extracted with ether. The extract is washed with 0.1 N sodium hydroxide and water and the washed extract is evaporated to dryness. The residue is chromatographed on glass plates coated with silica gel in the solvent system benzene : ethylacetate 3 : 2. Material in the urine chromatographing like authentic testosterone is eluted, acetylated, and the products of acetylation are rechromatographed on thin-layer plates in the solvent mixture benzene : ethylacetate 3 : 1. This treatment should separate etiocholanolone from testosterone and epitestosterone. Again, urinary material behaving like testosterone is eluted and radioactivity in a part of this eluate is determined. The sample recovery up to this point varies between 39—66%; the loss of testosterone and epitestosterone appears similar. To the rest of the eluate is added 1 µg each of testosterone and androsterone and the mixture is chromatographed on a 1.5 m QF-1 column. The column is operated at 200° C in a Pye Panchromatograph with an argon ionization detector. Quantification of steroids is done by cutting out the peaks of testosterone, androsterone and the double peak of testosterone and epitestosterone acetates from the gas chromatography tracings. These pieces of paper are then weighed and unknown steroid concentrations are computed by the method of Stein and Moore (1948). The error of measurement using from 0.4—0.6 µg of authentic testosterone and epitestosterone in different proportions is ± 10% for testosterone and − 18—1% for epitestosterone. Within an epitestosterone/testosterone ratio from 0.5—10, the error of testosterone measurement varied within ± 10% and that of epitestosterone from − 11—1%. By this method a sizeable excretion of epitestosterone is measured (Table 14).

Table 14. *Range of excretion of conjugated epitestosterone and testosterone in normal adult men and women*

Authors	Micrograms per 24 h			
	Testosterone		Epitestosterone	
	Men	Women	Men	Women
BROOKS 1964	33—120	7—18	27—330	27—53
DE NICOLA et al., 1966	17—173	15—13	9—396	7—20
TAMM and VOIGT, 1966	29—57 *		12—36	
SPARAGANA, 1965	59—202		0—52	

* One subject only.

A more exacting quantification of testosterone and epitestosterone could probably be achieved if these steroids were separated prior to gas phase analysis. Thus it is the recommendation of BROOKS that if this method is to be used for the measurement of testosterone production rates by the principle of isotope dilution, the separation of epitestosterone and testosterone must be accomplished by a suitable system of paper chromatography.

This type of separation is used by DE NICOLA et al. (1966) for separate estimation of epitestosterone and testosterone in the same sample of urine. In this method, hydrolysis and extraction of the hydrolysate are done in much the same way as in the method of FUTTERWEIT et al. (1965 b) except that known amounts of triated epitestosterone and carbon[14] labeled testosterone are added to the urine after hydrolysis. The residue from the extraction is chromatographed twice in the solvent mixture benzene : ethylacetate 3 : 2 on glass plates coated with Anasil for the first TLC separation and on glass plates coated with silica gel GF for the second TLC separation. The testosterone-epitestosterone area of the sample chromatogram is eluted and chromatographed on paper in the solvent mixture ligroin (50) : methanol(35) : water(15). In this system of paper chromatography testosterone and epitestosterone separate; they are eluted individually from the paper strip and 10% of each eluate is counted for radioactivity and the remainder of each sample is separated with a 5 ft × 1/8 in. glass column packed with 3% SE-30 (column temperature of 230° C). Steroid quantification is done by a flame ionization detector. Again, as in the study of BROOKS, the excretion of epitestosterone is higher than that of testosterone (Table 14).

The data of Tables 13 and 14 clearly demonstrate the need for measuring urinary testosterone in samples not contaminated with epitestosterone. In the method of SANDBERG and co-workers (1964), epitestosterone should be separated from testosterone by gradient elution and gas phase chromatography. Moreover, in this method only testosterone glucosiduronate is measured since free testosterone is removed from the urine prior to hydrolysis with β-glucuronidase. To the hydrolyzed urine radioactive testosterone is added, and the ether extract of the urine is chromatographed on a Florisil column (COMACHO and MIGEON, 1963). The testosterone fraction from this column is exposed to gradient elution chromatography as described by LAKSHMANAN and LIEBERMAN (1954) and the measurement of radioactivity in fractions from the column serves to locate testosterone. A known amount of epitestosterone is added to the testosterone fraction and TMSi derivatives of the mixture are formed. The derivatives are then chromatographed on a 6 ft × 0.6 cm glass column filled with 2%/o XE-60. This column is operated at 216° C and an argon ionization detector is used for compound quantification. On this column, testosterone TMSi has a relative retention time to that of epitestosterone TMSi of 1.25 (see also Chapter 1).

The recovery of known amounts (10—200 µg) of testosterone added to female urine and processed by this method varies between 81—120 %. When an extract of a urinary sample is divided in two parts after gradient elution chromatography and one-half is assayed by this method while the other half is assayed by the method of CAMACHO and MIGEON (1963), (involving additional purification by two systems of paper chromatography and spectrophotometric measurement of testosterone) data from such double assays agree well except for testosterone concentrations of less than 5 µg/24 h urine.

In their investigations of testosterone production rates in man, KORENMAN and his co-workers (KORENMAN et al., 1963); KORENMAN et al., 1964 b; KORENMAN and LIPSETT, 1964) used gas phase chromatography for the isolation and quantification of urinary testosterone. After hydrolysis and extraction of the urine, the extract is purified by extensive paper and thin-layer chromatography. Testosterone and epitestosterone are separated on paper strips in the solvent mixture of ligroin(100) : methanol(70) : water(30). The purified sample of urinary testosterone is finally separated with a 6 ft × 0.34 cm glass column packed with 1% SE-30 (HAAHTI, 1961). The gas chromatograph is equipped with an argon ionization detector, and the column is maintained at 207° C with detector and flash heater temperatures of 250° C. A high state of purity of urinary testosterone is achieved prior to gas phase chromatography. The concentrations of testosterone in the urinary extracts before such chromatography and measured by a fluorometric assay are the same as those recorded after gas phase chromatography and measurement of hormone concentrations by the argon ionization detector (HAAHTI, 1961; KORENMAN et al., 1963). This method appears excellently suited for accurate measurement of testosterone production rates in man.

In the technique of NICHOLS and co-workers (1966), the sum of free testosterone and testosterone glucosiduronate are measured in human urine. Following enzymic hydrolysis of the urine, testosterone-^{14}C is added and the sample is extracted with methylenedichloride. After washing the extract with sodium hydroxide solution and water, the extract is evaporated to dryness and the residue is applied to an alumina column (10 cm × 1) which is eluted successively with ethanol in methylenedichloride at concentrations of 0.2, 0.5 and 1%. The latter fraction is collected and the solvents are evaporated. The residue is chromatographed on glass plates coated with silica gel in the solvent system acetone : methanol (1 : 1, v/v). ^{14}C is located on the sample lane, the zone is eluted and the eluate evaporated. The residue is chromatographed on paper in the solvent mixture ligroin(100) : methanol(80) : water(20) and ^{14}C material in the sample located by strip scanning. The zone is eluted, the eluate evaporated and the residue is rechromatographed on an alumina column (10 cm × 1). Fractions are eluted successively with ethanol in hexane at concentrations of 0.5, 1 and 2%. The 2% fraction from the column is collected and evaporated. The residue is separated with a 6 ft × ¼ in. glass column packed with 2% SE-30. Steroid quantification is done with an argon ionization detector. The gas volume containing testosterone is collected from this column, condensed and assayed for concentration of ^{14}C. When sixty-three 24 h samples of urine, containing a total of from 4—130 µg testosterone, were analyzed in duplicate by this method, the mean difference between duplicates was 3.4 µg and at testosterone concentrations below 20 µg/24 h, a mean difference between duplicates of 1.5 µg was observed in thirty-one samples. In spite of the fact that too polar a solvent is used for initial extraction of the hydrolyzed urine, the method is worth further exploration since it separates testosterone from its epimere and gives absolute recovery data.

Another method for urinary testosterone which should give absolute recovery data is the method of SPARAGANA (1965). Hydrolysis and extraction of urine are done as described by IBAYASHI et al. (1964) except that free testosterone is removed by ether extraction prior to hydrolysis and 20 µg Δ^1-testosterone are added to the urine after hydrolysis as an internal standard. The ether extract of the hydrolysate is chromatographed on glass plates coated with silica gel in the solvent system methylenedichloride(10) : methanol(1). The areas corresponding to testosterone ($R_f·439$) and Δ^1-testosterone ($R_f·488$) are eluted, and the eluates acetylated and then oxidized with chromiumtrioxide. The products from these reactions are chromatographed (TLC) in the solvent mixture benzene(4) : acetone(1) and the distinct ultraviolet spot on the sample chromatogram produced by Δ^1-testosterone acetate is eluted and subjected to gas phase chromatography on a 12 ft glass column packed with 3% SE-30 on Gas Chrom P. This column is contained in a Perkin Elmer gas chromatograph equipped with a flame ionization detector. The conditions of gas phase chromatography are: column temperature, 220° C; injection block temperature, 290° C; and carrier gas-flow, 30 ml/min. On this column testosterone acetate ($R_f·736$) and epitestosterone acetate ($R_f·681$) do separate.

The recovery of testosterone and epitestosterone added to urine is high and similar. Moreover, the detector response to the acetates of Δ^1-testosterone, epitestosterone and testosterone are related in a linear fashion. When testosterone was determined by this method in ten identical aliquots, a mean concentration of 9.3 µg/100 ml was found with a standard deviation of ±.47 and a coefficient of variance of 5%. The uncertainty of measuring urinary epitestosterone is rather large by this method (coefficient variance of 9.2%). This can in part be due to the fact that an unknown compound in the purified extract of urine is eluted so close to epitestosterone during gas phase chromatography that a double peak is produced. It is also possible that this double peak is the reason for the low levels of this steroid found in the urine of nine normal males ranging in age from 20—48 years. In this group of subjects the range of epitestosterone excretion varied from

0—52 µg per 24 hr and that of testosterone from 59—202 µg/24 h. These data on epitestosterone excretion do not confirm the observations of BROOKS (1964) and of DE NICOLA et al. (1966) (Table 14).

PANICUCCI (1966) adds labeled testosterone to 100 ml urine, hydrolyzes the sample both with β-glucuronidase and by solvolysis and the ether extract of the hydrolysate is processed as described (page 256). Finally, in the technique of VERMEULEN (1966), Girard partition, paper chromatography (Bush A system), acetylation, and TLC are employed as means of sample purification prior to gas phase chromatography. This method is reported to have a sensitivity of about 1 µg conjugated testosterone per 24 h sample of urine.

Conclusion

The sensitive detector devices of the gas chromatograph should place gas phase chromatography in a most favorable position as an armamentarium for estimating testosterone in the urine from normal males and females (Table 9). Extensive purification is needed before the urine extract is ready for such chromatography and few column systems have hitherto been reported separating testosterone from its epimere. Thus, in most methods separating testosterone from epitestosterone, the step of paper chromatography in an adequate solvent system is incorporated. This will increase the time of assay. Since testosterone and epitestosterone can be separated on glass plates coated with aluminum oxide (MATHEWS et al., 1962; LORIAUX et al., 1966) and since this method of separation is less time-consuming than paper chromatography (DRAY, 1965), this TLC separation should be further explored in gas phase chromatography methods for specific estimation of testosterone in urine. Aluminum oxide heated at 750—850° prior to use in TLC appears to be a most adequate support medium for separation of the epimeres (HALPAAP et al., 1967). Steroid separation can be achieved with this support medium in the solvent system benzene/ether 3 : 2 (HALPAAP et al., 1967).

In a recent method for urinary testosterone, HORN et al. (1966) hydrolyze urine samples containing a known amount of radioactive testosterone with β-glucuronidase. Following extraction of the hydrolysate in the standard fashion, testosterone in this extract is purified by one thin-layer chromatogram and one paper chromatogram. The testosterone is then enzymatically converted to estradiol-17β which is purified on paper in the solvent system O-dichlorobenzene : formamide : methanol (AXELROD, 1954). Estradiol-17β is eluted, quantitated by fluorometry and the content of ^{14}C in the estradiol-17β measured. Epitestosterone can be excluded as a contaminant in these estimations since it is not converted to estradiol-17β by the enzyme systems. Moreover, testosterone and its epimere are separated from each other by the chromatographic systems used prior to enzymic conversion of testosterone to estradiol-17β. This reviewer has already expressed his opinion on evaluating methodology by comparing levels of testosterone in urinary samples from normal subjects by different methods. Data on excretion of testosterone in normal men by the method of HORN et al. compares favorably with the data of VERMEULEN and VERPLANCKE (1963) and with the data of VOIGT et al. (1964). In these two latter methods, the sum of testosterone and epitestosterone is measured. Moreover, the method of HORN et al. (1966) gives similar testosterone values in male urine as the methods of KORENMAN et al. (1963, 1964 a) and ZURBRÜGG and co-workers (1965). In these latter methods, epitestosterone is separated from testosterone by paper chromatography or by gradient elution column chromatography. Finally, the normal male excretion of testosterone is lower by the method of HORN et al. than by the methods of FUTTERWEIT et al. (1963) and of IBAYASHI et al. (1964) determining in both methods the sum of epitestosterone and testosterone, but also lower than those found by SPARAGANA (1962) and by SANDBERG et al. (1964), where considerable evidence has been presented that testosterone is clearly separated from epitestosterone. If these preliminary data are correct, it would be of paramount importance to establish purity of urinary testosterone in all methods before the final analysis. The hardheaded observer may also note that lower testosterone excretion values are recorded by the method of HORN et al. than by four methods using gas phase chromatography, although the data collected hitherto by these four gas phase chromatography methods do not form a coherent and logical body of evidence, and the true state of affairs may be much different from what emerges from preliminary data (Table 13). Conversion of testosterone to TMSi ether prior to gas phase chromatography and the selection of a proper phase for such chromatography appear to be the solution for adequate estimation of testosterone in human urine (see also Chapter 1).

Table 15. *Range of excretion of free and conjugated testosterone in urine of normal adult male and female subjects*

Authors	Endpoint Analysis	Free		Micrograms per 24 h "Glucosiduronate"		"Sulphate"	
		M	F	M	F	M	F
DULMANIS et al., 1964	Double isotope	3—6	2—4	39—383	26—139	3—165	3—62
VAN DER MOLEN et al., 1966a	Electron capture or ionization detection	0.65—1.53	0.52—1.20	23—67	2.5—9.2	3—12	0.8—4.5
DESSYPRIS et al., 1966	Ionization detection					6—10	

M: male subjects
F: female subjects

The following points in testosterone methodology must also be settled: the level of free testosterone in urine (SPARAGANA et al., 1962; HORTON et al., 1963; CAMACHO and MIGEON, 1964; DULMANIS et al., 1964) and the nature of the testosterone conjugates excreted in the urine (SPARAGANA et al., 1962; HORTON et al., 1963; CAMACHO and MIGEON, 1964; DULMANIS et al., 1964; DESSYPRIS et al., 1966; DRAY and LEDRU, 1966) (Table 15). The fact that following β-glucuronidase hydrolysis of urine additional testosterone can be released by pH 1 hydrolysis, does not necessarily indicate that testosterone is also excreted as a sulphate since the degree of hydrolysis of conjugated steroids in human urine with the enzyme β-glucuronidase appears to very from specimen to specimen (EIKNES, 1968). If, however, the preliminary levels of testosterone "sulphate" recorded in human urine can be proven to be the incontestably true values, estimation of this testosterone fraction in urine from women may be important (Table 15).

Finally, it would be desirable if testosterone glucosiduronate of high specific radioactivity could become commercially available. This compound should be added to urine prior to hydrolysis in order to check the total recovery of steroid through any given method including completeness of enzymic hydrolysis and destruction of hormone during hydrolysis. The method of computing recovery of radioactive testosterone used by NICHOLS et al. (1966) appears to be the method of choice in certain of the techniques using gas phase chromatography.

Only one method has been published for the estimation of Δ^4-androstenedione in human urine (SCHUBERT and FRANKENBERG, 1964). This method employs ultraviolet spectrophotometry for the final analysis. In the urine from nine normal males ranging in age from 18—44 years, from 14—85 µg Δ^4-androstenedione/24 h were excreted. With this excretion rate the technique of gas phase chromatography with sensitive detectors could favorably be applied to the accurate measurement of this hormone in normal urine (see page 266).

2. 17-Ketosteroids in Urine

The excretion of these compounds in human urine is sizeable and the only advancement gas phase chromatography can offer methodology in this field is through time-saving separation of the individual 17-KS. The separate quantification of some of these steroids (dehydroepiandrosterone, androsterone, etiocholanolone, 11-ketoetiocholanolone, 11-hydroxyetiocholanolone and 11-hydroxyandrosterone) may often be of help in diagnosing endocrine disorders, and in the following discussion only methods estimating many 17-ketosteroids in the same sample as urine will be considered. The interest in ratio estimation of urinary 17-KS has become more and more prevailing in endocrine research over the last five years. Up to that time estimation of total excretion of 17-KS (determined as DHEA equivalents) was used as an index both of adrenal and testicular function and adequate methods are indeed available for accurate measurement of total urinary 17-ketosteroids (Table 16). Moreover, if urine samples are hydrolyzed by the same method and their content of 17-KS assayed either by spectrophotometric methods or following gas phase chromatography on a hybrid column (0.60% XE-60 and 0.35% SE-30, 210° C) using a flame ionization detector, considerable agreement between the results from either method of analysis is observed (HEYNS and DeMOOR, 1966).

The advent of methods in the early 1950's for the measurement of urinary adrenocorticoids and the recent development of methods for the measurement of urinary testosterone have made estimation of total urinary 17-ketosteroids obsolete, though it should be remembered that much fundamental work in the field of clinical endocrinology is based on estimation of excretion of total 17-KS by the ZIMMERMANN reaction.

The *major* urinary 17-KS can be separated by gas phase chromatography either as free compounds (COOPER and CREECH, 1961; HAAHTI et al., 1961; SPARAGANA et al., 1962; DePAOLI et al., 1963), as trifluoroacetates (VANDEN HEUVEL et al., 1962), as trimethylsilyl ethers (VANDEN HEUVEL et al., 1962; HARTMAN and WOTIZ, 1963; KIRSCHNER and LIPSETT, 1963; FRANCE et al., 1965), or as ethylene-thioketal derivatives (ZMIGROD and LINDNER, 1966).

The problem of adequate hydrolysis of 17-KS conjugates has already been discussed. Most methods employ β-glucuronidase and acid hydrolysis, or some type of solvolysis for steroid sulphates. Hydrolysis of both conjugates in one step (JACOBSOHN and LIEBERMAN, 1962; DePAOLI et al., 1963) has up to now found limited use when measuring individual 17-KS in urine (BERRETT and McNEIL, 1966). It would be of interest to apply this form of hydrolysis to conjugated 17-KS extracted from alkalinized urine with n-butanol (LEHNERT et al., 1966).

19*

Table 16. *Estimation of total 17-ketosteroid in the same sample of dialyzed human urine* *

Hydrolysis	Extraction	Purification of extract	Method of analysis	μg(as DHEA)/10 ml of urine
10 vol. % conc. H_2SO_4, 25 min at 100° C	Ether	NaOH	Zimmermann reaction in KOH	81, 92, 89, 78, 75, 86
10 vol. % conc. H_2SO_4, 20 min at 93° C	Ether	NaOH, H_2O	Zimmermann reaction in KOH	67, 66, 69, 66, 69, 64, 70, 66
25 vol. % glacial acetic acid 33 vol. % conc. HCl, 30 min at 100° C	Ether	NaOH Phosphate buffer	Zimmermann reaction in KOH	86, 86, 86
20 vol. % conc. HCl, 30 min at 100° C	Ethylene-dichloride	NaOH, H_2O	Zimmermann reaction in KOH	60, 66, 67, 74
10 vol. % conc. HCl, 15 min at 100° C	Ether	NaOH, H_2O	Zimmermann reaction in KOH	Mean: 87.8 ± 4.3 (one standard deviation) for 7 individual samples
10 vol. % 11 M. H_2SO_4, 20 min at 95° C	Ether	NaOH, H_2O	Zimmermann reaction in KOH	81, 78, 76, 76, 73, 73, 81, 78, 79, 79
10 vol. % conc. HCl, 15 min at 100° C	Petroleum ether: benzene (1:1)	NaOH, H_2O	m-Dinitrobenzene in 40% benzyltrimethyl ammonium methoxide	101, 101, 101

Table 16 (continued)

Hydrolysis	Extraction	Purification of extract	Method of analysis	μg(as DHEA)/10 ml of urine
33 vol. % conc. HCl, 10 min at 100° C	Ethylene-dichloride	NaOH, H_2O	m-Dinitrobenzene in tetraethyl-ammonium hydroxide	68, 67, 68, 68
20 vol. % H_2SO_4, 15 min at 100° C	Ethylene-dichloride	NaOH, H_2O	Zimmermann reaction in KOH	66, 67, 68, 70
10 vol. % 10% $CuSO_4$ 10 vol. % 25% HCl, 30 min at 100°	Ether	NaOH, H_2O	Zimmermann reaction in KOH	80, 82, 74, 78
0.01 M perchloric acid in tetrahydro-furane 4 h at 24° C	Ether	H_2O	Zimmermann reaction in KOH	72, 75, 76, 77

* The samples of lyophilized, dialyzed urine were prepared by Warner-Chilcott Company, Morris Plains, N. Y. The assays were conducted in different laboratories in Europe, Australia, Japan and U.S.A. Different concentrations of sodium hydroxide were used for purification of the extract of hydrolyzed urine, and the Zimmermann reaction was carried out in different ways with respect to concentration of reagents and time of development.

KIRSCHNER and LIPSETT (1963, 1964) hydrolyze steroid glucosiduronates with β-glucuronidase and steroid sulphates by solvolysis (BURSTEIN and LIEBERMAN, 1958). The liberated steroids are extracted with ether and the extract chromatographed on glass plates coated with silica gel G in the solvent mixture benzene(40) : ethylacetate(60). On a separate lane is chromatographed a mixture of steroid standards: androsterone, pregnanediol and pregnanetriol. Elution from the sample chromatogram is done according to the chromatographic behavior of the steroid standards: Zone I, the area between androsterone and pregnanediol and a Zone II, the area between pregnanediol and pregnanetriol.

Zone I is eluted and the eluate is evaporated. The steroids in this residue (major compounds: DHEA, androsterone and etiocholanolone) are subjected to trimethylsilyl ether formation. This mixture of steroid TMSi ethers is then chromatographed on a 6 ft 2% XE-60 column. The column is operated at 195° C and steroid quantification is done by an argon ionization detector. The response of the detector is linear from 0.5—2 µg of the TMSi steroid ethers in question. In the range of from 2—4 µg of compound, the response curve is also linear, though exhibiting a higher slope than for the 0.5—2 µg range.

The TMSi ethers of androsterone, etiocholanolone and DHEA do separate on 2% XE-60 as well as on a 1% NGS column. The TMSi ethers of androsterone and epietiocholanolone show the same elution time on both columns. It is somewhat unlikely, however, that epietiocholanolone is present in normal urine from either sex (KIRSCHNER et al., 1963). If epiandrosterone should be present in the urine, it is advisable to do gas phase chromatography with a 1% QF-1 column (KIRSCHNER and LIPSETT, 1963) since the TMSi ether of this steroid will not separate from the TMSi ether of DHEA either on 2% XE-60 or on the 1% NGS column.

Zone II from the original TLC separation is also eluted, the eluate is evaporated and the steroids in this residue (major compounds: 11β-hydroxyandrosterone, 11β-hydroxyetiocholanolone and 11-ketoetiocholanolone) subjected to TMSi ether formation. This mixture of steroid TMSi ethers is chromatographed, as already described, on a 2% XE-60 column where 11-ketoetiocholanolone, 11β-hydroxyandrosterone and 11β-hydroxyetiocholanolone TMSi ethers separate well. Also, the 1% NGS column can be used for such separation. The TMSi ether of 17-hydroxypregnenolone may interfere, however, when eluting 11-hydroxyetiocholanolone TMSi ether. The reproducibility of separation by gas phase chromatography as well as the recovery of steroids through the method are most satisfactory in the technique of KIRSCHNER and LIPSETT. Moreover, no artefacts of the steroids to be determined appear to be produced by this method. This is of paramount importance when separating steroids by gas phase chromatography.

At an excretion range (mg/24 h) of from 0.67—7.0 for etiocholanolone, 0.25—5.2 for DHEA and 0.88—4.9 for androsterone, the following coefficients of variation are recorded: 4.7% for androsterone, 5.0% for etiocholanolone and 5.1% for DHEA. This coefficient is slightly higher for 11-hydroxyetiocholanolone (7%) and for 11-ketoetiocholanolone (10%) at excretion levels of 0.45 and 0.22 mg/24 h respectively.

In the technique of SPARAGANA and co-workers (1963) for urinary 17-ketosteroid estimation, no thin-layer chromatography is done prior to gas phase chromatography and the individual 17-KS are separated as the free compounds on two different gas chromatography columns. Moreover, this method incorporates the use of an internal standard, 11β-hydroxyandrostenedione, and compound recovery for each individual sample can be computed. This is a distinct advantage in the technique of SPARAGANA et al.

After addition of the internal standard, the urine is extensively hydrolyzed first with β-glucuronidase and then by ether extraction of low pH's for 5 days. The extracted 17-KS are separated by the Girard reaction and adrenal steroids with a dihydroxyacetone side chain are removed from the neutral ketonic fraction by partition between 50% methanol and benzene. This step is most necessary since ketonic corticoids are not well separated from 17-KS by the Girard reaction (WHEELER, 1962). Such corticoids will undergo pyrolysis when exposed to gas phase chromatography (VANDEN HEUVEL and HORNING, 1960) and these products will interfere with the accurate measurement of urinary $C_{19}O_3$ 17-KS (see Chapter 5).

The purified extract is analyzed by GLC with a 12 ft glass column packed with 3% SE-30 and operated at 220° C. Steroid quantification is done by flame ionization detection. With this column, androsterone and DHEA are eluted together but the free forms of etiocholanolone, 11-ketoetiocholanolone, 11β-hydroxyetiocholanolone and 11β-hydroxyandrosterone are adequately separated. Androsterone and

DHEA can be separated by digitonin precipitation prior to gas phase chromatography; these two steroids will also separate on a 12 ft 1.5% NGS column, where etiocholanolone and androsterone are eluted together. In light of these difficulties, the method is probably best applied to separation and estimation of $C_{19}O_3$ urinary 17-KS, though at high levels of urinary pregnanediol the method is apt to over-estimate 11β-hydroxyandrosterone. The level of excretion of this compound in five normal females is much higher by this method than estimated by KIRSCHNER and LIPSETT in nine normal women (KIRSCHNER and LIPSETT, 1964).

The recovery of individual 17-KS through the method of SPARA-GANA et al. is good and the internal standard appears well suited for its intended purpose. It should, however, be stressed that this internal standard will not indicate degree of hydrolysis of conjugated 17-KS in the urine. As in methods for estimation of conjugated testosterone, there is also in this field of steroid technology a need for authentic 17-KS conjugates of high specific radioactivity in order to permit measurement of completeness of hydrolysis by the different methods proposed for this purpose. Also, 11β-hydroxyandro-stenedione *can* be present in human urine (SALAMON and DOBRINER, 1953).

The agreement in steroid concentration in quadruplicate samples of the same urine is adequate when assayed by the technique of SPARAGANA et al.; so is the agreement between the sum of individual 17-KS estimated by this method and total excretion of ZIMMERMANN chromogens estimated by a routine technique. At low levels of urinary 17-KS (TALBOT et al., 1942; HOLTZ, 1957), the latter method will give higher values than the method using gas phase chromatography. In urine from normal women and men, the range of excretion of androsterone, etiocholanolone and DHEA is much the same by the method of SPARAGANA et al. as that reported by KIRSCHNER and LIP-SETT (1964).

SPARAGANA and co-workers record no measurable level of DHEA in the urine of a healthy male subject showing normal excretion range for the other 17-KS studied. Admittedly, this observation could be due to dehydroepiandrosterone destruction during hydrolysis. It has been claimed, however, that certain diseased states are associated with low or no excretion of DHEA in human subjects (SONKA et al., 1965). It would be of considerable interest to determine if lack of DHEA excretion also occurs in normal subjects. Several methods employing gas phase chromatography are well suited for such investigations (COOPER and CREECH, 1961; HARTMAN and WOTIZ, 1963; NAIR et al., 1964; FRANCE et al., 1965; THOMAS, 1965; BERRETT and McNEIL, 1966; THOMAS and BULBROOK, 1966), where the detector devices of the gas chromatograph should give decisive answers not obtainable by colorimetric techniques. At extremely low levels of urinary 17-KS, estimation of chloromethyldimethylsilyl ethers of such steroids by an electron capture cell may become a useful technique (THOMAS, 1966). Samples containing these steroids must be in a high state of purity prior to gas phase chromatography. The technique of gas phase chromatography may also shed light on the real excretion of 17-KS in animal species like the dog (GLENN and HEFTMANN, 1952) and the cow (WRIGHT, 1958). An interesting introduction to some of the problems in this field of research can be found in a recent publication by HEITZMAN and THOMAS (1965) estimating steroids in the urine of the pregnant cow. The method of hydrolysis used in this work, however, leaves much to be desired.

PANICUCCI (1966) hydrolyzes 50 ml urine with β-glucuronidase and by solvolysis. The hydrolysate is extracted with ether, phenolic steroids are removed, and the purified extract is chromatographed on glass plates coated with silica gel G in the solvent system chloroform : ethanol (24 : 1). Material chromatographing like authentic 17-KS are eluted, their TMSi ethers are formed and the ethers are chromatographed on a 6 ft 3% NGS column maintained at 220° C. The recovery of known amounts of 17-KS carried through the method is better than 75%.

As can be seen from Table 17, there is considerable agreement in the excretion range of $C_{19}O_3$ 17-KS in normal men and women regardless of hydrolytic procedures and methods of separation used — gradient elution or gas phase chromatography. This reviewer has already expressed his opinion on comparing methods by data on steroid concentrations in a modest number of "normal" subjects. The methods using gas phase chromatography (KIRSCHNER and LIPSETT, 1963; SPARAGANA et al., 1963; FRANCE et al., 1965; PANICUCCI, 1966) show, however, lower average excretion of DHEA, androsterone and etiocholanolone than methods using gradient elution chromatography. This difference is, in particular, apparent with regard to DHEA excretion where KIRSCHNER and LIPSETT (1963, 1964) find an average

Table 17. *Range of excretion (mg/24 h) of 17-ketosteroids in normal human subjects*

Sex	N	Purification	End point analysis	DHEA	Andros-terone	Etiocho-lanolone	11-hydroxy androsterone	11-hydroxy etiocho-lanolone	11-keto etiocho-lanolone	Reference
M	7	TLC, TMSi derivative formation, gas phase chromato-graphy	Argon ionization detector	0.20—1.71	2.1—3.8	1.4—5.4	0.16—0.89	0.22—0.67	0.42—1.41	KIRSCHNER and LIPPSETT, 1963
F	9			0.20—1.13	0.9—2.6	0.6—2.2	0.05—0.48	0.10—1.18	0.25—0.85	KIRSCHNER and LIPPSETT, 1964
M	4	Girard T, methanol: benzene partition, gas phase chromato-graphy	Flame ionization detector	0.02—1.90	2.4—4.4	2.2—4.4	0.60—0.90	0.20—0.40	0.20—0.40	SPARAGANA et al., 1963
F	5			0.10—0.70	0.8—2.6	0.7—3.5	0.50—1.10	0.30—0.80	0.20—0.50	
M	?	TLC, TMSi formation, gas phase chromato-graphy	Argon ionization detector	0.93—3.12	1.54—5.10	1.46—5.62	0.10—0.53	0.47—0.93	0.12—0.36	PANICUCCI, 1966

Table 17 (continued)

Sex	N	Purification	End point analysis	DHEA	Andros-terone	Etiocho-lanolone	11-hydroxy androsterone	11-hydroxy etiocho-lanolone	11-keto etiocho-lanolone	Reference
M	10	Gradient elution	Zimmermann's reaction	0.36—8.15	3.19—5.97	1.45—4.89	0.77—1.92	0.29—1.03	0.40—1.70	VESTERGAARD and CLAUSSEN 1962
F	10	chromatography		0.57—5.26	1.71—4.60	1.73—3.38	0.54—1.05	0.43—0.74	0.54—1.51	
M	5	Gradient elution	Zimmermann's reaction	0.25—2.57	2.13—5.70	3.11—5.19	0.36—0.46	0.15—0.52	0.48—0.94	KELLIE and WADE, 1957
F	6	chromatography		0.81—2.14	2.93—4.08	4.10—6.20	0.16—0.58	0.09—0.56	0.55—1.35	

excretion of 0.56 mg/24 h in normal women, SPARAGANA et al. 0.50 mg per 24 h while VESTERGAARD and CLAUSEN observed an average excretion of 2.01 mg/24 h, a mean concentration higher than that reported by KELLIE and WADE (1957) also using gradient elution chromatography for steroid separation and the ZIMMERMANN reaction for DHEA quantification. This latter mean excretion figure (1.4 mg/24 h) is close to the mean value for excretion of DHEA in normal women of 1.11 found by RIVERA et al. (1965) using a gas phase chromatography technique for steroid separation.

The data of Thomas (1965) may shed light on some of the problems inherent to the measurement of urinary 17-KS by the technique of gas phase chromatography. In this work, urinary 17-KS are hydrolyzed much in the same way as by KIRSCHNER and LIPSETT except that in the publication of THOMAS, the conjugated urinary 17-KS are extracted prior to hydrolysis (THOMAS and BULBROOK, 1964). After hydrolysis of this extract, the free 17-KS are chromatographed on paper, eluted and converted to their TMSi ethers. These ethers are chromatographed on a 7 ft column of Gas Chrom P coated with 2% XE-60. Solid sample application to the column is used, but further details on gas phase chromatography on the 2% XE-60 column are not given except that an argon ionization detector is used for steroid quantification. When the concentration of DHEA, androsterone, and etiocholanolone are estimated in the same sample after this type of purification and after gradient elution (KELLIE and WADE, 1957) with ZIMMERMANN reaction as end point analysis, the gas phase chromatography method gives the lowest levels of etiocholanolone and DHEA and the highest ones of androsterone. Comparing steroid levels in the same urinary extract following purification by gradient elution and by gas phase chromatography on a hybrid column of 0.6% Hi-Eff 8B and 0.6% JXR, the differences between means for androsterone and for DHEA concentrations in fourteen experiments had the same t and p values: 0.04 and >0.2 respectively. These values were 2.88 and <0.01 for etiocholanolone. In an extension of this work, THOMAS and BULBROOK (1966) found a correlation coefficient exceeding 0.9 when DHEA, androsterone and etiocholanolone were purified in the same samples of urine by gradient elution or by gas phase chromatography. Still, these authors discuss the possibility that small divergences from absolute agreement may exist between the two methods.

From these data the problem of stability of etiocholanolone TMSi during gas phase chromatography arises. On the other hand, degree of purity of 17-KS after gradient elution chromatography must be considered, though substantial evidence has been presented in support of homogeneity of steroid isolated by this procedure (KELLIE and WADE, 1957). Finally, the accuracy of measurement of individual 17-KS in small amounts by the ZIMMERMANN reaction enters this rather thorny problem (TALBOT et al., 1942). Since in the work of THOMAS (1965) all urinary specimens were hydrolyzed by the same method, his work is not open to the criticism of different degree of hydrolysis of conjugated 17-KS by different methods as is the case with the data of Table 17.

Conclusion

From the foregoing discussion it must be concluded that adequate methods have been developed for the estimation of many 17-keto-steroids in the same sample of urine by the technique of gas phase chromatography. Again the advantage of this technique is speed of execution and precision of measurement. In a recent essay, BUSH (1966 a) discusses an automated technique for the estimation of urinary steroids. This method does not depend on gas phase chromatography with sensitive detectors for final analysis (BUSH, 1966 b), but on paper chromatography and spectrophotometric estimations. With knowledge of the accuracy, specificity, sensitivity and precision of the technique of BUSH (1966 a) for the estimation of urinary 17-KS, it would be of interest to compare the cost per analysis in the gas phase chromatography technique of THOMAS and BULBROOK (1966) and in the technique of BUSH (1966 a). The belief widely current in certain research circles that gas phase chromatography is potentially more satisfactory with regard to speed of analysis may be a pardon-able misinterpretation. However that may be, sensitive and accurate estimation of the different 17-ketosteroids in the same sample of urine is probably a significant contribution of gas phase chromatography to technology in this field of endocrine research.

The work from the author's own laboratory reviewed in this chapter was supported in part by U.S. Public Health Service Grants Nos. AM-06651, T01 CA 5000 and 5-K3-GM-15-354.

References

AAKVAAG, A., and K. B. EIK-NES: Metabolism *in vivo* of steroids in the canine ovary. Biochim. biophys. Acta 111, 273 (1965).

ACEVEDO, H. F., and J. CORRAL-GALLARDO: Epitestosterone: An *in vitro* metabolite of Δ⁴-androstenedione in a sclerocystic ovary. J. clin. Endocr. 25, 1675 (1965).

ATTAL, J., S. M. HENDELES, J. A. ENGELS, and K. B. EIK-NES: Elution of steroids after thin-layer chromatography. J. Chromatog. 27, 167 (1967).

AXELROD, L. R.: The chromatographic fractionation and identification of compounds related to the estrogens. Rec. Progr. Horm. Res. 9, 69 (1954).

BAGGETT, B., L. L. ENGEL, L. L. FIELDING, K. SAVARD, R. I. DORFMAN, F. L. ENGEL, and H. T. MCPHERSON: Production of hydrocortisone by a human testicular tumor. Fed. Proc. 16, 149 (1957).

BAULIEU, E.-E.: Three sulfate esters of 17-ketosteroids in the plasma of normal subjects and after administration of ACTH. J. clin. Endocr. 20, 900 (1960).

— Studies of conjugated 17-ketosteroids in a case of adrenal tumor. J. clin. Endocr. 22, 501 (1962).

—, and P. MAUVAIS-JARVIS: Studies on testosterone metabolism. I. Conversion of testosterone-17α-³H to 5α- and 5β-androstane-3α,17β-diol-17α-³H: a new "17β-hydroxyl pathway". J. biol. Chem. 239, 1569 (1964 a).

— — Studies on testosterone metabolism. II. Metabolism of testosterone-4-¹⁴C and androst-4-ene-3,17-dione-1,2-³H. J. biol. Chem. 239, 1578 (1964 b).

BERNSTEIN, S., and R. H. LENHARD: The absorption spectra of steroids in concentrated sulfuric acid. I. Method and data. J. org. Chem. 18, 1146 (1953).

BERRETT, C., and C. MCNEIL: The quantitation of major 17-ketosteroid fractions by gas-liquid chromatography. Clin. Chem. 12, 399 (1966).

BRINCK-JOHNSEN, B., and K. EIK-NES: Effect of human chorionic gonadotropin on the secretion of testosterone and 4-androstene-3,17-dione by the canine testis. Endocrinology 61, 676 (1957).

BROOKS, R. V.: A method for the simultaneous estimation of testosterone and epitestosterone in urine. Steroids 4, 117 (1964).

—, and G. GIULIANI: Epitestosterone: Isolation from human urine and experiments on possible precursors. Steroids 4, 101 (1964).

BROWNIE, A. C., H. J. VAN DER MOLEN, E. E. NISHIZAWA, and K. B. EIK-NES: Determination of testosterone in human peripheral blood using gas-liquid chromatography with electron capture detection. J. clin. Endocr. 24, 1091 (1964).

BURGER, H. G., J. R. KENT, and A. E. KELLIE: Determination of testosterone in human peripheral and adrenal venous plasma. J. clin. Endocr. 24, 432 (1964).

BURSTEIN, S., and S. LIEBERMAN: Hydrolysis of ketosteroid hydrogen sulfates by solvolysis procedures. J. biol. Chem. **233**, 331 (1958).

BUSH, I. E.: Use of thiosemicarbazide in microestimation and recognition of steroid ketones. Fed. Proc. **12**, 186 (1953) (Abstract).

— Automation of steroid analysis. Science **154**, 77 (1966 a).

— Development of automated method for large number steroid analyses. Excerpta Medica Found. Int. Congress Series **111**, 136 (1966 b).

CALLOW, N. H. : The isolation of two transformation products of testosterone from urine. Biochem. J. **33**, 559 (1939).

CAMACHO, A. M., and C. J. MIGEON: Isolation, identification and quantitation of testosterone in the urine of normal adults and in patients with endocrine disorders. J. clin. Endocr. **23**, 301 (1963).

— — Studies on the origin of testosterone in the urine of normal adult subjects and patients with various endocrine disorders. J. clin. Invest. **43**, 1083 (1964).

CAWLEY, L. P., B. O. MUSSER, W. FAUCETT, S. BECKLOFF, and H. LEARNED: Evaluation of hydrolytic products of 17-ketosteroids by means of gas-liquid chromatography. Clin. Chem. **11**, 1009 (1965).

CERESA, F., and C. A. CRAVETTO: A method for the simultaneous assay of 17-hydroxycorticosteroids and 17-ketosteroids both in their free and conjugated forms on the same plasma sample. Acta endocr. **29**, 321 (1958).

CHAPDELAINE, A., P. C. MacDONALD, O. GONZALEZ, E. GURPIDE, R. L. VANDE WIELE, and S. LIEBERMAN: Studies on the secretion and interconversion of the androgens. IV: Quantitative results in a normal man whose gonadal and adrenal function were altered experimentally. J. clin. Endocr. **25**, 1569 (1965).

CLARK, S. J., and H. H. WOTIZ: Separation and detection of nanogram amounts of steroids. Steroids **2**, 535 (1963).

CLAYTON, G. W., A. M. BONGIOVANNI, and C. PAPADATOS: Preliminary investigations into the nature of neutral 17-ketosteroids in human plasma. J. clin. Endocr. **15**, 693 (1955).

COHN, G. L., P. K. BONDY, and C. CASTIGLIONE: Studies on pyrogenic steroids. I. Separation, identification, and measurement of unconjugated dehydroepiandrosterone, etiocholanolone, and androsterone in human plasma. J. clin. Invest. **40**, 400 (1961).

CONRAD, S. H., V. MAHESH, and W. HERRMANN: Quantitative paper chromatography of conjugated 17-ketosteroids in plasma. J. clin. Invest. **40**, 947 (1961).

— M. C. LINDBERG, and W. L. HERRMANN: Significance of plasma dehydroisoandrosterone and androsterone sulfates in the diagnosis of virilizing disorders. Amer. J. Obst. Gynecol. **91**, 449 (1965).

COOPER, J. A., and B. G. CREECH: The application of gas-liquid chromatography to the analysis of urinary 17-ketosteroids. Anal. Biochem. **2**, 502 (1961).

CONNELL, G., and K. B. EIK-NES: Unpublished (1967).

COPPAGE, W. S., and A. E. COONER: Testosterone in human plasma. New Engl. J. Med. 273, 902 (1965).

DE MOOR, P., and W. HEYNS: Gas chromatographic determination of dehydroepiandrosterone sulfate and androsterone sulfate in human plasma. In: Androgens in normal and pathological conditions. A. VERMEULEN and D. EXLEY (eds.). Excerpta Medica Found. Int. Congress Series 101, 54 (1966).

DE NEVE, L., and A. VERMEULEN: The determination of 17-oxosteroid sulphates in human plasma. J. Endocr. 32, 295 (1965).

DE NICOLA, A. F., R. I. DORFMAN, and E. FORCHIELLI: Urinary excretion of epitestosterone and testosterone in normal individuals and hirsute and virilized females. Steroids 7, 351 (1966).

DE PAOLI, J. C., E. NISHIZAWA, and K. B. EIK-NES: Hydrolysis of conjugated 17-ketosteroids. J. clin. Endocr. 23, 81 (1963).

DESSYPRIS, A., M. A. DROSDOWSKY, N. L. McNIVEN, and R. I. DORFMAN: Identification of testosterone sulfate in urine of normal adult subjects. Proc. Soc. exp. Biol. Med. 121, 1128 (1966).

DIXON, R., V. VINCENT, and N. KASE: Biosynthesis of steroid sulfates by normal human testis. Steroids 6, 757 (1965).

DORFMAN, L.: Ultraviolet absorption of steroids. Chem. Rev. 53, 47 (1953).

DORFMAN, R. I.: Etioallocholanol-3(β)-17-one (Isoandrosterone) as a metabolite of testosterone in the human male. Proc. Soc. exp. Biol. Med. 46, 351 (1941).

—, and R. A. SHIPLEY: Androgens — Biochemistry, physiology and clinical significance. New York: John Wiley & Sons, Inc. 1956.

—, and F. UNGAR: Metabolism of steroid hormones. New York and London: Academic Press 1965.

DRAY, M. F., et Y. ADAM: L'Estimation dans le plasma des 17 cetosteroides sulfo-conjugues, de la dehydro-epiandrosterone, de l'etiocholanolone et de l'androsterone. Rev. franç. Etud. Clin. Biol. 7, 71 (1962).

— Mesure de la testosterone du plasma veineux peripherique chez l'homme adulte par une technique de double dilution isotopique. Bull. Soc. Chim. Biol. 47, 2145 (1965).

— et M.-J. LEDRU: Metabolisme de l'epitestosterone. Absence d'interconversion peripherique de l'epitestosterone et de la testosterone et existence d'une production de sulfate d'epitestosterone, chez l'homme adulte normal. C. R. Acad. Sci. (Paris) 262, 679 (1966).

DULMANIS, A., J. P. COGHLAN, M. WINTOUR, and B. HUDSON: The estimation of testosterone in biological fluids: II. Testosterone in urine. Aust. J. exp. Biol. Med. Sci. 42, 385 (1964).

EBERLEIN, W. R.: A transesterification method for the measurement of plasma 17-ketosteroid sulfates. J. clin. Endocr. 23, 990 (1963).

EIK-NES, K. B.: In: Methods in hormone research. R. I. DORFMAN (ed.). New York: Academic Press. In press, 1968.

EIK-NES, K. B.: Factors influencing the secretion of testosterone in the anesthetized dog. Ciba Found. Colloq. on Endocrinology 16, 120 (1967).

—, G. W. OERTEL, R. NIMER, and F. H. TYLER: Effect of human chorionic gonadotropin on plasma concentrations of 17-hydroxycorticosteroids, dehydroepiandrosterone and androsterone in man. J. clin. Endocr. 19, 1405 (1959).

—, and P. F. HALL: Isolation of dehydroepiandrosterone-C^{14} from dogs infused with cholesterol-4-C^{14} by the spermatic artery. Proc. Soc. exp. Biol. Med. 111, 280 (1962).

— — Secretion of steroid hormones *in vivo*. Vitam. and Horm. 23, 153 (1965).

—, H. J. VAN DER MOLEN, and A. C. BOWNIE: In: Steroid Hormone Analysis, Vol. 1. H. E. CARSTENSEN (ed.) New York: M. Dekker, Inc. 1967, p. 319.

EWING, L. L., and K. B. EIK-NES: On the formation of testosterone by the perfused rabbit testis. Canad. J. Biochem. 44, 1327 (1966).

EXLEY, D.: The ultramicro-determination of testosterone using gas-liquid chromatography with electron capture detection. In: Androgens in normal and pathological conditions. A. VERMEULEN and D. EXLEY (eds.). Excerpta Medica Found. Int. Congress Series 101, 11 (1966).

FINKELSTEIN, M.: Fluorometric determination of micro amounts of oestrone-oestradiol and oestriol in urine. Acta endocr. 10, 149 (1952).

—, S. HESTRIN, and W. KOCH: Estimation of steroid estrogens by fluorimetry. Proc. Soc. exp. Biol. Med. 64, 64 (1947).

—, E. FORCHIELLI, and R. I. DORFMAN: Estimation of testosterone in human plasma. J. clin. Endocr. 21, 98 (1961).

FORCHIELLI, E., G. SORCINI, M. S. NIGHTINGALE, N. BRUST, R. I. DORFMAN, W. H. PERLOFF, and G. JACOBSON: Testosterone in human plasma. Anal. Biochem. 5, 416 (1963).

—, G. S. RAO, I. R. SARDA, N. B. GIBREE, P. E. POCHI, J. S. STRAUSS, and R. I. DORFMAN: Effect of ethinylestradiol on plasma testosterone levels and urinary testosterone excretion in man. Acta endocr. 50, 51 (1965).

FOTHERBY, K., and J. A. STRONG: The hourly excretion of steroids after a short intravenous infusion of ACTH. J. Endocr. 19, 389 (1960).

FRANCE, J. T., R. RIVERA, N. L. MCNIVEN, and R. I. DORFMAN: Determination of androsterone, etiocholanolone and dehydroepiandrosterone in urine by gas-liquid chromatography. Steroids 5, 687 (1965).

FRITZ, G. R., and E. KNOBIL: The measurement of testosterone in plasma by competitive protein binding analysis. Fed. Proc. 26, 757 (1967).

FUTTERWEIT, W., N. L. MCNIVEN, L. NARCUS, C. LANTOS, M. DROS-DOWSKY, and R. I. DORFMAN: Gas chromatographic determination of testosterone in human urine. Steroids 1, 628 (1963).

— —, R. GUERRA-GARCIA, N. GIBREE, M. DROSDOWSKY, G. L. SIEGEL, L. J. SOFFER, I. M. ROSENTHAL, and R. I. DORFMAN: Testosterone in human urine. Steroids 4, 137 (1964).

FUTTERWEIT, W., G. L. SIEGEL, R. FREEMAN, S. I. GRIBOFF, M. DROSDOWSKY, N. GIBREE, R. I. DORFMAN, and L. J. SOFFER: Gas chromatography of steroids in biological fluids. M. B. LIPSETT (ed.) New York: Plenum Press 1965 a, 19.

—, R. FREEMAN, G. L. SIEGEL, S. I. GRIBOFF, R. I. DORFMAN, and L. J. SOFFER: Clinical applications of a gas chromatographic method for the combined determination of testosterone and epitestosterone glucuronide in urine. J. clin. Endocr. 25, 1451 (1965 b).

GANDY, H. M., and R. E. PETERSON: Plasma levels of unconjugated Δ^4-androstene-3,17-dione, dehydroisoandrosterone, etiocholanolone, androsterone and testosterone in man. 46th Meeting, American Endocrine Society, 1964. (Abstract).

GARDNER, L. I.: Plasma neutral 17-ketosteroids. I. Technique of estimation. J. clin. Endocr. 13, 941 (1953).

GERDES, H., and W. STAIB: Fluorescence of testosterone and some other steroids in sulphuric acid. Steroids 6, 793 (1965).

GIBREE, N. B., E. FORCHIELLI, J. S. STRAUSS, P. E. POCHI, and R. I. DORFMAN: Testosterone in the urine of castrated men. Proc. Soc. exp. Biol. Med. 119, 1019 (1965).

GLENN, E. M., and E. HEFTMANN: Urinary excretion of neutral 17-ketosteroids by normal dogs. Proc. Soc. exp. Biol. Med. 77, 147 (1951).

GOLDFIEN, A., J. JONES, M.-E. YANNONE, and B. WHITE: In: Gas chromatography of steroids in biological fluids. M. B. LIPSETT (ed.). New York: Plenum Press 1965, p. 35.

GUERRA-GARCIA, R., S. C. CHATTORAJ, L. J. GABRILOVE, and H. H. WOTIZ: Studies in steroid metabolism XX. "The determination of plasma testosterone using thin-layer and gas-liquid chromatography." Steroids 2, 605 (1963).

—, A. VELASQUEZ, and J. WHITTEMBURY: Urinary testosterone in high altitude natives. Steroids 6, 351 (1965).

HAAHTI, E.: Major lipid constituents of human skin surface with special reference to gas-chromatographic methods. Scand. J. clin. Lab. invest. Suppl. 59, 13 (1961).

HAAHTI, E. O. A., W. J. A. VANDEN HEUVEL, and E. C. HORNING: Separation of urinary 17-ketosteroids by gas chromatography. Anal. Biochem. 2, 182 (1961).

HADD, H. E., and R. K. RHAMY: Isolation of testosterone-($17\beta \rightarrow 1\beta$-oside)-D-glucopyranosuronic acid from human blood. J. clin. Endocr. 25, 876 (1965).

HALPAAP, H., W. REICH, and K. IRMSCHER: Factors influencing TLC separation of testosterone and 17-epitestosterone. In: Workshop on testosterone. J. TAMM and K. D. VOIGT (eds.). To be published (1967).

HARTMAN, I. S., and H. H. WOTIZ: A method for the simultaneous separation of $C_{19}O_2$ and $C_{19}O_3$ 17-ketosteroids and progesterone metabolites by gas chromatography. Steroids 1, 33 (1963).

HEITZMAN, R. J., and G. H. THOMAS: Evaluation by gas chromatography of the urinary steroids of the pregnant dairy cow. J. Endocr. **33**, 455 (1965).

HEYNS, W., and P. DE MOOR: Validation of the gas chromatographic determination of some urinary steroids by comparison with spectro-photometric methods. In: Androgens in normal and pathological conditions. A. VERMEULEN and D. EXLEY (eds.). Excerpta Medica Found. Int. Congress Series **101**, 42 (1966).

HOLLANDER, N., and V. P. HOLLANDER: The micro determination of testosterone in human spermatic vein blood. J. clin. Endocr. **18**, 966 (1958).

HOLTZ, A. H.: 17α-ketosteroids and pseudo-ketosteroids in the urine of cattle. Acta endocr. **26**, 75 (1957).

HORN, H., M. STATTER, and M. FINKELSTEIN: Estimation of testosterone in human urine. Steroids **7**, 118 (1966).

HORNING, E. C., and W. J. A. VANDEN HEUVEL: Gas chromatography. Ann. Rev. Biochem. **32**, 709 (1963).

HORTON, R.: Estimation of androstenedione in human peripheral blood with ^{35}S-thiosemicarbazide. J. clin. Endocr. **25**, 1237 (1965).

—, J. M. ROSNER, and P. H. FORSHAM: Urinary excretion pattern of in-jected H^3-testosterone. Proc. Soc. exp. Biol. Med. **114**, 400 (1963).

—, and K. MANN: Estimation of androstenedione and testosterone in plasma with ^{35}S-thiosemicarbazide. Excerpta Medica Found. Int. Congress Series **111**, 131 (1966).

HUDSON, B., and G. W. OERTEL: Determination of dehydroepiandrosterone and total neutral 17-ketosteroids in human plasma. Anal. Biochem. **2**, 248 (1961).

—, J. COGHLAN, A. DULMANIS, M. WINTOUR, and I. EKKEL: The estimation of testosterone in biological fluids. Aust. J. exp. biol. med. Sci. **41**, 235 (1963).

—, J. P. COGHLAN, A. DULMANIS, and M. WINTOUR: The measurement of testosterone in biological fluids in the evaluation of androgen activity. Proc. 2nd Int. Congr. Endocrinol. London, 1964. Excerpta Medica Found. Int. Congress Series **83**, Vol. II, 1127 (1964).

IBAYASHI, H., M. NAKAMURA, S. MURAKAWA, T. UCHIKAWA, T. TANIOKA, and K. NAKAO: The determination of urinary testosterone using thin-layer chromatography and gas chromatography. Steroids **3**, 559 (1964).

— —, T. UCHIKAWA, S. MURAKAWA, S. YOSHIDA, K. NAKAO, and S. OKI-NAKA: C_{19} Steroids in canine spermatic venous blood following gonado-tropin administration. Endocrinology **76**, 347 (1965).

ISMAIL, A., and R. A. HARKNESS: The estimation of testosterone in urine. Acta endocr., Suppl. 10, Abstract No. 15, 47 (1965).

ISMAIL, A. A. A., and R. A. HARKNESS: The urinary excretion of testosterone by normal men and women. J. Endocr. **34**, XVII (1966).

JACOBSOHN, G. M., and S. LIEBERMAN: Studies on the chemical cleavage of the urinary glucuronosides of the 17-ketosteroids. J. biol. Chem. **237**, 1469 (1962).

Kellie, A. E., and A. P. Wade: The analysis of urinary 17-oxo steroids by gradient elution. Biochem. J. **66**, 196 (1957).

Kirschner, M. A., M. B. Lipsett, and H. Wilson: Metabolism of exogenous dehydroepiandrosterone in man. Acta endocr. **43**, 387 (1963).

— — Gas-liquid chromatography in the quantitative analysis of urinary 11-deoxy-17-ketosteroids. J. clin. Endocr. **23**, 255 (1963).

— — The analysis of urinary steroids using gas-liquid chromatography. Steroids **3**, 277 (1964).

— —, and D. R. Collins: Plasma ketosteroids and testosterone in man: A study of pituitary-testicular axis. J. clin. Invest. **44**, 657 (1965).

Kliman, B., and C. Briefer: Collection of carbon-14 in gas-liquid chromatography with application to the analysis of testosterone in human plasma. In: Steroid gas chromatography. J. K. Grant (ed.). Endocr. Mem. No. 16. London: Cambridge Univ. Press. In press, 1967.

Koenig, V. L., F. Melzer, C. M. Szego, and L. T. Samuels: A colorimetric reaction for testosterone. J. Biol. Chem. **141**, 487 (1941).

Korenman, S. G., H. Wilson, and M. B. Lipsett: Testosterone production rates in normal adults. J. clin. Invest. **42**, 1753 (1963).

—, and M. B. Lipsett: Is testosterone glucuronoside uniquely derived from plasma testosterone? J. clin. Invest. **43**, 2125 (1964).

—, T. E. Davis, H. Wilson, and M. B. Lipsett: A simplified procedure for the estimation of testosterone production rates. Steroids **3**, 203 (1964 a).

—, H. Wilson, and M. B. Lipsett: Isolation of 17α-hydroxy-androst-4-en-3-one (epitestosterone) from human urine. J. biol. Chem. **239**, 1004 (1964 b).

Lakshmanan, T. K., and S. Lieberman: An improved method of gradient elution chromatography and its application to the separation of urinary ketosteroids. Arch. Biochem. Biophys. **53**, 258 (1954).

Lamb, E. J., W. J. Dignam, R. J. Pion, and H. H. Simmer: Plasma androgens in women. I. Normal and non-hirsute females, oophorectomized and adrenalectomized patients. Acta endocr. **45**, 243 (1964).

Landowne, R. A., and S. R. Lipsky: The electron capture spectrometry of haloacetates: A means of detecting ultramicro quantities of sterols by gas chromatography. Anal. Chem. **35**, 532 (1963).

Lehnert, G., W. Mucke und H. Valentin: Über eine Methode zur Gaschromatographischen Analyse von 11-Desoxy-17-Ketosteroiden im Harn und ihre Ergebnisse beim Menschen. Endokrinologie **46**, 241 (1966).

Levvy, G. A.: Glucuronide metabolism, with special reference to the steroid hormones. In: Vitamins and hormones. R. S. Harris, G. F. Marrian, and K. V. Thimann (eds.). New York: Academic Press, 14: 267 (1956).

Lim, N. Y., and J. F. Dingman: Measurement of testosterone excretion and production rate by glass paper chromatography. J. clin. Endocr. **25**, 563 (1965).

—, and R. V. Brooks: A modification of the ^{35}S-thiosemicarbazide method for the estimation of plasma testosterone. Steroids **6**, 561 (1965).

Lim, N. Y., and J. F. Dingman: Estimation of androstenedione in peripheral plasma with ³⁵S-thiosemicarbazide. Excerpta Medica Found. Int. Congress Series 111, 238 (1966).

Lindner, H. R.: Androgens in the bovine testis and spermatic vein blood. Nature 183, 1605 (1959).

Lipsett, M. B., G. D. Coffman, and W. E. Nixon: Lack of activity of dehydroepiandrosterone sulphate in metabolic balance studies. J. clin. Endocr. 25, 993 (1965).

Lobotsky, J., H. I. Wyss, E. J. Segre, and C. W. Lloyd: Plasma testosterone in the normal woman. J. clin. Endocr. 24, 1261 (1964).

Loriaux, D. L., J. R. Lehman, R. H. Kaufman, and M. W. Noall: Evidence that testosterone and dehydroepiandrosterone sulphate do not contribute to urinary epitestosterone in the Stein-Leventhal syndrome. Steroids 8, 377 (1966).

Lucas, W. M., W. F. Whitmore, and C. D. West: Identification of testosterone in human spermatic vein blood. J. clin. Endocr. 17, 465 (1957).

Madigan, J. J., E. E. Zenno, and R. Pheasant: Determination of testosterone propionate in vegetable oil solution. Anal. Chem. 23, 1691 (1951).

Mahesh, V. B., and R. B. Greenblatt: The *in vivo* conversion of dehydroepiandrosterone and androstenedione to testosterone in the human. Acta endocr. 41, 400 (1962).

Martin, R. P.: A note on the specificity of the Koenig colour reaction as modified by Oertel. Acta endocr. 40, 263 (1962).

Mathews, J. S., A. L. Pereda, and A. Aguilera: Steroids. CCXV. The quantitative analysis of steroids by thin layer chromatography. J. Chromat. 9, 331 (1962).

McKenna, J., and A. E. Rippon: The extraction of plasma 3-hydroxy-17-oxo steroid sulphates and the measurement of the constituent dehydroepiandrosterone sulphate and androsterone sulphate. Biochem. J. 95, 107 (1965).

McKerns, K. W., and E. Nordstrand: Stimulation of the rat ovary by gonadotropins and separation of steroids by gas chromatography. Biochim. biophys. acta 104, 237 (1965).

Migeon, C. J: Identification and isolation of androsterone from peripheral human plasma. J. biol. Chem. 218, 941 (1956).

— In: Hormones in human plasma. H. N. Antoniades (ed.). Boston: Little, Brown and Company 1960, p. 297.

—, and J. E. Plager: Identification and isolation of dehydroisoandrosterone from peripheral human plasma. J. biol. Chem. 209, 767 (1954 a).

— — Neutral 17-ketosteroids in human plasma. Rec. Progr. Horm. Res. 9, 235 (1954 b).

—, A. R. Keller, B. Lawrence, and T. H. Shepard: Dehydroepiandrosterone and androsterone levels in human plasma. Effect of age and sex; day to day and diurnal variations. J. clin. Endocr. 17, 1051 (1957).

MORER-FARGAS, F., und H. NOWAKOWSKI: Die Testosteronausscheidung im Harn bei männlichen Individuen. Acta endocr. **49**, 443 (1965).

NAIR, P. P., I. J. SARLOS, D. SOLOMON, and D. A. TURNER: Simultaneous separation of 17-ketosteroids and estrogens by biphase gas chromatography. Anal. Biochem. **7**, 96 (1964).

NAKAGAWA, K., N. L. McNIVEN, E. FORCHIELLI, A. VERMEULEN, and R. I. DORFMAN: Determination of testosterone by gas-liquid chromatography using an electron capture detector. I. Responses of halo-alkyl derivatives. Steroids **7**, 329 (1966).

NICHOLS, T., C. A. NUGENT, and F. H. TYLER: Glucocorticoid suppression of urinary testosterone excretion in patients with idiopathic hirsutism. J. clin. endocr. **26**, 79 (1966).

NISHINA, T., Y. SAKAI, and M. KIMURA: A specific method for the determination of Δ^4-3-ketosteroids with p-nitrophenylhydrazine. Steroids **4**, 255 (1964).

NISHIZAWA, E. E., and K. B. EIK-NES: On the secretion of progesterone and Δ^4-androstene-3,17-dione by the canine ovary in animals stimulated with human chorionic gonadotropin. Biochim. biophys. acta **86**, 610 (1964).

OERTEL, G. W.: Determination of plasma testosterone. Acta endocr. **37**, 237 (1961).

—, and K. B. EIK-NES: Determination of dehydroepiandrosterone in human blood plasma. J. biol. Chem. **232**, 543 (1958).

— — Isolation and identification of testosterone in systemic blood from normal human male adults. Proc. Soc. exp. Biol. Med. **102**, 553 (1959).

— — Isolation and identification of 4-pregnen-17α-ol-3,20-dione and 5-pregnen-3β-ol-20-one from human blood plasma. Arch. Biochem. Biophys. **93**, 392 (1961).

—, and E. KAISER: Determination of dehydroepiandrosterone, androsterone, etiocholanolone, and "11β-hydroxyetiocholanolone" in plasma. Clin. chim. acta **7**, 221 (1962).

O'GATA, A., und S. HIRANO: Maennliches Sexualhormon aus dem Hoden der Schweine. Proc. Imp. Acad. **9**, 345 (1933).

PANICUCCI, F.: Gas chromatographic determination of plasma and urinary androgens (testosterone and 17-ketosteroids) in normal men. In: Androgens in normal and pathological conditions. A. VERMEULEN and D. EXLEY (eds.). Excerpta Medica Found. Int. Congress Series **101**, 25 (1966).

PEARLMAN, W. H., and E. CERCEO: The estimation of saturated and α,β-unsaturated ketonic compounds in placental extracts. J. biol. Chem. **203**, 127 (1953).

PEILLON, F., et J. RACADOT: Actions comparees de la testosterone, de la dehydroepiandrosterone (DHA) et du sulfate de dehydroepiandrosterone sur la fonction gonadotrope hypophysaire de la ratte prepubre. Ann. Endocr. (Paris) **26**, 419 (1965).

Pochi, P. E., J. S. Strauss, G. S. Rao, I. R. Sarda, E. Forchielli, and R. I. Dorfman: Plasma testosterone and estrogen levels, urine testosterone excretion, and sebum production in males with acne vulgaris. J. clin. Endocr. 25, 1660 (1965).

Rapp, J. P., and K. B. Eik-Nes: The effect of front size on electron capture detector sensitivity. J. Gas Chromatogr. 4, 376 (1966).

Reich, H., K. F. Crane, and S. J. Sanfilippo: The reaction of steroid ketones with 2,4-dinitrophenylhydrazine. J. org. Chem. 18, 822 (1953).

Resko, J. A., and K. B. Eik-Nes: Diurnal testosterone levels in peripheral plasma of human male subjects. J. clin. Endocr. 26, 573 (1966).

Riondel, A., J. F. Tait, M. Gut, S. A. S. Tait, E. Joachim, and B. Little: Estimation of testosterone in human peripheral blood using S^{35}-thiosemicarbazide. J. clin. Endocr. 23, 620 (1963).

Rivarola, M. A., and C. J. Migeon: Determination of testosterone and androst-4-ene-3,17-dione concentration in human plasma. Steroids 7, 103 (1966).

Rivera, R., R. I. Dorfman, and E. Forchielli: A method for the simultaneous determination of individual 17-ketosteroids, pregnanediol and pregnanetriol. Excerpta Medica Found. Int. Congress Series 99, E 159 (1965).

Rosner, J. M., and N. F. Conte: Evaluation of testicular function by measurement of urinary excretion of testosterone. J. clin. Endocr. 26, 735 (1966).

— —, J. H. Briggs, P. Y. Chao, E. M. Sudman, and P. H. Forsham: Determination of urinary testosterone by chromatography and colorimetry: Findings in normal subjects and in patients with endocrine diseases. J. clin. Endocr. 25, 95 (1965).

Sachs, L.: A sulphuric acid reagent for the colorimetric determination of testosterone. Nature 201, 296 (1964).

Saez, J. M., S. Saez, and C. J. Migeon: Identification and measurement of testosterone in the sulfate fraction of plasma of normal subjects and patients with gonadal and adrenal disorders. Steroids 9, 1 (1967).

Saier, E. L., E. Campbell, H. S. Strickler, and R. C. Grauer: A simplified method for the simultaneous determination of 17-ketosteroids, dehydroepiandrosterone, and 17-hydroxycorticosteroids in serum. J. clin. Endocr. 19, 1162 (1959).

Salamon, I. I., and K. Dobriner: Studies in steroid metabolism. XVI. Isolation of 11β-hydroxy-Δ^4-androstene-3,17-dione. J. biol. Chem. 204, 487 (1953).

Sandberg, D. H., N. Ahmad, W. W. Cleveland, and K. Savard: Measurement of urinary testosterone by gas-liquid chromatography. Steroids 4, 557 (1964).

—, J. Sjövall, K. Sjövall, and D. A. Turner: Measurement of human serum bile acids by gas-liquid chromatography. J. Lipid Res. 6, 182 (1965 a).

SANDBERG, D. H., N. AHMAD, M. ZACHMANN, and W. W. CLEVELAND: Measurement of plasma 11-deoxy-17-ketosteroid sulfates by gas-liquid chromatography. Steroids 6, 777 (1965 b).

SAROFF, J., W. R. SLAUNWHITE, and A. A. SANDBERG: Assay of non-conjugated testosterone (T), androstenedione (Δ) and DHEA (D) in human plasma using Bromine-82. Excerpta Medica Found. Int. Congress Series 111, 116 (1966).

SCHILLER, S., R. I. DORFMAN, and M. MILLER: Metabolism of the steroid hormones: The metabolism of testosterone in a normal woman. Endocrinology 36, 355 (1945).

SCHUBERT, K., und K. WEHRBERGER: Isolierung von Testosteron aus normalem Harn. Naturwissenschaften 47, 281 (1960).

—, und G. FRANKENBERG: Die Bestimmung von Testosteron und Δ⁴-Androstenedion-(3,17) im Harn. Z. Physiol. Chem. 336, 91 (1964).

—, K. WEHRBERGER, and G. FRANKENBERG: 6β-Hydroxytestosterone and 11β-hydroxytestosterone in human urine. Steroids 3, 579 (1964).

SHORT, R. V.: Progesterone in blood. I. The chemical determination of progesterone in peripheral blood. J. Endocr. 16, 415 (1958).

SIMMER, H., I. SIMMER und O. ZELLMER: Androgene im peripheren Venenblut von gesunden und an Spätgestosen erkrankten Schwangeren. Klin. Wschr. 37, 966 (1959).

SJÖVALL, J., and R. VIHKO: Determination of androsterone and dehydroepiandrosterone sulfates in human serum by gas-liquid chromatography. Steroids 6, 597 (1965).

— — Identification of 3β,17β-dihydroxyandrost-5-ene, 3β,20α-dihydroxypregn-5-ene and epiandrosterone in human peripheral blood. Steroids 7, 447 (1966).

SJÖVALL, .K, J. SJÖVALL, K. MADDOCK, and E. C. HORNING: Estimation of dehydroepiandrosterone sulfate in human serum by gas-liquid chromatography. Anal. Biochem. 14, 337 (1966).

SOMMERVILLE, I. F., and G. N. DESHPANDE: The quantitative determination of progesterone and pregnanediol in human plasma. J. clin. Endocr. 18, 1223 (1958).

SONKA, J., P. GREGOROVA, M. JIPANEK, and Z. MATYS: Detekt dehydroeipiandrosteronu-novy' syndrom? Cas. Lek. Ces. 104, 268 (1965).

SPARAGANA, M.: Quantitative gas chromatographic analysis of urinary testosterone and epitestosterone. Steroids 5, 773 (1965).

—, W. B. MASON, and E. H. KEUTMANN: Preliminary isolation of 17-ketosteroids from urine for analysis by gas chromatography. Anal. Chem. 34, 1157 (1962).

—, E. H. KEUTMANN, and W. B. MASON: Quantitative determination of individual $C_{19}O_2$ and $C_{19}O_3$ urinary 17-ketosteroids by gas chromatography. Anal. Chem. 35, 1231 (1963).

STEIN, W. H., and S. MOORE: Chromatography of amino acids on starch columns. Separation of phenylalanine, leucine, isoleucine, methionine, tyrosine, and valine. J. biol. Chem. 176, 337 (1948).

SURACE, M., M. LUISI, E. MONETA, V. MARESCOTTI, and F. POLVANI: Plasma testosterone determination of women in normal and pathological conditions using horizontal thin-layer and gas-liquid chromatography. In: Androgens in normal and pathological conditions. A. VERMEULEN and D. EXLEY (eds.). Excerpta Medica Found. Int. Congress Series 101, 16 (1966).

—, e F. POLVANI: Determinazione gas-chromatografica del testosterone plasmatico nella policistosi ovarica. Ann. Obstet. Ginec. 88, 103 (1966).

TAIT, J. F.: Personal communication to this author, November, 1966.

TALBOT, N. B., R. A. BERMAN, and E. A. MACLACHLAN: Elimination of errors in the colorimetric assay of neutral urinary 17-ketosteroids by means of a color correction equation. J. biol. Chem. 143, 211 (1942).

TAMM, J., and K. D. VOIGT: The excretion in human urine of free and conjugated testosterone and epitestosterone following intravenous infusions of testosterone, epitestosterone and androstenedione. Excerpta Medica Found. Int. Congress Series 111, 141 (1966).

—, I. BECKMANN, and K. D. VOIGT: Determination of neutral steroids in human blood. Acta endocr. Suppl. 31, 219—225 (1957).

—, K. D. VOIGT, and U. VOLKWEIN: Water soluble steroid conjugates. I. Extraction, separation, and estimation. Steroids 2, 271 (1963).

THOMAS, B. S.: The specificity of a gas chromatographic method for the determination of urinary androsterone, etiocholanolone and dehydroepiandrosterone. In: Gas chromatography of steroids in biological fluids. M. B. LIPSETT (ed.). New York: Plenum Press 1965, p. 1.

— Preparation and gas chromatography of steroid chloromethyldimethylsilyl ethers. Chem. Communic., p. 408 (1966).

—, and R. D. BULBROOK: A rapid method for estimation of total 11-deoxy-17-oxosteroids in urine. J. Chromatog. 14, 28 (1964).

— — Routine assay of urinary dehydroepiandrosterone, androsterone and aetiocholanolone in urine by gas-liquid chromatography. In: Androgens in normal and pathological conditions. A. VERMEULEN and D. EXLEY (eds.). Excerpta Medica Found. Int. Congress Series 101, 49 (1966).

UMBERGER, E. J.: Isonicotinic acid hydrazide as a reagent for determination of Δ^4-3-ketosteroids. Determination of progesterone and testosterone propionate in oil solutions. Anal. Chem. 27, 768 (1955).

VANDE WIELE, R. L., P. C. MACDONALD, E. GURPIDE, and S. LIEBERMAN: Studies on the secretion and interconversion of the androgens. Rec. Prog. Horm. Res. XIX, 275 (1963).

VANDEN HEUVEL, W. J. A., and E. C. HORNING: Gas chromatography of adrenal cortical steroid hormones. Biochem. biophys. Res. Comm. 3, 356 (1960).

— — Gas chromatographic characterization of steroid ketones as N,N-dimethylhydrazones. Biochim. biophys. acta 74, 560 (1963).

—, J. SJÖVALL, and E. C. HORNING: Gas chromatographic behavior of trifluoracetoxy steroids. Biochim. biophys. acta 48, 596 (1961).

VANDEN HEUVEL, W. J. A., B. G. CREECH, and E. C. HORNING: Separation and estimation of the principal human urinary 17-ketosteroids as trimethyl ethers Anal. Biochem. **4**, 191 (1962).

VAN DER MOLEN, H. J., and D. GROEN: Determination of progesterone in human peripheral blood using gas-liquid chromatography with electron capture detection. J. clin. Endocr. **25**, 1625 (1965).

— — Quantitative determination of submicrogram amounts of steroids in blood using electron capture and flame ionization detection following gas-liquid chromatography. In: Steroid gas chromatography. J. K. GRANT (ed.). Endocr. Memoir No. 16. London: Cambridge Univ. Press. In press (1967).

—, and K. B. EIK-NES: Steroids in canine spermatic venous blood. Excerpta Medica Found. Int. Congress Series **111**, 264 (1966).

—, D. GROEN, and J. H. VAN DER MAAS: Steroid monochloroacetates. Physical-chemical characteristics and use in gas-liquid chromatography. Steroids **6**, 195 (1965).

— —, and A. PETERSE: Measurement of testosterone in plasma and urine using gas-liquid chromatography. In: Androgens in normal and pathological conditions. A. VERMEULEN and D. EXLEY (eds.). Excerpta Medica Found. Int. Congress Series **101**, 1 (1966 a).

—, J. H. VAN DER MAAS, and K. B. EIK-NES: On the presence of testosterone in peripheral blood from normal men. Clin. chim. acta **14**, 11 (1966 b).

VERMEULEN, A.: Urinary excretion of testosterone. In: Androgens in normal and pathological conditions. A. VERMEULEN and D. EXLEY (eds.). Excerpta Medica Found. Int. Congress Series **101**, 71 (1966).

—, and J. C. M. VERPLANCKE: A simple method for the determination of urinary testosterone secretion in human urine. Steroids **2**, 453 (1963).

VESTERGAARD, P., and B. CLAUSSEN: Hydrolysis of urinary 17-ketosteroid conjugates and estimation of the individual 17-ketosteroids by gradient elution chromatography. Acta endocr. Suppl. **64**, 3 (1962).

—, E. RAABO, and S. VEDSÖ: Determination of urinary testosterone in men, women and children. Clin. chim. acta **14**, 540 (1966).

VIHKO, R.: Gas chromatographic-mass spectrometric studies on solvolyzable steroids in human peripheral plasma. Acta endocr. Suppl. **109**, 1 (1966).

VOIGT, K. D., U. VOLKWEIN und J. TAMM: Eine Methode zur Bestimmung der Testosteron-Ausscheidung im Urin. Klin. Wschr. **42**, 642 (1964).

WASSERMANN, G. F., and K. B. EIK-NES: Unpublished (1967).

WEST, C. D., H. REICH, and L. T. SAMUELS: Urinary metabolites after intravenous injection of human subjects with testosterone. J. biol. Chem. **193**, 219 (1951).

WHEELER, O. H.: The irard reagents. Chem. Rev. **62**, 205 (1962).

WILSON, H.: Absorption spectra of Δ^5-3β-hydroxysteroids in several sulfuric acid reagents. Anal. Biochem. **1**, 402 (1960).

WRIGHT, A. A.: The excretion of steroids by animals. Vet. Res. **70**, 662 (1958).

ZANDER, J.: Methods in hormone research, Vol. 1. R. I. DORFMAN (ed.). New York: Academic Press 1962.

ZMIGROD, A., and H. R. LINDNER: Gas-chromatographic separation of ketosteroids as ethylene-thioketal derivatives. Steroids 8, 119 (1966).

ZURBRÜGG, R. P., R. D. B. JACOBS, and L. I. GARDNER: Urinary testosterone: A method utilizing column chromatography. J. clin. Endocr. 25, 315 (1965).

Chapter 5

Gas Phase Chromatography
of Corticosteroids in Biological Samples

E. BAILEY

I. Introduction

The analytical procedures available for the separation and estimation of corticosteroids from biological fluids fall far short of what
is desired. Gas chromatographic techniques are of potential value in
this field and the progress made in their application is here reviewed.
For the purpose of this chapter corticosteroids are defined as cortisol,
corticosterone and aldosterone together with their C-21 metabolites,
but some mention will also be made of cortisol analogues in clinical
use.

The first report on gas phase chromatography (or gas liquid chromatography of corticosteroids was that of VANDENHEUVEL and
HORNING (1960). Using an SE-30 column at 222° they showed that
corticosteroids with a 17α,21-dihydroxy-20-oxo side-chain (cortisol,
cortisone, and 11-deoxycortisol) lost this side-chain through thermal
degradation. The only peaks which were observed had the retention
times of the corresponding 17-ketosteroid (17-KS) derivatives. The
structure of these degradation products was confirmed by recovering
them from the gas effluent and studying their infrared spectra. They
also showed that corticosteroids with a 21-hydroxy-20-oxo side-chain
(corticosterone and deoxycorticosterone) decomposed during GLC.
Deoxycorticosterone gave two major peaks and corticosterone four.
Corticosteroids with the 17,20,21-trihydroxy side-chain (e. g. cortols
and cortolones) have also been shown to decompose during GLC and
to give peaks for their 17-KS derivatives but in low yield. We have
found that prednisolone and its metabolites have the same gas chromatographic characteristics as cortisol and that dexamethasone, beta-

methasone and triamcinolone decompose to at least two products. As a consequence of this thermal degradation that occurs under the conditions necessary for GLC, attempts have been made to separate and measure corticosteroids as 1. their thermal degradation products, 2. their direct oxidation products, *i. e.* 17-KS, 17-aldehydes, and 3. other derivatives made prior to GLC. These three approaches will be considered for each of the three groups of corticosteroids.

II. Cortisol, Prednisolone and Some of Their Metabolites

1. Thermal Decomposition Products

KIRSCHNER and FALES (1962) chromatographed cortisone and found that the peak area for the derived 17-KS (adrenosterone) varied directly with the amount of cortisone injected in the range of 2—8 µg. The response of the detector (mass/area), however, was only 20% of that expected had all the cortisone been degraded to adreno-sterone. BAILEY (1964) chromatographed cortisol, cortisone, predni-solone and prednisone (2—8 µg) and found linear mass/area response for the 17-KS formed but under the conditions used this response ranged from 40 to 50% of the theoretical maximum. These divergent results suggest that the percent of injected corticosteroid degraded to 17-KS varies with the GLC conditions. If the conditions could be accurately controlled it would still be necessary to show that the mass/area response was constant in the presence of other substances that might be present in biological extracts. GOTTFRIED (1965 a), in a study of the thermal degradation of cortisol, cortisone and 11-deoxycortisol, was unable to obtain a linear mass/area response for these corticosteroids in the range of 0.25—2 µg. LEUTSCHER and GOULD (1964) used the 17-KS peaks derived from tetrahydrocortisone (THE), tetrahydrocortisol (THF), and allo-tetrahydrocortisol (allo-THF) to monitor the separation of these steroids in urine extracts fol-lowing liquid-liquid partition chromatography. CRANE and HARRIS (1965) reported their experiences in attempting to use GLC for the final separation and measurement (via thermal decomposition) of urinary cortisol and some of its metabolites. They were unable to show that this method satisfied the usual criteria for steroid assays. In summary, although the direct GLC separation, with thermal alteration of structure, of cortisol, prednisolone and some of their metabolites having the 17α,21-dihydroxy-20-one side-chain may be of use in some circumstances, it is not likely to prove of value for accurate measurement owing to the low yield of 17-KS obtained during GLC and the uncertainties that attend the extent of degradation in the presence of other compounds present in biological extracts.

2. Oxidation Products

BAILEY (1964, 1965, 1967) developed methods for the measurement of cortisol, prednisolone and their unconjugated 17-hydroxycorticosteroid (17-OHCS) metabolites in biological fluids based on GLC of their preformed 17-KS. Prior to oxidation with sodium bismuthate the corticosteroids were separated into groups by thin-layer chromatography (TLC) such that no two steroids in any group would be oxidized to the same 17-KS. The methods have been applied to the measurement of a) cortisol and its unconjugated 17-OHCS metabolites in 4 hr urine specimens collected at a rate of urine flow of 3 to 5 ml per min. between 8 a.m. — 12 noon, b) prednisolone and its unconjugated 17-OHCS metabolites in 12 hr urine specimens collected following the oral administration of 5 mg of prednisolone phosphate, and c) cortisol in plasma, synovial fluid and amniotic fluid. When cortisol and its metabolites were to be measured prednisone and prednisolone were added as internal standards to the urine before extraction. For prednisolone assays cortisol and 20β-dihydrocortisol were added.

a) Extraction

For urine the method used was essentially that of FRANTZ, KATZ and JAILER (1961) and extracts were partitioned between light petroleum (essentially equivalent to hexane) and 70% aqueous methanol to remove lipids.

b) Thin-layer Chromatography

Extracts and appropriate standards as markers were chromatographed on silica gel GF 254 (Merck). The solvent system used for cortisol and its metabolites was chloroform : ethanol : water (174 : 26 : 2) and that for prednisolone and its metabolites ethyl acetate : ethylene dichloride : methanol (120 : 70 : 10). From the cortisol plate four fractions were eluted (Fig. 1) which could contain the following corticosteroids: F1, cortisone and prednisone; F2, cortisol, prednisolone, 20-dihydrocortisone, 6-hydroxycortisone and tetrahydrocortisone; F3, tetrahydrocortisol, 20-dihydrocortisol and 6-hydroxycortisol; F4, cortolones and cortols. From the prednisolone plate three fractions were eluted (Fig. 2) which could contain F1, prednisone, cortisol and prednisolone; F2, 6-hydroxyprednisolone; F3, 20-dihydroprednisone, 20-dihydrocortisol and 20-dihydroprednisolone.

c) Bismuthate Oxidation

The cortisol fractions 1, 2 and 3 (Fig. 1) and the prednisolone fractions 1, 2 and 3 (Fig. 2) were oxidized with 25 mg of sodium

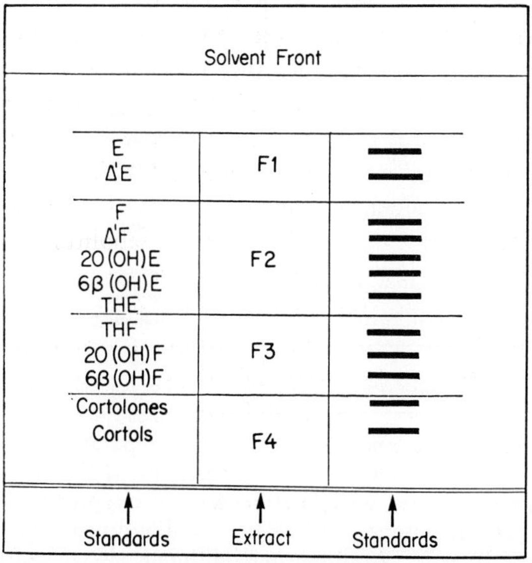

Fig. 1. A diagrammatic representation of the separations effected on the TLC plate in the cortisol assay. E, cortisone. Δ^1E, prednisone, F, cortisol. Δ^1F, prednisolone. 20(OH)E, 20-dihydrocortisone. 6β(OH)E, 6β-hydroxycortisone. THE, tetrahydrocortisone. THF, tetrahydrocortisol. 20(OH)F, 20-dihydrocortisol 6β(OH)F, 6β-hydroxycortisol

bismuthate in 1 ml of 15% aqueous acetic acid. Under these conditions quantitative conversion of the 17-OHCS to their respective 17-KS derivatives was obtained. Cortisol fraction 4 (Fig. 1) was oxidized with periodic acid to cleave selectively the glycerol side-chain of the 20-dihydro derivatives.

d) Trimethylsilyl (TMSi) Ether Formation

The oxidized F3 from the cortisol plates and F2 from the prednisolone plates were treated with hexamethyldisilazane and trimethylchlorosilane in chloroform to decrease the polarity of the 6-hydroxylated 17-KS. This markedly reduced their retention times on the XE-60 column used for GLC and decreased the risk of losses through column adsorption.

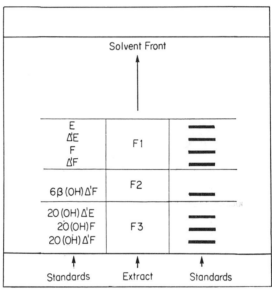

Fig. 2. A diagrammatic representation of the separations effected on the TLC plate in the prednisolone assay. E, cortisone. Δ^1E, prednisone, F, cortisol. Δ^1F, prednisolone. $6\beta(OH)\Delta^1$F, 6β-hydroxyprednisolone. 20(OH)Δ^1E, 20-dihydroprednisone. 20(OH)F, 20-dihydrocortisol. 20(OH)Δ^1F, 20-dihydroprednisolone

e) Gas Phase Chromatography

For routine assays a gas chromatograph equipped with a flame ionization detector and modified to incorporate a closed solid injection system (BAILEY, 1967) was employed. The columns, 213 cm or 152 cm in length and of 4 mm internal diameter were packed with 1% XE-60 on 100—120 mesh Gas Chrom Q. Column and detector temperatures were 230—240° and the carrier gas inlet pressure was 29 p.s.i. Fig. 3 shows chromatograms of the cortisol plate (Fig. 1)

F1, F2 and F3 both with and without TMSi formation. Fig. 4 shows chromatograms of the prednisolone plate (Fig. 2) F1, F2 TMSi, F3.

The *specificity* of the methods with respect to each steroid depicted in Figs. 3 and 4 appears to be high when working with urine from normal male and female subjects, and so far no interfering substances have been detected in the urine of 50 patients. However,

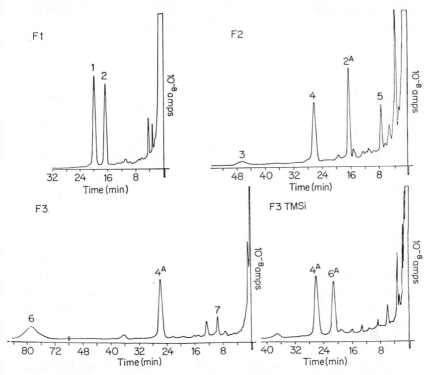

Fig. 3. Chromatograms from a 4 hr normal urine specimen. The peaks are of the 17-KS derived from 1, prednisone (added as internal standard); 2, cortisone; 3, 6-hydroxycortisone; 4, cortisol; 2A, 20-dihydrocortisone; 5, tetrahydrocortisone; 6, 6-hydroxycortisol; 4A, 20-dihydrocortisol; 7, tetrahydrocortisol; Peak 6A, 6-TMSi ether derivative of the 17-KS derived from 6β-hydroxycortisol. (F1, F2 and F3 are from Fig. 1)

it should not be assumed that there are no drugs, synthetic hormones or abnormal metabolites that could interfere. The specificity is based on Rf values of the steroids in the TLC systems, the relative retention time values (RRT) of the 17-KS on polar and non-polar columns, the RRT values of derivatives e. g. TMSi ethers and methyloximes, and on the finding that the addition of the relevant standards to extracts resulted in a symmetrical increase in height of the observed peaks. It should moreover be noted that following side-chain cleavage the derived 17-KS in each group will be unambiguous and further that if any one fraction overlaps its neighbour this will be apparent on the gas chromatogram if a sufficient amount of the relevant steroid is chromatographed. Finally, peaks for prednisolone metabolites did not occur in urine extracts unless prednisolone was given.

f) Reproducibility

When 6 normal 4 hr urine specimens were combined, divided into 6 equal aliquots of 450 ml, and assayed, the S.D. $\times \frac{n}{n-1}$ was approximately $\pm 7\%$ for the steroids of the cortisol assay. When a single specimen of urine obtained from a subject receiving prednisolone phosphate was assayed 8 times the S.D. for the steroids measured (Fig. 2) ranged from $\pm 5\%$ to $\pm 10\%$.

g) Accuracy

The quantity of each steroid was measured by reference to the peak given by a standard added before extraction. When such standards are chemically and physically very similar to the steroids to be measured the accuracy should be high. Had standards of 6β-hydroxycortisol and 6β-hydroxyprednisolone been in adequate supply they would have been used as internal standard/recovery steroids for each other.

h) Recovery

Recovery of the internal standards used ranged from 76.4% to 82.2% for the cortisol assay and from 60.1% to 84.2% for the prednisolone assay. The recoveries of added tritiated cortisol, up to the stage of GLC, were in the same range.

For the assay of cortisol in plasma, synovial fluid and amniotic fluid, modifications of the urine assay were made. Prednisolone was used as the internal standard and extraction was effected with ethyl acetate. Extracts were chromatographed on TLC plates in the system chloroform : ethanol : water (174 : 26 : 2) and the area containing cortisol and prednisolone was eluted. The 17-KS derived from bismuthate oxidation were chromatographed on TLC plates in the system chloroform : ethanol (95 : 5) and following elution their TMSi

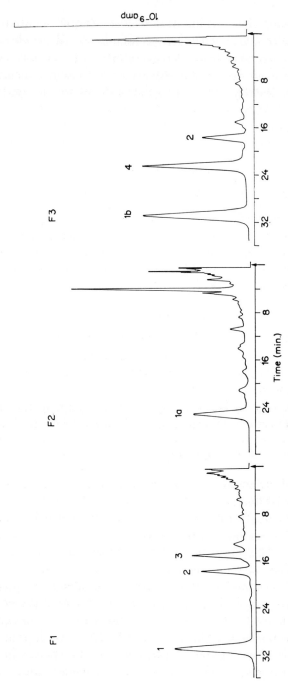

Fig. 4. Chromatograms of urine from a normal individual given 5 mg of prednisolone phosphate. The peaks in F1 are the 17-KS derived from, 1, prednisolone; 2, prednisone; 3, cortisone (added as internal standard); in F2, 1ᵃ, the 6-TMSI of the 17-KS derived from 6-hydroxyprednisolone; in F3, the 17-KS derived from 1ᵇ, 20-dihydroprednisolone; 4, 20-dihydro-cortisol (added as internal standard) and 2, 20-dihydroprednisone. (F1, F2 and F3 are from Fig. 2)

ethers were formed using pyridine as the solvent. Gas phase chromatography was carried out on a 1% XE-60 column with the same operating conditions described above. Recovery of tritiated cortisol up to
the stage of GLC and the overall recovery of prednisolone including
GLC was approximately 40%. Fig. 5 shows the use of the modified

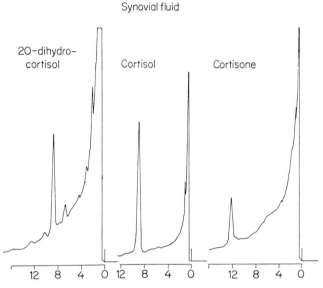

Fig. 5. Chromatograms of the TMSi ethers of the 17-KS derived from
cortisol and 20-dihydrocortisol and of the 17-KS derived from cortisone in
synovial fluid obtained from the knee of an untreated rheumatoid arthritic
man. Internal standards (see text) are omitted

method for the estimation of cortisol, cortisone and 20-dihydro-
cortisol in synovial fluid.

SPARAGANA (1965), using a similar approach to that of BAILEY
(1964), described a method for the estimation of urinary glucosiduronate conjugated THE, THF and allo-THF. Following hydrolysis and
extraction a preliminary purification was made on TLC plates in the
system benzene : acetone (70 : 150). 20β-Dihydrocortisol and prednisolone were chromatographed as markers for the separation of the
THE, THF, allo-THF region from the regions of the more polar
cortols and cortolones and the less polar 17-KS. The appropriate
region was oxidized with sodium bismuthate and the 17-KS reaction
products were chromatographed on a 366 cm column packed with

3% SE-30 coated on silanized 80—100 mesh Gas Chrom P (column temp., 220°; carrier gas flow, 33 ml/min; flame ionization detector). The peak areas were measured by reference to a peak derived from a known amount of prednisolone that had been added to the urine. It was found that the 17-KS derived from THE, THF and allo-THF

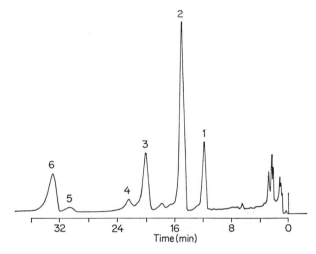

Fig. 6. A chromatogram of SPARAGANA's THE-THF fraction from a normal 24 hr urine specimen. The peaks represent 1, etiocholanolone thought to be derived from pregnanetriol; 2, 3, 4, 5 and 6, the 17-KS derived from THE, THF, allo-THF, cortisol and prednisolone (added as internal standard) respectively

gave similar molar responses and that these were 1.2 times that given for the 17-KS derived from prednisolone. Fig. 6 shows a gas chromatogram of the THE, THF, allo-THF fraction from a normal urine using this method. Evidence for the specificity of the assay was based on the findings that the addition of standards of THE, THF and allo-THF to the initial urine resulted in the appropriate increase in peak heights without change in peak symmetry and that when TMSi and acetate derivatives were formed of the final extract the expected displacement in retention times on SE-30 and XE-60 columns occurred. Further evidence for the specificity of this assay was given in a later publication (SPARAGANA, 1966). The relevant peaks were "trapped" from the gas effluent and their identity was confirmed by infrared spectroscopy. The reproducibility of the assay was good and the overall recovery was stated to be approximately 60%. The results for the individual steroids measured were similar to those reported by others using techniques not involving GLC. Fig. 7 is the gas chromatogram of the cortol and cortolone region from the TLC plate of a normal 24 hr specimen assayed by the method of SPARAGANA (1965). It is evident that this method could be used for the estimation

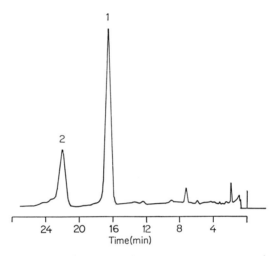

Fig. 7. Chromatogram of a normal 24 hr urine specimen hydrolysed by β-glucuronidase and fractionated by TLC as in the method of SPARAGANA. The peaks are of the 17-KS derived from 1, cortols and 2, cortolones

of cortols and cortolones in urine. However since the method involves removing the side-chain chemically prior to GLC, it does not allow measurement of the isomeric forms of these corticosteroids. TSUDA et al. (1966) have reported RRT values for the oxidation products of a number of corticosteroids with SE-30, QF-1 and XE-60 stationary phases.

3. Group Assay

Assays for groups of urinary "17-OHCS" are used extensively to assess the function of the adrenal cortex. In recent years they have been displaced to some extent by comparatively simple and rapid fluorometric assays of plasma "hydrocortisone". Plasma assays assess only a concentration at a moment in time and the fluorometric methods may lack sufficient accuracy due to unpredictable background values. There remains therefore a need for an accurate means of measuring adrenocortical activity over a period of time. The group assays for urinary 17-OHCS based on the Porter-Silber reaction and those based on the Zimmermann reaction after side-chain cleavage, lack the needed selectivity, e. g. they do not distinguish between cortisol and prednisolone metabolites. As commonly performed they also lack sufficient sensitivity. With this in mind the application of gas chromatography to the problem has been studied in this laboratory. Murphy et al. (1963) showed the value of GLC for monitoring adrenal suppression induced by the administration of 16-methylene prednisolone. Groups of unconjugated cortisol metabolites and of cortisol metabolites released by β-glucuronidase hydrolysis were separated by paper chromatography, oxidized with sodium bismuthate, and gas chromatographed as their 17-KS. More recently Murphy and West (1966) have reported a GLC method for the routine measurement of urinary "17-OHCS". The essential features of the method are potassium borohydride reduction of 10 ml of a 24 hr urine specimen, followed by oxidation with sodium metaperiodate (both reactions being carried out at 60°). Following the addition of 5 N NaOH extraction is effected with ethylene dichloride and the dried extract is acetylated. Aliquots of the final extract are gas chromatographed on a 120 cm × 4 mm (i. d.) column packed with 0.6% XE-60 coated on 100—120 mesh silanized Celite. (Column and detector temp., 232°; argon inlet pressure, 30 p.s.i.; flow rate, approximately 50 ml/min; detector, argon ionization.) The procedure converts free and glucosiduronate-conjugated THE, THF, cortols and cortolones to 11β-hydroxyetiocholanolone acetate and converts the allo-compounds to 11β-hydroxyandrosterone acetate. Both compounds appear in a single peak which is measured, as the "17-OHCS", against known amounts of THE that have been taken through the assay procedure. Corticosteroids not reduced in ring A, such as prednisolone metabolites, do not interfere with the assay (see Fig. 8). On the XE-60 column the "17-OHCS" peak has a minor peak or shoulder on its rising edge which has been shown by Murphy (personal communication) to be derived from urinary 11-oxygenated etiocholanolone and androsterone. He has also shown that when TMSi ethers are employed in the assay instead of acetates the "17-OHCS" are resolved by GLC into their 5α and 5β isomers. The urinary 11-oxygenated etiocholanolone and androsterone are reduced in the assay to 3α,11β,17-trihydroxy-5β and 5α androstanes and so give 3,17-di-TMSi ethers that have, on

GLC, short retention times. This modified procedure of MURPHY is providing results of considerable significance and is clinically attractive as 20 or more assays can be done every 2 days. The published assay of MURPHY and WEST (1966) is of interest in pregnancy (Fig. 9) as it provides a "pregnanediol" peak which may be of use in the diagnosis

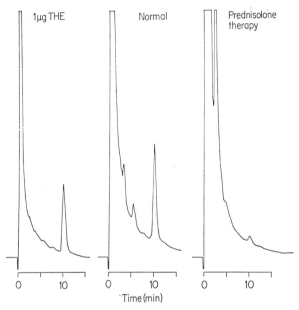

Fig. 8. Chromatograms given by the MURPHY and WEST (1966) "17-OHCS" assay procedure. Left:—an assay of standard THE; center:—an assay of 1/8000th of a normal 24 hr urine specimen; right:—an assay of 1/8000th of a 24 hr specimen from a patient receiving 10 mg of predniso-lone daily

of early pregnancy and also a peak more polar than the "17-OHCS" peak which rises throughout pregnancy and is at term larger than the "17-OHCS" peak. This "unknown" peak is at least partly due to 6-hydroxylated progesterone metabolites. In the assay of MURPHY and WEST (1966) the reproducibility was measured by assaying one hundred 24-hr urine specimens in duplicate. The mean percentage deviation of the duplicates (about their means) was 3.5% (range 0—10%). The sensitivity was such that 1 mg 17-OHCS could be measured in a 24-hr specimen with a precision of approximately ±25%. Evidence for the specificity was that when adrenal activity was suppressed the 17-

OHCS measured fell to below 1 mg/24 hr. So far no metabolites of endogenous or therapeutic origin have been found that interfere with the assay. The accuracy was assessed by assaying twenty-three 24-hr specimens and then adding the equivalent of 20 mg of THE per specimen to aliquots and repeating the assay. The initial assays ranged

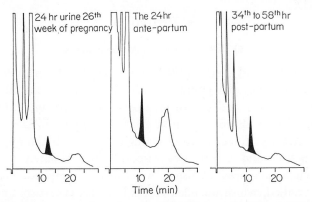

Fig. 9. Chromatograms given by the MURPHY and WEST (1966) "17-OHCS" assay procedure. The assay of 24 hr urine specimes from a normal pregnant subject—left:—in the 26th week (1/8000th gas chromatographed); center:—the 24 hr before labour (1/5333rd chromatographed); right:—from the 34th to the 58th hr post-partum (1/5333rd chromatographed). The black peak is that for the "17-OHCS"; the peak to its left has the retention time of pregnanediol diacetate; the asymmetric peak to its right is at least in part produced from polar progesterone metabolites (see text)

from 10—40 mg "17-OHCS" and the recovery of added THE was $95\% \pm 9$ (S.D.). It is anticipated that GLC assays for urinary cortisol metabolites will replace those in use at present owing to the greater specificity, sensitivity, accuracy and reproducibility that they may provide and also because of their ability to give information about several steroids simultaneously.

In a detailed and interesting analysis of the common 17-OHCS, 17-KS and progesterone metabolites of neutral urine extracts MENINI and NORYMBERSKI (1965) showed that much qualitative and quantitative information could be obtained with the help of GLC. The quantitative study involved reduction with borohydride, side-chain cleavage with bismuthate or periodate, Girard separation, oxidation of the ketonic and non-ketonic fractions with tert-butylchromate and GLC of the two fractions on a 120 cm × 4 mm i. d. column packed with 1% SE-30 on 100—120 mesh silanized Gas Chrom P. (Column and detector temp., 220°; carrier gas flow, 30 ml/min; detector, argon ionization.) In the ketonic fraction THF, THE, the cortols and cortolones were measured as 5β-pregnane-3,11,17-trione. They did not attempt, however, to develop a routine assay for these steroids using GLC.

4. Derivatives

a) Bismethylenedioxy Derivatives

KIRSCHNER and FALES (1962) prepared the bismethylenedioxy (BMD) derivatives of a number of 17-OHCS having the dihydroxy-acetone side-chain and gas chromatographed them on a 183 cm × 3.4 mm i. d. 1% SE-30 column at 235°. Cortisone BMD was found to be thermally stable. It gave a single peak with the appropriate retention time and a mass/area response approximately twice that given when unaltered cortisone was chromatographed. Other 17-OHCS studied, which included cortisol, 11-deoxycortisol and tetra-hydrocortisone, gave less satisfactory results due to the occurrence of shoulders or small peaks in addition to the major peak. No other reports of the use of BMD derivatives for assay procedures have been published up to the present time.

b) 17β-Carbomethoxy Derivatives

MERITS (1962) oxidized cortisol, cortisone and 11-deoxycortisol to their 17β-carboxylic acids with periodic acid and then prepared their methyl esters with diazomethane. He found that these "17β-carbomethoxy" derivatives gave single peaks on GLC and that "infrared absorption spectra and melting point determinations of the compounds, before and after separation on the column, showed no differences". He also found that they could be separated from each other and from similar derivatives of corticosterone, 11-deoxycortico-sterone and the γ-lactone of aldosterone when chromatographed on a 180 cm × 6 mm i. d. 0.3% neopentyl glycol adipate column at 220°. Their retention times were very long, e. g., the retention time of the cortisol carbomethoxy derivative was approximately 1 hr.

c) Acetates

BROOKS (1965) studied the effect of acetylation upon the gas chromatographic stability of a number of corticosteroids using 1%

SE-30 columns at 225°. He showed that 21-acetoxy-17α-hydroxy-20-ketones gave major peaks which, from their relative retention times, were likely to have been due to D-homosteroid transformations. 17α,21-Diacetoxy-20-ketones were considerably more stable but generally gave two peaks. One was due to the unaltered derivative and this was the predominant peak when new columns were used. The other was due to 21-acetoxy-Δ^{16}-20-ketones and was predominant when old columns were used. These observations, together with the finding that cortisone diacetate and tetrahydrocortisone triacetate could be vacuum sublimed at 190° and 200° respectively without decomposition, suggest that the degradation products resulted from catalytic reactions taking place at the top of the column. WOTIZ and CLARK (1966) suggested that cortisone-21-acetate might have been gas chromatographed unchanged if a higher concentration of stationary phase had been used but concluded that corticosteroid acetates were generally unsuitable derivatives for GLC assays owing to their adsorption on non-polar columns. On polar columns their retention times would be excessively long. RAPP and EIK-NES (1965) gas chromatographed the acetates and chloroacetates of cortisol, cortisone and 11-deoxycortisol using an electron capture detector. Under the conditions of this investigation the derivatives did not give sufficiently well defined peaks for measurement.

d) Heptafluorobutyrate Derivatives

EXLEY and CHAMBERLAIN (1967) prepared the 3-enol heptafluorobutyrates of a number of C-19 and C-21 steroids and showed that in general they were more sensitive to electron capture detection than heptafluorobutyrate derivatives of sterols. The corticosteroid derivatives decomposed on GLC but they suggested that the major peak might prove suitable for measurement down to 1 mμg or less. It might be better to oxidize the 17-OHCS to their 17-KS and then form the 3-enol heptafluorobutyrates which these investigators found to be stable during GLC. The method proposed for the estimation of adrenal steroids in plasma included a preliminary purification in two TLC systems and one paper chromatography system.

e) O-Methyloxime or Methoxime (MO) Derivatives

FALES and LUUKKAINEN (1965) prepared O-methyloxime derivatives of many naturally occurring steroids by reacting them with methoxylamine hydrochloride in pyridine and allowing the reaction to proceed overnight. They measured the relative retention times of these derivatives on SE-30 and NGS columns and characterized many of them with the help of mass spectrometry. It was observed in this work that the 3,20-disubstituted derivatives of cortisol and cortisone lost their side-chain on GLC. The mass/area responses given by the formed 17-KS were no greater than those obtained when the unaltered corticosteroids

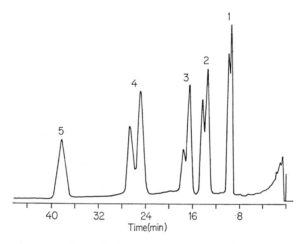

Fig. 10. Peaks 1 and 2 are the 3,17-dimethoxime derivatives of 11-keto and 11β-hydroxyandrostenedione. Peaks 3 and 4 are the 3-methoxime derivatives of 11-oxo and 11β-hydroxyandrostenedione resulting from the GLC of the 3,20-dimethoxime derivatives of cortisone and cortisol respectively. Peak 5 is adrenosterone. Conditions: 213 cm$\times$4 mm 1^0/$_0$ XE-60 column at 210°; carrier gas inlet pressure, 30 p.s.i.; flame ionization detector

were gas chromatographed. The chemical stability and excellent gas chromatographic properties of the O-methyloxime derivatives of 17-KS led us to use these derivatives to confirm further the identity of the 17-KS derived from corticosteroids by bismuthate oxidation in the assay procedures for cortisol and prednisolone metabolites already described. We found that 3-keto and Δ^4-3-keto-O-methyloximes each gave two peaks when chromatographed on polar columns. This was due to the formation of two stereoisomeric derivatives as was noted by GARDINER and HORNING (1966) and by LUUKKAINEN and by FALES (personal communications). LUUKKAINEN found that there was a relationship between the relative quantities of the isomers and the structure of the 17-KS chromatographed, a finding that we have confirmed. Fig. 10 shows the peaks of the 3-methoxime and 3,17-dimethoxime of 11-ketoandrostenedione and 11β-hydroxyandrostenedione. (The 3-methoxime peaks resulted from the GLC of the 3,20-dimethoxime derivatives of cortisol and cortisone.)

f) Trimethylsilyl Ether Derivatives

Attempts to stabilize the cortisol side-chain by TMSi ether formation have not been successful. ROSENFELD (1964, 1965), however, showed that the TMSi ether derivatives of the C-20 epimeric cortols and cortolones could be gas chromatographed without decomposition. He prepared the TMSi ethers by reacting the four steroids with hexamethyldisilazane and trimethylchlorosilane in pyridine and separated the reaction products on a 180 cm × 4 mm 3% QF-1 column at 220°. He noted that the β-epimers underwent some decomposition during preparation of their TMSi ethers. He applied the method to the non-ketonic fractions of extracts of β-glucoronidase-hydrolysed urine. ROSENFELD also investigated the composition of the TMSi ether derivatives formed in chloroform and those formed in pyridine. From evidence based on infrared spectroscopy, analysis for carbon, hydrogen and silicone and retention data on QF-1 and SE-30 columns, he concluded that when the derivatives were prepared in pyridine all the hydroxyl groups reacted but in chloroform the 11β-hydroxyl group of the cortols did not react.

g) O-Methyloxime-trimethylsilyl Ether Derivatives

In a recent publication GARDINER and HORNING (1966) have reported that the MO-TMSi derivatives of cortisol, cortisone and related 17-OHCS can be gas chromatographed without thermal degradation. This is an important advance in the GLC of corticosteroids. The MO derivatives were prepared by reaction with methoxylamine hydrochloride in pyridine (FALES and LUUKKAINEN, 1965) and the TMSi ether derivatives were prepared by adding hexamethyldisilazane to the mixture and allowing the reaction to proceed overnight. They applied this technique to the neutral fractions of extracts from enzymic hydrolysed normal urine and chromatographed an aliquot of the extract, equivalent to approximately 1/1000th of a 24 hr urine specimen, on a 366 cm × 4 mm 1% SE-30 column programmed from 190—250°. The resulting chromatogram revealed peaks for most of the common neutral C-19 and C-21 urinary steroids. The identity of many of the peaks was ascertained by mass spectrographic analysis of the gas effluent. They deduced from these analyses that 11β-hydroxy, 17α-hydroxy and 11-keto groups did not participate in derivative formation. The 17-OHCS metabolites identified were THE, THF, β-cortolone, cortol and allo-THF with cortolone in a

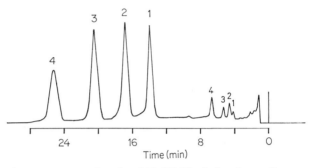

Fig. 11. Chromatograms for the MO-TMSi derivatives of pure 1, THE; 2, 11-deoxycortisol; 3, cortisone and 4, cortisol. For the identity of peaks 1, 2, 3 and 4 see text

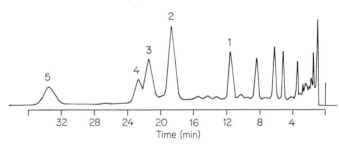

Fig. 12. Chromatogram of the THE-THF region separated by TLC from a normal 24 hr urine specimen after β-glucuronidase hydrolysis. Peak 1 has the retention time of pregnanetriol TMSi ether. Peaks 2, 3, 4 and 5 are the O-methyloxime/TMSi ether derivatives of THE, THF, allo-THF and prednisolone (added as internal standard) respectively

single peak; β-cortol was not seen. This comparatively simple procedure may provide a screening technique for a wide range of neutral urinary steroids. For the accurate measurement of individual corticosteroids in biological fluids some preliminary purification would, of course, be necessary. Fig. 11 shows the gas chromatogram of the MO-TMSi ether derivatives of THE, 11-deoxycortisol, cortisone and cortisol on a 366 cm $\times$ 4 mm 1% SE-30 column at 250° with a carrier gas inlet pressure of 30 p.s.i. The four small peaks seen are due to incomplete TMSi ether formation at the 21-position. The side-chains have been lost during GLC and the peaks represent$_1$ the 3-TMSi ether derived from THE, and $_2$, $_3$ and $_4$ the 3-MO derivatives from 11-deoxycortisol, cortisone and cortisol. Fig. 12 shows the gas chromatogram on a 1% SE-30 column of the MO-TMSi ether derivatives of THE, THF, allo-THF and prednisolone (internal standard) from a single TLC separation of an extract from a normal 24 hr urine specimen after β-glucuronidase hydrolysis. Column conditions as in Fig. 11.

h) Acetonides

(Isopropylidenedioxy derivatives.) ADLERCREUTZ et al. (1966) investigated the gas chromatographic properties of steroidal acetonides formed by the reaction of cis-diols with acetone in the presence of an acid catalyst. They referred to the use of these derivatives in the isolation of both neutral and phenolic steroids. The C-20,21 acetonides formed from corticosteroids having the glycerol side-chain were found to be stable to GLC. We (BAILEY, 1967) have prepared the C-20,21 acetonides of the 20-dihydro derivatives of cortisol, cortisone, 11-deoxycortisol, the cortols and cortolones, prednisolone and prednisone and have gas chromatographed them on SE-30, SE-52, JXR, XE-60 and QF-1 columns. They were found to have good gas chromatographic properties and to give single peaks with a mass/area response similar to that given by equivalent amounts of the 17-KS derived from the parent corticosteroid. They were stable when stored in benzene and did not decompose when chromatographed on TLC plates. When hydrolysed the parent corticosteroid could be obtained in quantitative yield. The acetonides were prepared by dissolving the steroid or extract in 2 ml dry acetone containing 1 mg p-toluene-sulphonic acid. 50 mg of dried calcium chloride was added and the reaction mixture was shaken for 4 hr. The calcium chloride was then removed by centrifugation and following the addition of several drops of pyridine the reaction mixture was taken to dryness. The residue was dissolved in ethylene chloride, washed with alkali and water, filtered through sodium sulphate and finally evaporated to dryness. The extracts were dissolved in benzene for GLC. Urine extracts were prepared as for the cortisol and prednisolone studies (see page 318) and chromatographed on TLC plates in the system ethyl acetate :

methanol : water (170 : 20 : 5) and the area containing the 20-dihydro derivatives was eluted. Moisture was removed from the extract prior to acetonide formation by evaporation from benzene : acetone mixture. Fig. 13 shows a gas chromatogram from a 4 hr urine specimen

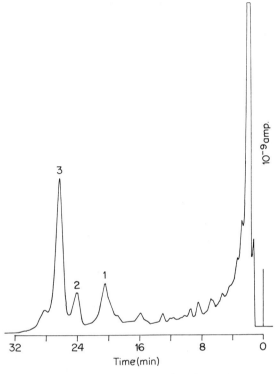

Fig. 13. Gas chromatogram from a normal 4 hr urine specimen. The asymmetric peak 1 contains the C-20,21 acetonides of 20α and 20β-dihydrocortisone. Peaks 2 and 3 are the C-20, 21 acetonides of 20β and 20α-dihydrocortisol respectively. For details see text

of a normal individual on a 366 cm × 4 mm 1% SE-30 column at 250° with a carrier gas inlet pressure of 40 p.s.i. It will be noted that the 20α and 20β isomers of 20-dihydrocortisol are separated but the corresponding isomers of 20-dihydrocortisone are only partially resolved. The RRT values of the derivatives of standards on a 1% SE-30 column were: 20β-dihydrocortisone, 3.39, 20α-dihydrocortisone, 3.45, 20β-dihydrocortisol, 4.10, 20α-dihydrocortisol, 4.54 (androst-4-ene-3,11,17-trione = 1, 6.1 min). When gas chromatographed on a 1% XE-60 column these derivatives followed the same order of elution but the isomers of 20-dihydrocortisone were contained in a single symmetrical peak. The separation factor for the 20α and 20β isomers of 20-dihydrocortisol was, however, greater than on the SE-30 phase. The findings for prednisolone (pure standards and urine extracts) were similar and attempts to separate the isomers of

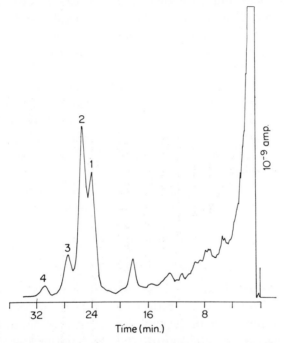

Fig. 14. Gas chromatogram from a normal 24 hr urine specimen after β-glucuronidase hydrolysis. Peaks 1, 2, 3 and 4 are the C-20,21 acetonide derivatives of β-cortolone, cortolone, β-cortol and cortol respectively. For details see text

20-dihydrocortisone and 20-dihydroprednisone on the following columns were unsuccessful: 2% QF-1, 2% JXR and 1.5% SE-52. Fig. 14 shows a gas chromatogram on a 1% SE-30 column of the C-20,21 acetonides of cortols and cortolones from a single TLC separation of an extract of a normal 24 hr urine specimen after β-glucuronidase hydrolysis. The conditions were the same as in Fig. 13. Similar separations were obtained on 2% JXR and 1.5% SE-52 columns.

III. Corticosterone and its Metabolites

17-Deoxycorticosteroids break down during GLC to give several peaks that cannot be used for measurement.

1. Oxidation Products

Periodic acid and bismuthate both oxidize corticosterone and those of its metabolites that have the 20,21-ketol side-chain to 17β-carboxylic acids which are not volatile and therefore not suitable for gas chromatography except by conversion to esters. Similar oxidations of the 20-dihydro metabolites of corticosterone that have the 20,21-glycol side-chain yield the C-17 aldehydes that can be gas chromatographed without decomposition. EXLEY (1965) used gas chromatography as an aid to the identification of these corticosterone metabolites in urine. He found (personal communication) that the C-17 aldehydes derived from 20-dihydrotetrahydrocorticosterone and 20-dihydroallotetrahydrocorticosterone gave well defined peaks on a 122 cm × 4 mm 1% SE-30 column at 220° but that their mass/area responses were poor by comparison with those given by 17-KS.

2. Derivatives

a) 17β-Carbomethoxy Derivatives

As has already been noted the 17β-carbomethoxy derivatives of 17-deoxycorticosteroids are satisfactory for use in gas chromatography. The procedure of MERITS (1962) has been applied by KITTINGER (1964) to the problem of separating and measuring steroids synthesized by rat adrenal incubated with ACTH. The ethylene dichloride extracts obtained from the incubation fluid were treated with periodic acid an an aliquot of the oxidized extracts gas chromatographed on a 244 cm × 5 mm column packed with 0.75% SE-30 coated on silanized 120—140 mesh Gas Chrom P (column temp., 245°; carrier gas inlet pressure, 38 p. s. i.; argon ionization detector). Peaks were obtained which had the retention times of unaltered progesterone and 11-hydroxyprogesterone and of the γ-lactones of aldosterone and 18-hydroxydeoxycorticosterone (the periodic acid oxidation products of these two steroids). Another aliquot was reacted with diazomethane to form methyl esters of the α-ketolic steroids that had been oxidized to 17β-carboxylic acids. GLC, under identical

conditions, gave an additional peak for the derivative of 11-dehydro-
corticosterone but the peaks for the 11-deoxycorticosterone and corticosterone derivatives were superimposed on those from progesterone
and 11β-hydroxyprogesterone. The peak areas for the overlapping
steroids were measured by subtraction. This is the only report of the
application of MERITS' procedure to an assay problem, but in this
laboratory MAVIS GREAVES (unpublished results) has used the carbomethoxy derivatives for the measurement of high concentrations of
urinary corticosterone and 11-dehydrocorticosterone after a preliminary separation of these steroids by paper chromatography.

b) Acetates

BROOKS (1965) found that 21-acetoxy-20-ketones with saturated
ring A *(e. g.* tetrahydrocorticosterone) were suitable for quantitative
gas chromatography but that the 21-acetoxy derivative of corticosterone itself was not. No assay procedure has been reported in
which tetrahydrocorticosterone has been estimated as its 21-acetate.
RAPP and EIK-NES (1965) using an electron capture detector found
that deoxycorticosterone acetate gave a single peak which could be
measured down to 0.005 μg. Corticosterone acetate, however, although
more sensitive to electron capture, gave a peak which was too broad
to be of value. In a subsequent paper RAPP and EIK-NES (1966)
described in detail the estimation of deoxycorticosterone, as its acetate,
in rabbit adrenal venous blood and in the incubation media of rat
adrenals. The methylene dichloride extracts were run on paper in a
hexane : benzene : formamide system; the appropriate regions were
eluted, the steroids were acetylated and re-run on thin-layer plates
with the solvent system benzene : acetone (3 : 1). Suitable aliquots
in toluene were gas chromatographed on a 91 cm × 4 mm column
packed with 1% XE-60 on Gas Chrom Q and operated at 210—215°.
An electron capture detector was employed using a pulsed system. The
carrier gas was high purity nitrogen at 30 p. s. i. Measurement was
effected by the addition just prior to GLC of a known amount of a
suitable internal standard — 20β-dihydroprogesterone chloroacetate
— together with a recovery, measured up to the stage of GLC, of
tritiated deoxycorticosterone added before extraction. In adrenal vein
plasma containing 27 μg/100 ml of deoxycorticosterone they could
measure 0.02 μg. Fig. 15 shows the peaks given by deoxycorticosterone
(as acetate) from rabbit adrenal venous blood and the internal stan-

dard of 0.02 µg 20β-dihydroprogesterone chloroacetate. It is not known whether deoxycorticosterone exists in peripheral human blood but higher precision, sensitivity and accuracy than in the methods of

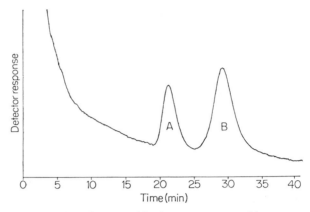

Fig. 15. GLC recording for 20β-dihydroprogesterone chloroacetate (A) and deoxycorticosterone acetate (B). Pooled rabbit adrenal venous blood (3 ml) was processed by the method of RAPP and EIK-NES (1966). Reprinted with the permission of the authors and Analytical Biochemistry

RAPP and EIK-NES would probably be required for the application of this technique to the measurement of deoxycorticosterone in human plasma. The method of RAPP and EIK-NES may be useful when measuring the specific activity of deoxycorticosterone products derived from radioactive precursors. An example of this application is given in their paper. EXLEY and CHAMBERLAIN (1967) in the paper referred to above suggested that 17-deoxycorticosteroids might be measured at the mµg level by electron capture detection of their 3-enol heptafluorobutyrates.

c) Trimethylsilyl Ether Derivatives

GOTTFRIED (1965 b) attempted to prepare the TMSi ethers of corticosterone and its 11-deoxy and 11-dehydro derivatives but found that more than one compound was formed and that these gave several peaks when gas chromatographed. He prepared, however, the 21-20-ditrimethylsilyl ether derivative of 20-dihydrocorticosterone and it gave a single peak of GLC with a good mass/area response. He found, moreover, that this derivative could be purified by TLC without decomposition.

d) O-Methyloxime-trimethylsilyl Ether Derivatives

GARDINER and HORNING (1966) in the publication referred to previously observed peaks for the MO-TMSi derivative of tetra-hydro-11-deoxycorticosterone and allo-tetrahydrocorticosterone. We have confirmed that this derivative (the 21-TMSi, 20-methoxime) stabilizes the corticosterone side-chain. In the procedure used the 11-hydroxyl function did not react but we have found that it will do so if, following methoxime formation, the TMSi derivatives are prepared in pyridine using trimethylchlorosilane as a catalyst.

e) Acetonides

Corticosterone metabolites that have the C-20,21 glycol side-chain form C-20,21 acetonides which are stable to GLC. We (unpublished results) have prepared acetonide derivatives of 20β-dehydrocorticosterone, 20β-dihydro-11-dehydrocorticosterone, 20β-dihydrodeoxycorticosterone and 20β-dihydrotetrahydrocorticosterone and have gas chromatographed them on several polar and nonpolar columns. They were found to have good gas chromatographic properties and gave in each case a single peak.

IV. Aldosterone

Aldosterone decomposes on GLC to a least three products which cannot be used for measurement.

1. Oxidation Products

MERITS (1962) showed that the γ-lactone of aldosterone prepared by periodic acid oxidation was stable to gas chromatography, as did KLIMAN and FOSTER (1962) who prepared it by chromic acid oxidation. KITTINGER (1964) measured aldosterone and 18-hydroxy-deoxycorticosterone as their γ-lactones in methylene dichloride extracts of rat adrenal incubates.

RAPP and EIK-NES (1966) have described in detail a procedure for isolating and measuring sub-microgram amounts of aldosterone from rabbit adrenal vein blood and adrenal incubates. Methylene dichloride extracts were chromatographed in the Bush B5 paper chromatographic system; the aldosterone regions were eluted and oxidized with periodic acid to convert the aldosterone to its γ-lactone. The products were further purified by TLC in the system benzene : acetone (3:1), and the region containing the aldosterone γ-lactone was eluted and suitable aliquots in toluene were gas chromatographed on a 91 cm × 4 mm 0.3% XE-60 column using an electron capture detector. (Other GLC conditions were as for the deoxycorticosterone assay described above.) In the absence of a suitable internal standard, measurement was effected by reference to a known amount of aldosterone γ-lactone injected onto the column 10 min after the sample. Recovery up to the stage of GLC was estimated by addition of a trace amount of tritiated aldosterone before extraction. Fig. 16 shows the peaks obtained for

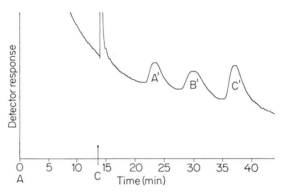

Fig. 16. Gas chromatographic recording of aldosterone-γ-lactone. Pooled rabbit adrenal venous blood (6 ml) was processed by the method of RAPP and EIK-NES (1966). The purified sample was injected at point A. At point C, 0.04 μg of aldosterone-γ-lactone was injected. The first peak (A') is γ-lactone from sample injection; the middle peak (B') is from the lactone of 18-hydroxydeoxycorticosterone which is inconsistently present in such samples; the last peak (C') is aldosterone-γ-lactone from the standard injected. Reprinted with the permission of the authors and Analytical Biochemistry

aldosterone γ-lactone, derived from rabbit adrenal venous blood; the standard was injected 10 min later. When aldosterone, corticosterone and deoxycorticosterone were measured in the same sample a paper chromatographic separation in the Bush B1 system preceded the B5 chromatogram. It was possible to measure all three hormones using 3—6 ml of adrenal venous blood containing 1 μg/100 ml of aldosterone, and relatively large quantities of deoxycorticosterone and corticosterone. In one sample of adrenal vein plasma a separate GLC

peak was seen that corresponded to the lactone of 18-hydroxyde-
hydrocorticosterone. In discussion they commented on the fact that,
unlike other aldosterone derivatives, the γ-lactone could be rapidly
and quantitatively formed and that it was stable on GLC and
sensitive to electron capture detection. The very low concentrations
of aldosterone found in normal human peripheral vein blood would
not be measurable by the method of Rapp and Eik-Nes.

2. Derivatives

a) Acetates

Vandenheuvel and Horning (1960) found that the 21-acetate
of aldosterone decomposed when gas chromatographed at 222° on an
SE-30 column. Wotiz et al. (1961) and Kliman and Foster (1962)
studied the GLC characteristics of the 18,21-diacetate. Both found
that it could be prepared quantitatively and that it gave a single
symmetrical and reproducible peak that could be used for quantification down to at least 0.4 µg. Wotiz et al. (1961) recovered the
compound from the gas effluent and found that it was the unaltered
diacetate, as would be expected from its GLC chraracteristics. Kliman
and Foster (1962), however, found that the product recovered from
the column was similar to the 21-monoacetate on infrared analysis
"but was not identical as shown by paper chromatography and the
failure of the compound to be reacetylated to the diacetate". The
resolution of this problem would not appear to affect the usefulness
of the diacetate for the measurement of aldosterone by GLC provided
that a relatively high concentration of aldosterone is present in the
original sample.

Kliman (1965) investigated the use of gas chromatography in the assay of urinary aldosterone extracted at pH 1. Using a 183 cm × 3.4 mm
2% SE-30 column at 245° and a radium ionization detector he was
able to measure 0.05 µg of aldosterone-18,21-diacetate as a reference
compound. His problem was to find a practical means of extracting
at least this amount from urine in sufficiently pure form for direct
analysis by GLC. When he extracted 250 ml of normal urine and used
three preliminary purification procedures (two paper chromatographic
systems and one TLC system), the resolving power of the column and
the mass/area response to the derivative were not adequate for
reasonably accurate measurement and the results deviated a good deal

from those found using the double isotope analysis of KLIMAN and PETERSEN (1960). He did, however, arrive at a means for measuring accurately normal and subnormal levels of urinary aldosterone extracted at pH 1. A trace of 4-^{14}C-aldosterone was added to 15 ml of urine prior to its extraction at pH 1 with methylene chloride. Acetylation was effected with tritiated acetic anhydride and the diacetate purified by one paper chromatogram and one two-dimensional TLC separation. Following GLC on a 2% SE-30 column the aldosterone diacetate peak from the gas effluent was trapped in p-terphenyl crystals using a Packard 830 Gas Fraction Collector. The aldosterone content of the specimen was computed from the relative quantities of ^{14}C and tritium determined by liquid scintillation counting. He found the accuracy, precision and sensitivity to be similar to that of the double isotope method. The GLC method may be more convenient than the double isotope method referred to above, but the part played by the gas chromatograph was to help in the isolation of the diacetate, not to measure it.

CARR and WOTIZ (1963) developed a method for the GLC measurement of tetrahydroaldosterone from urine hydrolysed by treatment with a *Helix pomatia* preparation. The urine extract was acetylated and the tetrahydroaldosterone triacetate partially separated by paper chromatography in a modified BUSH system. Pure tetrahydroaldosterone triacetate was found to give a single peak on a 183 cm 3% SE-30 column at 250° and the partially purified extracts gave discrete peaks that were used to measure the increased excretion of tetrahydroaldosterone occasioned by ACTH administration and salt deprivation. Insufficient data were given for the assessment of the accuracy, precision and sensitivity of their method. As previously mentioned corticosteroid acetates are not ideal for GLC owing to their tendency to be adsorbed on the column.

b) Trimethylsilyl Ether Derivatives

GOTTFRIED (1965 b) prepared the TMSi ether of aldosterone in pyridine and showed that it could be gas chromatographed at 275° on a 3.8% SE-30 column to give a single peak. A drawback in the use of this derivative is its tendency to decompose. EXLEY and CHAMBERLAIN (1967) in the paper referred to above suggested that aldosterone might be measured at the mμg level by the electron capture detection of its 3-enol heptafluorobutyrate.

V. Conclusion

In summary it may be said that GLC has already made assays possible for cortisol, prednisolone and their individual metabolites and for groups of 17-OHCS metabolites, and that these methods are an advance over those previously available. It has provided the basis for assays of corticosterone and its C-21 metabolites that could prove superior to those in use at present. GLC, however, has not yet led to the development of assays for aldosterone and its metabolites, in urine or blood plasma, that are an obvious advance over those presently in use.

References

ADLERCREUTZ, H., S. LAIHO, and T. LUUKKAINEN: Preparation of steroid derivatives for gas chromatography including studies on gas chromatographical properties of steroidal acetonides. Meeting on gas chromatographic determination of hormonal steroids. Rome 22nd.—23rd. September, 1966.
APPLEBY, J. I., G. GIBSON, J. K. NORYMBERSKI, and R. D. STUBBS: Indirect analysis of corticosteroids. I. The determination of 17-hydroxycorticosteroids. Biochem. J. 60, 453 (1955).
BAILEY, E.: The use of gas-liquid chromatography in the assay of some corticosteroids in urine. J. Endocr. 28, 131 (1964).
— The estimation of unconjugated cortisol metabolites in urine by gas chromatography. In: Gas chromatography of steroids in biological fluids. M. B. LIPSETT (ed.). New York: Plenum Press 1965, p. 57.
— The estimation of cortisol, prednisolone and some of their metabolites in biological fluids using gas-liquid chromatography. In: Gas chromatography of steroids. Memoir, Society for Endocrinology 1967 [16, 183 (1967)].
— The gas-liquid chromatographic analysis of some C-20,21-dihydroxycorticosteroids as C-20,21-acetonides. Steroids 10, 527 (1967).
BROOKS, C. J. W.: Studies of acetylated corticosteroids and related 20-oxopregnane derivatives by gas chromatography. Anal. Chem. 37, 636 (1965).
CARR, H. F., and H. H. WOTIZ: The measurement of urinary tetrahydroaldosterone by gas-liquid partition chromatography. Biochim. biophys. Acta 71, 178 (1963).

Thanks are due to Dr. H. F. WEST for help and encouragement in the preparation of this chapter. Thanks are also due to the Journal of Endocrinology for permission to reproduce Figs. 8 and 9, and to Analytical Biochemistry for permission to reproduce Figs. 15 and 16.

CHAMBERLAIN, J., B. A. KNIGHTS, and G. H. THOMAS: Analysis of steroid metabolites by gas chromatography. J. Endocr. **26**, 367 (1963).

CRANE, M. G., and J. J. HARRIS: Urinary corticoids by gas chromatography. In: Gas chromatography of steroids in biological fluids. M. B. LIPPSETT (ed.). New York: Plenum Press 1965, p. 73.

EXLEY, D.: Urinary excretion of C-20 reduction products of corticosterone. Biochem. J. **94**, 271 (1965).

—, and J. CHAMBERLAIN: Properties of steroidal 3 enol heptafluorobutyrates. Steroids **10**, 509 (1967).

FALES, H. M., and T. LUUKKAINEN: O-Methyloximes as carbonyl derivatives in gas chromatography, mass spectrometry and nuclear magnetic resonance. Anal. Chem. **37**, 955 (1965).

FRANTZ, A. G., F. H. KATZ, and J. W. JAILER: 6β-Hydroxycortisol and other polar corticosteroids: measurement and significance in urine. J. clin. Endocr. **21**, 1290 (1961).

GARDINER, W. L., and E. C. HORNING: Gas-liquid chromatographic separation of C_{19} and C_{21} human urinary steroids by a new procedure. Biochim. biophys. Acta **115**, 524 (1966).

GOTTFRIED, H.: Studies of the thermal decomposition of corticosteroids during gas chromatography. Steroids **5**, 385 (1965 a).

— A specific method for the gas chromatographic determination of aldosterone and adrenocortical steroids in gas chromatography of steroids in biological fluids. In: Gas chromatography of steroids in biological fluids. M. B. LIPSETT (ed.). New York: Plenum Press 1965 b, p. 89.

KIRSCHNER, M. A., and H. M. FALES: Gas chromatographic analysis of 17-hydroxycorticosteroids by means of their bis-methylenedioxy derivatives. Anal. Chem. **34**, 1548 (1962).

KITTINGER, G. W.: Quantitative gas chromatography of 17-deoxycorticosteroids and other steroids produced by the rat adrenal gland. Steroids **3**, 21 (1964).

KLIMAN, B., and R. E. PETERSEN: Double isotope derivative assay of aldosterone in biological extracts. J. biol. Chem. **235**, 1639 (1960).

—, and D. W. FOSTER: Analysis of aldosterone by gas-liquid chromatography. Anal. Biochem. **3**, 403 (1962).

— Analysis of aldosterone in urine by double isotope dilution and gas-liquid chromatography. In: Gas chromatography of steroids in biological fluids. M. B. LIPSETT (ed.). New York: Plenum Press 1965, p. 101.

LUETSCHER, J. A., and R. G. GOULD: Gas-liquid chromatography of the tetrahydro-derivatives of cortisol isolated from urine. J. Chromatog. **13**, 350 (1964).

MENINI, E., and J. K. NORYMBERSKI: An approach to the systematic analysis of urinary steroids. Biochem. J. **95**, 1 (1965).

MERITS, I.: Gas-liquid chromatography of adrenal cortical steroid hormones. J. Lipid Res. **3**, 126 (1962).

MURPHY, D., E. BAILEY, and H. F. WEST: 16-Methylene-prednisolone adrenal suppression shown by gas chromatography. Lancet **II**, 809 (1963).

MURPHY, D., and H. F. WEST: Urinary 17-hydroxycorticosteroids measured by gas-liquid chromatography. J. Endocr. 36, 331 (1966).

RAPP, J. P., and K. B. EIK-NES: Gas chromatography with electron capture detection of some corticosteroid derivatives. J. Gas Chromatogr. 3, 235 (1965).

— — Determination of deoxycorticosterone and aldosterone in biological samples by gas chromatography with electron capture detection. Anal. Biochem. 15, 386 (1966).

ROSENFELD, R. S.: Gas chromatography of some C-21 metabolites of cortisol. Steroids 4, 147 (1964).

— Gas chromatography of cortols and cortolones. In: Gas chromatography of steroids in biological fluids. M. B. LIPSETT (ed.). New York: Plenum Press 1965, p. 67.

SPARAGANA, M.: Determination of urinary tetrahydrocortisone, tetrahydrocortisol and 3α-allo-tetrahydrocortisol by gas chromatography. Steroids 6, 583 (1965).

— Infrared microspectrophotometry of urinary steroids separated by gas chromatography. Steroids 8, 219 (1966).

TSUDA, K., N. IKEKAWA, Y. SATO, and R. WATANUKI: Gas chromatographic analysis of oxidation products of adrenal corticosteroids. Anal. Biochem. 16, 183 (1966).

VANDENHEUVEL, W. J. A., and E. C. HORNING: Gas chromatography of adrenocortical steroid hormones. Biochem. biophys. Res. Commun. 3, 356 (1960).

WOTIZ, H. H., I. NAUKKARINEN, and H. E. CARR: Gas chromatography of aldosterone. Biochim. biophys. Acta 53, 449 (1961).

—, and S. J. CLARK: Gas chromatography in the analysis of steroid hormones. New York: Plenum Press 1966.

Trivial and Systematic Names of Steroids

Adrenosterone: androst-4-ene-3,11,17-trione

Aldosterone: 11β,21-dihydroxypregn-4-ene-18-al-3,20-dione

Aldosterone γ-lactone: 17 → 18 lactone of 11β-hydroxy-3-one-18-al-androst-4-ene-17-oic acid 18—11 hemiacetal

Allopregnanediol: 3α,20α-dihydroxy-5α-pregnane

Allotetrahydrocorticosterone (allo-THB): 3α,11β,21-trihydroxy-5α-pregnan-20-one

Allotetrahydrocortisol (allo-THF): 3α,11β,17α,21-tetrahydroxy-5α-pregnan-20-one

Androstanedione: 5α-androstane-3,17-dione

Androstenediol: 3β,17β-dihydroxyandrost-5-ene

Δ⁴-Androstenedione: androst-4-ene-3,17-dione

Androsterone: 3α-hydroxy-5α-androstan-17-one

Betamethasone: 16β-methyl-9α-fluoro-11β,17α,21-trihydroxypregn-1,4-diene-3,20-dione

Cholestanone: 5α-cholestan-3-one

Coprostan-3α-ol: 3α-hydroxy-5β-cholestane

Corticosterone (compound B): 11β,21-dihydroxypregn-4-ene-3,20-dione

Cortisol (compound F): 11β,17α,21-trihydroxypregn-4-ene-3,20-dione

Cortisone (compound E): 17α,21-dihydroxypregn-4-ene-3,11,20-trione

Cortol: 3α,11β,17α,20α,21-pentahydroxy-5β-pregnane

β-Cortol: 3α,11β,17α,20β,21-pentahydroxy-5β-pregnane

Cortolone: 3α,17α,20α,21-tetrahydroxy-5β-pregnan-11-one

β-Cortolone: 3α,17α,20β,21-tetrahydroxy-5β-pregnan-11-one

11-Dehydrocorticosterone: 21-hydroxypregn-4-ene-3,11,20-trione

Dehydroepiandrosterone (DHEA): 3β-hydroxyandrost-5-ene-17-one

11-Dehydroestradiol-17α: 3,17α-dihydroxyestra-1,3,5(10),11-tetraene

11-Deoxycorticosterone: 21-hydroxypregn-4-ene-3,20-dione

11-Deoxycortisol: 17α,21-dihydroxypregn-4-ene-3,20-dione

21-Deoxycortisol: 11β,17α-dihydroxypregn-4-ene-3,20-dione

Dexamethasone: 16α-methyl-9α-fluoro-11β,17α,21-trihydroxypregn-1,4-diene-3,20-dione

20-Dihydroallotetrahydrocorticosterone: 3α,11β,20β,21-tetrahydroxy-5α-pregnane

20β-Dihydro-11-dehydrocorticosterone: 20β,21-dihydroxypregn-4-ene-3,11-dione

20β-Dihydrocorticosterone: 11β,20β,21-trihydroxypregn-4-ene-3-one
20-Dihydrocortisol (20(OH)F): 11β,17α,20,21-tetrahydroxypregn-4-ene-3-one
20-Dihydrocortisone (20(OH)E): 17α,20,21-trihydroxypregn-4-ene-3,11-dione
20β-Dihydrodeoxycorticosterone: 20β,21-dihydroxypregn-4-ene-3-one
20-Dihydroprednisolone (20(OH)Δ¹F): 11β,17α,20,21-tetrahydroxypregn-1,4-diene-3-one
20-Dihydroprednisone (20(OH)Δ¹E): 17α,20,21-trihydroxypregn-1,4-diene-3,11-dione
3α-Dihydroprogesterone: 3α-hydroxypregn-4-ene-20-one
3β-Dihydroprogesterone: 3β-hydroxypregn-4-ene-20-one
20α-Dihydroprogesterone: 20α-hydroxypregn-4-ene-3-one
20β-Dihydroprogesterone: 20β-hydroxypregn-4-ene-3-one
3-Dihydroprogesterones: 3α and 3β-hydroxypregn-4-ene-20-one
20-Dihydroprogesterones: 20α and 20β-hydroxypregn-4-ene-3-one
20β-Dihydrotetrahydrocorticosterone: 3α,11β,20β,21-tetrahydroxy-5β-pregnane

Epiandrosterone: 3β-hydroxy-5α-androstan-17-one
Epicoprostanol: 3β-hydroxy-5β-cholestane
16-Epiestriol: 3,16β,17β-trihydroxyestra-1,3,5(10)-triene
16,17-Epiestriol: 3,16β,17α-trihydroxyestra-1,3,5(10)-triene
17-Epiestriol: 3,16α,17α-trihydroxyestra-1,3,5(10)-triene
Epietiocholanolone: 3β-hydroxy-5β-androstan-17-one
Epitestosterone: 17α-hydroxyandrost-4-ene-3-one
Estradiol-17α: 3,17α-dihydroxyestra-1,3,5(10)-triene
Estradiol-17β: 3,17β-dihydroxyestra-1,3,5(10)-triene
Estriol: 3,16α,17β-trihydroxyestra-1,3,5(10)-triene
Estrone: 3-hydroxyestra-1,3,5(10)-triene-17-one
Etiocholanolone: 3α-hydroxy-5β-androstan-17-one
Δ⁹-Etiocholanolone: 3α-hydroxy-5β-androst-9-ene-17-one

11β-Hydroxyandrostenedione: 11β-hydroxyandrost-4-ene-3,17-dione
11β-Hydroxyandrosterone: 3α,11β-dihydroxy-5α-androstan-17-one
6-Hydroxycortisol (6(OH)F): 6,11β,17α,21-tetrahydroxypregn-4-ene-3,20-dione
6-Hydroxycortisone (6(OH)E): 6,17α,21-trihydroxypregn-4-ene-3,11,20-trione
18-Hydroxydehydrocorticosterone γ-lactone: 17 → 18 lactone of 18-hydroxyandrost-4-ene-3,11-dione-17-oic acid
18-Hydroxydeoxycorticosterone: 18,21-dihydroxypregn-4-ene-3,20-dione
6α-Hydroxyestradiol-17β: 3,6α,17β-trihydroxyestra-1,3,5(10)-triene
6β-Hydroxyestradiol-17β: 3,6β,17β-trihydroxyestra-1,3,5(10)-triene
11β-Hydroxyestradiol: 3,11β,17β-trihydroxyestra-1,3,5(10)-triene
16α-Hydroxyestrone: 3,16α-dihydroxyestra-1,3,5(10)-triene-17-one

11β-Hydroxyetiocholanolone: 3α,11β-dihydroxy-5β-androstan-17-one
6-Hydroxyprednisolone (6(OH)Δ^1F): 6,11β,17α,21-tetrahydroxypregn-
   1,4-diene-3,20-dione
17α-Hydroxypregnanolone: 3α,17α-dihydroxy-5β-pregnan-20-one
17α-Hydroxypregnenolone: 3β,17α-dihydroxypregn-5-ene-20-one
11β-Hydroxyprogesterone: 11β-hydroxypregn-4-ene-3,20-dione
16α-Hydroxyprogesterone: 16α-hydroxypregn-4-ene-3,20-dione
17α-Hydroxyprogesterone: 17α-hydroxypregn-4-ene-3,20-dione
20α-Hydroxyprogesterone, 20α-reduced progesterone, 20α-dihydro-
   progesterone (20α-progesterone): 20α-hydroxypregn-4-ene-3-one
20β-Hydroxyprogesterone, 20β-reduced progesterone, 20β-dihydro-
   progesterone (20β-progesterone): 20β-hydroxypregn-4-ene-3-one
11β-Hydroxytestosterone: 11β,17β-dihydroxyandrost-4-ene-3-one

11-Ketoandrostenedione: androst-4-ene-3,11,17-trione
11-Ketoandrosterone: 3α-hydroxy-5α-androstan-11,17-dione
16-Ketoestradiol-17β: 3,17β-dihydroxyestra-1,3,5(10)-triene-16-one
11-Ketoetiocholanolone: 3α-hydroxy-5β-androstan-11,17-dione
11-Ketoprogesterone: pregn-4-ene-3,11,20-trione
2-Methoxyestrone: 2-methoxy-3-hydroxyestra-1,3,5(10)-triene-17-one
16-Methyleneprednisolone: 16-methylene-11β,17α,21-trihydroxypregn-
   1,4-diene-3,20-dione

19-Nortestosterone: 17β-hydroxy-19-norandrost-4-en-3-one

Prednisolone (Δ^1F): 11β,17α,21-trihydroxypregn-1,4-diene-3,20-dione
Prednisone (Δ^1E): 17α,21-dihydroxypregn-1,4-diene-3,11,20-trione
Pregnanediol: 3α,20α-dihydroxy-5β-pregnane
Pregnanediol-20β: 3α,20β-dihydroxy-5β-pregnane
Pregnanediols: 3α,20α-dihydroxy-5β-pregnane and 3α,20α-dihydroxy-
   5α-pregnane
Pregnanetetrol: 3α,11β,17α,20α-tetrahydroxy-5β-pregnane
Pregnanetriol: 3α,17α,20α-trihydroxy-5β-pregnane
Pregnanetriolone: 3α,17α,20α-trihydroxy-5β-pregnan-11-one
Pregnanolone: 3α-hydroxy-5β-pregnan-20-one
Pregnenolone (Δ^5-pregnenolone): 3β-hydroxypregn-5-ene-20-one
Pregnanolones: 3α or 3β-hydroxy 5α or 5β-pregnan-3-ones or 20α or
   20β-hydroxy 5α or 5β-pregnan-3-ones
Progesterone: pregn-4-ene-3,20-dione

Ring D α-ketols: Ring D with 17-hydroxy-16-one or 16-hydroxy-17-one
β-Sitosterol: 3β-hydroxystigmast-5-ene

Testosterone: 17β-hydroxyandrost-4-ene-3-one
Δ^1-Testosterone: 17β-hydroxyandrost-1,4-diene-3-one

Tetrahydroaldosterone: $3\alpha,11\beta,21$-trihydroxy-18-al-5β-pregnan-20-one
Tetrahydrocortisol (THF): $3\alpha,11\beta,17\alpha,21$-tetrahydroxy-$5\beta$-pregnan-20-one
Tetrahydrocorticosterone (THB): $3\alpha,11\beta,21$-trihydroxy-5β-pregnan-20-one
Tetrahydrocortisone (THE): $3\alpha,17\alpha,21$-trihydroxy-5β-pregnan-11,20-dione
Tetrahydro-11-dehydrocorticosterone (THA): $3\alpha,21$-dihydroxy-5β-
     pregnan-11,20-dione
Tetrahydrodeoxycorticosterone: $3\alpha,21$-dihydroxy-5β-pregnan-20-one
Triamcinolone: 9α-fluoro-$11\beta,16\alpha,17\alpha,21$-tetrahydroxypregn-1,4-diene-
     3,20-dione

Author Index

Page numbers in *italics* refer to the references

Bauld, W. S. see Givner, M. L.
146, 147
Baulieu, E.-E. 238, 268, 270, 302
—, and P. Mauvais-Jarvis 238, 302
Becker, R. S., see Wentworth, W. E.71
Beckloff, S., see Cawley, L. P. 303
Beckmann, I., see Tamm, J. 313
Bedford, A. R., see Cox, R. I. 146
Beer, C. T., and T. F. Gallagher
72, 145
Beerthuis, R. K., and J. H. Recourt
2, 65
Beling, C. G. 73, 74, 79, 94, 96, 97,
110, 133, 145
Bell, E. T., see Harkness, R. A. 228
—, see Loraine, J. A. 147, 231
Bel-van den Bosch, N., see Cejka, V.
66
Bender, S. R., see Kroman, H. S. 147
Beque, J., see Jayle, M. F. 229
Bergström 3
Berman, R. A., see Talbot, N. B.
234, 313
Bernstein, S., and R. H. Lenhard
251, 302
—, E. W. Cantrall, J. P. Dusza, and
J. P. Joseph 62, 65
Beroza, M., and M. C. Bowman 89,
145
Berrett, C., and C. McNeil 291, 297,
302
Besch, N. F., see Barry, R. D. 226
Biemann, K., P. Bommer, and D. M.
Desiderio 3, 65
Blair, A. J., see Carlson, I. H. 226
Blair, H. A. F., see Brown, J. B. 145
Bair, L. R., see Mason, L. H. 69
Bloch, E., and N. B. Gibree 72, 145
Bommer, P., see Biemann, K. 65
Bonanno, P., see Patti, A. A. 232
Bondy, P. K., see Cohn, G. L. 303
Bonelli, E. J., see Oaks, D. M. 232
Bongiovanni, A. M., and W. R.
Eberlein 222, 226
—, see Eberlein, W. R. 227
—, see Clayton, G. W. 303
Borth, R. 196, 226

Bowman, M. C., see Beroza, M. 145
Bowman, R. L., see Karmen, A. 68
Brago, C., see Goldfien, A. 228
Breuer, H. 72, 113,. 145
—, and G. Pangels 83, 145
Briefer, C., see Kliman, B. 68, 308
Briggs, J. H., see Rosner, J. M. 311
Briggs, L. H., L. D. Colebrook, H. M.
Fales, and W. C. Wildman 90,
145
Brink-Johnsen, B., and K. B.
Eik-Nes 244, 302
Brodie, A. H., N. Shimizu, S. A. S.
Tait, and J. F. Tait 49, 65
Brooks, C. J. W. 216, 217, 224, 226,
330, 339, 345
—, and L. Hanaineh 155, 164, 183,
188, 189, 191, 192, 197, 200, 224,
226
—, E. M. Chambaz, W. L. Gardiner,
and E. C. Horning 82, 145
—, —, and E. C. Horning 6, 18, 65
—, see Gardiner, W. L. 66
—, see Horning, E. C. 67
Brooks, R. V. 257, 279, 280, 281,
282, 283, 284, 287, 302
—, and G. Giuliani 276, 279, 280, 302
—, see Lim, N. Y. 308
Brown, J. B. 71, 76, 77, 80, 81, 94,
95, 98, 99, 100, 101, 103, 109,
110, 118, 129, 131, 145
—, and H. A. F. Blair 73, 74, 75,
99, 145
—, R. D. Bulbrook, and F. C. Greenwood 110, 146
—, see Fishman, J. 146
—, see Klopper, A. I. 230
—, see Roy, E. J. 148
Brownie, A. C. 266
—, H. J. van der Molen, E. E. Nishizawa, and K. B. Eik-Nes 20, 47,
52, 53, 65, 84, 131, 132, 146, 167,
171, 172, 226, 243, 245, 247, 248,
249, 250, 251, 252, 253, 254, 255,
257, 259, 260, 261, 263, 264, 266,
270, 274, 275, 277, 302
—, see Eik-Nes, K. B. 305

Horning, E. C., see Jaakonmaki, P. I. 67
—, see Luukkainen, T. *148*
—, see Sjövall, K. *312*
—, see Sweeley, C. C. *70*
—, see Vandenheuvel, W. J. A. *70, 234, 313, 314, 347*
Horning, M. G., K. L. Knox, C. E. Dalgliesh, and E. C. Horning *7, 19, 67*
—, A. M. Moss, and E. C. Horning *67*
—, see Horning, E. C. *67*
Horton, R. 236, 263, 264, 265, 280, *307*
—, and K. Mann 254, 264, *307*
—, J. M. Rosner, and P. H. Forsham 244, 258, 280, *307*
Hudson, B., J. P. Coghlan, A. Dulmanis, and M. Wintour 254, *307*
—, —, —, M. Wintour, and I. Ekkel 244, 250, 253, 254, 256, 257, 258, *307*
—, and G. W. Oertel 267, 269, *307*
—, see Wintour, M. *304*

Ibayashi, H., M. Nakamura, S. Murakawa, T. Uchikawa, T. Tanioka, and K. Nakao 257, 280, 281, 288, *307*
—, —, T. Uchikawa, S. Murakawa, S. Yoshida, K. Nakao, and S. Okinaka 272, *307*
Ikekawa, N., see Horning, E. C. *67*
—, see Tsuda, K. *234, 347*
Irmscher, K., see Halpaap, H. *306*
Ismail, A. A. A., and R. A. Harkness 159, 229, 244, 281, *307*
Isurugi, K., see Kinoshita, K. *229*
Ittrich, G. 77, *147*

Jaakonmaki, P. I., K. L. Knox, E. C. Horning, and M. G. Horning 63, *67*
—, K. A. Yarger, and E. C. Horning 64, *67*

Jaakonmaki, P. I., see Horning, E. C. *67*
Jacobs, R. D. B., see Zurbrügg, R. P. *315*
Jacobsohn, G. M., and S. Lieberman 267, 291, *307*
Jacobson, G., see Forchielli, E. *305*
Jailer, J. W., see Frantz, A. G. *346*
James, A. T., and A. J. P. Martin 1, *67*
—, see Martin, A. J. P. *69*
Jandorek, R. D., see Rosenfeld, R. S. *233*
Jansen, A. P. 204, 207, *209*
Jayle, M. F., et O. Crépy 152, *229*
—, R. Scholler, J. Beque et L. Hanns 152, *229*
—, see Lachèse, H. *230*
Jipanek, M., see Sonka, J. *312*
Joachim, E., see Riondel, A. *311*
Johnson, L., see Horning, E. C. *67*
Jones, G. E., D. Turner, I. J. Sarlos, A. C. Barnes, and R. Cohen 204, 207, 212, *229*
—, see Lau, H. L. *230*
—, see Turner, D. A. *234*
Joseph, J. P., see Bernstein, S. *65*

Kadrnka, F. O. 225
Kahn, L., and M. C. Goldberg 52, *67*
Kaiser, E., see Oertel, G. W. *310*
Karmen, A. *68*, 46
—, and H. R. Tritch 46, *67*
—, —, J. W. Winkelman, and R. L. Bowman 46, *68*
—, —, and B. Kliman 46, *68*
—, I. McCaffrey, and R. L. Bowman 46, *68*
Kase, N., see Dixon, R. *304*
Katz, F. H., see Frantz, A. G. *346*
Katzman, P. A., R. F. Straw, H. J. Buehler, and E. A. Doisy 72, *147*
Kaufman, R. H., see Loriaux, D. L. *305*
Keller, A. R., see Klein, P. D. *68*
—, see Migeon, C. J. *309*

Compound Index

Derivatives are not listed separately; this index lists parent steroids, either free or in derivative form.

24*

Steroid Technique Index

Steroid Assay Index

Monographs on Endocrinology

In Preparation:

BAULIEU, E., Bicêtre: Current Problems in the Metabolism of Steroid Hormones

BERSON, S. A., and R. YALOW, Bronx: Immunoassay of Protein Hormones

BORTH, R., Toronto: Reliability of Clinical Hormone Assays

CALDEYRO-BARCIA, R., Montevideo: Oxytocin

COPP, D. H., Vancouver: Calcitonin, Parathormone and Calcium Homeostasis

HORTON, E. W., London: Prostaglandins and Related Substances

JENSEN, E., Chicago: Estradiol Receptors and Hormonal Action

LUNENFELD, B., Tel-Hashomer: Gonadotropins

MCKENZIE, J. M., Montreal: The Pathogenesis of Graves' Disease

NEUMANN, F., H. STEINBECK, and W. ELGER, Berlin: Hormones in Sexual Differentiation

RENOLD, A. E., Geneva: Immunology and Diabetes

ROBERTS, S., Los Angeles: Subcellular Mechanisms in the Regulation of Corticosteroidogenesis

SHORT, R. V., Cambridge: The Corpus Luteum

STAUFFACHER, W., and A. E. RENOLD, Geneva: Pathophysiology of Diabetes mellitus

WESTPHAL, U., Louisville: Steroid-Protein Interactions

WILLIAMS-ASHMAN, H. G., Baltimore: Androgen Action

SPRINGER-VERLAG NEW YORK INC.

175 Fifth Avenue • New York, New York 10010

Monographs on Endocrinology

Volume 1   Sex Chromosomes and Sex-linked Genes

By Dr. **Susumu Ohno**
Department of Biology,
City of Hope Medical Center
Duarte/Calif. (USA)

With 33 figures
X, 192 pages 8vo. 1967
Cloth DM 38,—; US $ 9.50

A deeper insight into the biological problem at hand can usually be gained by treating it from a phylogenetic as well as an ontogenetic viewpoint.

In recent years, it became clear that even in man, various abnormal sex chromosome constitutions occur in association with abnormal sexual development. The above development and the discovery that the Barr sex chromatin body seen in interphase nuclei of female somatic cells of man and other mammals actually represents one of the two X-chromosomes which has been rendered inactive, greatly expanded an interest on the biological role of sex chromosomes, sex-linked genes and on what a great Drosophila geneticist, H. J. Muller, termed "the dosage compensation mechanism for sex-linked genes".

This book follows step by step the development of sex chromosomes during vertebrate evolution from an originally homologous pair of ordinary chromosomes, tracing the evolutional origin of sex-linked genes and the chromosomal sex-determining mechanism. An excursion into the phylogenetic past of the mammalian X-chromosome reveals the reason for the development by mammals of a unique dosage compensation mechanism for their X-linked genes.